Mental Wellness
for Women

Mental Wellness for Women

Rita Baron-Faust

with the

*Physicians of the New York University Medical
Center Women's Health Service and the
NYU School of Medicine Department of Psychiatry*

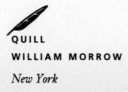

QUILL
WILLIAM MORROW
New York

Copyright © 1997 by Rita Baron-Faust

Library of Congress Cataloging-in-Publication Data

Baron-Faust, Rita.
   Mental wellness for women / Rita Baron-Faust.
     p. cm.
   Includes bibliographical references and index.
   ISBN 0-688-16113-8
   1. Women—Mental health. 2. Mental illness—Sex Factors.
  3. Women—Mental health—Sociological aspects. 4. Consumer education. I. Title.
   RC451.4.W6B375   1997
   616.89'0082—dc20   96-22903
                                      CIP

Printed in the United States of America

First Quill Edition 1998

1 2 3 4 5 6 7 8 9 10

BOOK DESIGN BY LEE FUKUI

www.williammorrow.com

To Dr. Anthony Grieco,
whose help and support over the years
have helped me to maintain
my own mental wellness

And to Alexander, who
brings me joy

Introduction

When we began the New York University Medical Center Women's Health Service in 1992, there were only a few dozen such programs across the country. Today, there are hundreds of facilities where women's diverse health needs can be met under one roof.

We started our own program with the goal of providing an interdisciplinary facility for women's health care in an academic environment, utilizing the best of our gynecological, medical, radiological and surgical staff. The program has since expanded to include Primary Care; a Maternal-Fetal Medicine Service to assist women with complicated pregnancies or who have experienced recurrent miscarriage and preterm deliveries; a comprehensive Oncology Service; Reproductive Services offering infertility evaluation and state-of-the-art in-vitro fertilization technology; advanced diagnostic and screening services for breast, ovarian and uterine cancer, osteoporosis, gynecological abnormalities and a Menopause Unit to serve the needs of mid-life women. However, continued research in these fields is vital. To this end, the Women's Health Service gathers patient data and participates in laboratory, biomedical and clinical research by the NYU School of Medicine and NYU Medical Center. The nonprofit WHS also participates in clinical trials in a number of fields, and continues to offer community outreach and education. We hope to eventually clone our program and assist other medical centers in developing their own comprehensive health programs for women.

Underlying all of our efforts, however, is the goal of preventive medicine. For while women outlive men, they still suffer more days of disability due to health problems than men, and the gender gap widens as women age. As physicians, we must begin to involve women at the earliest stages of their lives, to interest and educate them in good health and well-being. This includes mental health, the subject of the third in our ongoing series of women's health handbooks.

Mental health is a topic of vital importance to women, who suffer from depression, anxiety disorders, abuse and eating disorders in much higher numbers than men. For the first time, scientific research is looking at why this should be so, and how treatments can be tailored more effectively to women. We now know that mental disorders are not *mental weaknesses* but *medical problems* in the same sense as diabetes or coronary artery disease: They can be diagnosed and treated both with medication and behavioral interventions.

It is our hope that the cutting-edge scientific information contained in *Mental Wellness for Women* will help to erase the lingering stigma of mental illness and prompt more women to seek treatment. For we know most assuredly that a woman's mental well-being *cannot* be separated from her physical well-being.

—ROBERT H. MORRIS, M.D.
Director, Women's Health Service,
NYU Medical Center

Foreword

Unfortunately, the terms *mental health* and *mental illness* have become so ambiguous in their meaning that they are often confusing to the public. This is particularly worrisome concerning the mental health needs of women. Some of the special aspects and problems of women's health are unique to that sex, while others generalize to men as well. Furthermore, in recent years we are discovering what our forebears knew: that men and women are indeed different in real ways. As we understand more about the biology of human beings and the special needs of women, it becomes increasingly important to have a single comprehensive source for women on the various aspects of mental health and illness. This volume should fill that need.

Rita Baron-Faust describes the major mental illnesses, some of which affect women in disproportionate numbers. Some illnesses, such as schizophrenia, are found in men and women in approximately equal rates but with differing degrees of severity. The illness tends to run a more benign course in women. There is also evidence that the etiology of schizophrenic disorders tends to be different in women. Even when an illness occurs equally in both sexes, it may still differ in its manifestation, course or response to treatment.

Ms. Baron-Faust is to be complimented for not restricting this volume to the usual group of so-called women's issues, such as eating disorders, depression, anxiety and domestic violence. That is not to say that these issues are unimportant. They are treated, and treated intelligently in this volume. However, the author recognizes that mental health issues pertinent to women run the entire gamut, and are not restricted to those that are more visible at a particular time. Prevalence rates are scant comfort for the victims of an illness. The knowledge that in the past, alcoholism was uncommon in women as a group did little to help the individual woman who suffered from it.

The author has also recognized the important role of biologic systems in mental illness. One cannot have a significant mental disorder with normal brain functioning. This does not mean that attitudes cannot be dysfunctional, but there is a fundamental difference between a problematic attitude and a mental illness. Much of what is published about mental health is oversimplified and often misleading; a serious treatise on the subject has been needed for some time. This readable volume provides a comprehensive discussion of mental health issues, a resource that women both need and deserve.

—ROBERT CANCRO, M.D.
Lucius N. Littauer Professor of Psychiatry
Chairman, Department of Psychiatry
NYU School of Medicine, NYU Medical Center

Foreword

This well-written exploration of the current medical knowledge of psychiatric disorders is based on two empowering assumptions: First, that every woman should know this information in order to maintain her mental well-being, and second, that every woman *can* come to know about these ideas in much greater depth than has traditionally been presumed by the keepers of medical knowledge.

The medical community's expertise in identifying and treating mental illness has leaped forward, thanks to state-of-the-art technologies and new discoveries about the fascinating workings of our bodies at the molecular level. Yet information about these advances has not often been clearly or reliably provided to the public, creating many misperceptions.

Women continue to be viewed in our culture as "the emotional ones." It's a label that is outdated and it has resulted in some very repressive attitudes about women in our society. But that view has also enabled women to become attuned to their emotions in ways that men historically have not been permitted to do. This freedom to accept and recognize feelings leads to an ability in women to detect subtle changes in mood states and behavior—both in themselves and in others. Marketing surveys tell us that women have long been the primary decision-makers in most households. This fact, coupled with their often greater attunement to the emotional dynamics of the home, means that a woman may find herself the primary caretaker of the mental health of her family—a role that brings both rewards and burdens.

Many women find themselves alone when confronting their own emotional fluctuations and stresses. After a miscarriage, a woman may find herself consumed with self-blame. A woman who has prided herself on her unflappability throughout her professional life may be dismayed by sudden and debilitating attacks of anxiety. Perhaps a woman has been struggling with the symptoms of depression, but never realized that life didn't have to look so gray. The emphasis we place in American society on the self-sufficiency of the individual puts a heavy responsibility on a person needing to adapt to traumatic circumstances. Too few women who need treatment are being helped. Some are held back by fear, others by lack of access to care. This book offers ideas, support and information that can help women feel less alone and more aware of treatment options.

This book also creates an important bridge between women and health care providers. Most young medical professionals have never experienced serious mental (or physical) illness, which may make it hard for them to understand the intimate, subjective parameters of "being sick." Moreover, it's all too common for the diagnostic term "mental disorder" to be misinterpreted by patients as "crazy," a stigma that can pose a serious roadblock to recovery. When doctor and patient become partners in treatment, they create an atmosphere in which the prevention of serious complications and future illness are possible. Information contained in *Mental Wellness for Women* is the first step in forging that healing partnership and banishing the stigma.

Ms. Baron-Faust writes compellingly about her subject, clarifying ideas without oversimplifying them and offering an engrossing view of the workings of the human mind. Her book builds a base upon which women can participate in the medical decisions that affect their well-being. The symptoms of mental illness can be debilitating and the treatment challenging. With this book in hand, women can gain a new understanding of the many facets of the human psyche and can move past self-blame to help, hope and power.

—VEVA H. ZIMMERMAN, M.D.
Associate Dean, NYU School of Medicine
Associate Professor of Clinical Psychiatry

Acknowledgments

I am deeply grateful to New York University Medical Center, which has continued to support and nurture this project. The Department of Public Affairs, especially Dan Perkes and Lynn Odell, has helped immensely, as have Dr. Robert Morris and Dr. Anthony Grieco. I am especially indebted to Dr. Virginia Sadock, who has worked closely on the first outline and initial drafts of the manuscript, lending her insights and personal support.

Special thanks are also due to Dr. Robert Cancro, Dr. Veva Zimmerman and Dr. Bruce Rubenstein, whose knowledge, enthusiasm and backing have helped me immeasurably. My gratitude also goes to the physicians in the Department of Psychiatry and NYU Medical Center, who acted as medical advisers and helped me ensure the scientific accuracy of often new and evolving material.

Thanks are also due to Gus Cervini at the American Psychiatric Association, Pam Willenz of the American Psychological Association and to the National Institute of Mental Health; and the federal Substance Abuse and Mental Health Services Administration (SAMHSA), for allowing me access to their meetings and conferences. I am also grateful to the National Association for the Mentally Ill, especially NAMI executive director Laurie

Flynn; Sybil Shalo and Cynthia Amorese at Wang Associates Health Communications for providing transcripts of NAMI meetings and for their help in finding women to share their experiences; the task force and the faculty of the American Medical Women's Association (AMWA) Advanced Curriculum in Women's Health; Dr. Leah Dickstein, past president of the American Medical Women's Association; Dr. Carol Nadelson, editor in chief, American Psychiatric Press; Dr. Susan Blumenthal, deputy assistant secretary for women's health and assistant U.S. surgeon general; Sophia Glezos at NIMH's Office of Scientific Information for providing background materials and access to the resources at the institute; and Dr. Myrna Weissman, Dr. Michael Leibowitz, Dr. John Oldham and Claudia Bial of the New York State Psychiatric Institute for their continued help over the years.

Thanks also go to my longtime friends at the American Medical Association, including Dr. George Lundberg, editor of the *Journal of the American Medical Association*, Tom Toftey, Jeff Molter, Barry Cohn, Diane Cohn, Jill Stewart and all the others, who over the years have helped me access sources and provided me with the *Archives of General Psychiatry* to help me better keep track of this tremendously exciting field.

To my editor at William Morrow, Toni Sciarra, who has helped immeasurably to hone my writing skills over the past four years and taught me so much about the real world of publishing, and to my agent, Vicky Bijur, for her continued enthusiasm and advocacy.

Love and gratitude also go to my husband, Allen, for checking all the web sites, phone numbers, and not minding (too much) my out-of-town-conference trips and late hours; to my son, Alexander, for being such a good "helper" in the office; and to my mother, always my best critic, who reads every single word with a sharp eye and a sharper pencil.

Veva H. Zimmerman, M.D.
Associate Dean, NYU School of
Medicine
Associate Professor of Clinical
Psychiatry

Virginia A. Sadock, M.D.
Director, Program in Human
Sexuality and Sex Therapy
Clinical Professor of Psychiatry

Bruce E. Rubenstein, M.D.
Director, Behavioral Health
Programs
Clinical Instructor of Medicine

Anthony J. Grieco, M.D.
Medical Director, Cooperative Care
Professor of Clinical Medicine

**NYU Medical Advisers and
Peer Reviewers**

Machelle Harris Allen, M.D.
Director of Substance Abuse and
Domestic Abuse Service
NYU-Bellevue Hospital Center
Assistant Professor of Obstetrics
and Gynecology

Helen A. DeRosis, M.D.
Clinical Associate Professor of
Psychiatry

Melissa Ferguson, Ph.D.
Co-director, Eating Disorders
Program

Michael L. Fleisher, M.D.
Clinical Associate Professor of
Psychiatry
Faculty, NYU Psychoanalytic
Institute

Michael L. Freedman, M.D.
The Diane and Arthur Belfer
Professor of Geriatric Medicine
Director, Division of Geriatrics

Arnold J. Friedhoff, M.D.
Menas S. Gregory Professor of
Psychiatry
Director, Margaret S. Millhauser
Laboratory for Research in
Psychiatry and the Behavioral
Sciences

Marc A. Galanter, M.D.
Professor of Psychiatry
Director, Division of Alcoholism
and Drug Abuse
Coeditor, *Textbook of Substance
Abuse*, American Psychiatric Press

David L. Ginsberg, M.D.
Director of Outpatient Psychiatric
Services
Tisch Hospital
Medical Director, Eating Disorders
Program

Bruce S. Klutchko, M.D.
Clinical Assistant Professor of
Psychiatry
Director, Electroshock Service
NYU Medical Center

Carol Feit Lane, Ph.D.
Counselor, Women's Wellness
NYU Women's Health Service

Andrew McCullough, M.D.
Assistant Professor of Neurology
Director, Male Sexual Health
Program
NYU Medical Center

Margaret McHugh, M.D.
Clinical Associate Professor of
Pediatrics
Director, Child Protection Team
NYU-Bellevue Hospital

Reed C. Moskowitz, M.D.
Founder and Medical Director
Stress Disorders Medical Services

Lila E. Nachtigall, M.D.
Associate Professor, Obstetrics and
Gynecology
Director, Women's Wellness
NYU Women's Health Services

Nicholas A. Pace, M.D.
Assistant Professor of Clinical
Medicine
Vice Chairman, American Council
for Drug Education
Board of Directors of National
Council on Alcoholism and Drug
Dependence, Inc.

Eric D. Peselow, M.D.
Research Professor of Psychiatry
NYU School of Medicine

Barry Reisberg, M.D.
Professor of Psychiatry
Clinical Director
Aging and Dementia Research
Center

Norman Sussman, M.D.
Director, Psychopharmacology
Research and Consultation Service,
NYU-Bellevue Hospital Center
Clinical Associate Professor of
Psychiatry

Joyce A. Walsleben, Ph.D.
Research Assistant Professor of
Medicine
Director, Sleep Disorders Center

Herman J. Weinreb, M.D.
Assistant Professor of Neurology
Chief, Neurology Service
N.Y. Veterans Administration
Medical Center

Mary Zachary, M.D.
Instructor in Clinical Emergency
Medicine
Director, Women's Emergency
Care Program
NYU-Bellevue Hospital Center

Arthur Zitrin, M.D.
Professor of Psychiatry
Chairman, Dean's Committee on
Medical Ethics
NYU School of Medicine

The author also wishes to express gratitude to the following people, who provided information, insight and peer review on the newly evolving subject of women and mental health during the research and writing of this book.

Judith S. Beck, Ph.D.
Director
Beck Institute for Cognitive
Therapy and Research
Bala Cynwyd, PA

Mary C. Blehar, Ph.D.
Acting Chief
Mood, Anxiety, and Personality
Disorders Research Branch
National Institute of Mental Health

Sheila Blume, M.D.
Medical Director of Alcoholism,
Chemical Dependency, and
Compulsive Gambling Programs
South Oaks Hospital
Amityville, NY
Professor of Psychiatry
State University of New York
Stony Brook

Susan J. Blumenthal, M.D., M.P.A.
Deputy Assistant Secretary for
Women's Health
U.S. Assistant Surgeon General,
Department of Health and Human
Services

Robert N. Butler, M.D.
Brookdale Professor and Founding
Chairman
Department of Geriatrics and Adult
Development
Director, International Longevity
Center
Mount Sinai Medical Center, New
York

Larry Cahill, Ph.D.
Research Neurobiologist
Center for the Neurobiology of
Learning and Memory
Bonney Center, University of
California at Irvine

C. Robert Cloninger, M.D.
Wallace Renard Professor of
Psychiatry
Department of Psychiatry
Washington University
St. Louis, MO

Christine A. Courtois, Ph.D.
Clinical Director
The Center: Posttraumatic and
Dissociative Disorder Program
Washington, D.C.

Leah J. Dickstein, M.D.
Professor and Associate Chair for
Academic Affairs
Director, Division of Attitudinal
and Behavioral Medicine
Department of Psychiatry and
Behavioral Sciences
Associate Dean for Faculty and
Student Advisory
University of Louisville School of
Medicine, Louisville, KY

Park Dietz, M.D., Ph.D.
President, Threat Assessment
Group, Inc.
Newport Beach, CA

Adam Drewnowski, Ph.D.
Professor and Director, Program in
Human Nutrition
School of Public Health
University of Michigan, Ann Arbor

Carol J. Eagle, Ph.D.
Head, Child/Adolescent Psychology
Montefiore Medical Center,
Bronx, NY
Associate Professor of Psychiatry
Albert Einstein College of
Medicine, New York

Jean Endicott, Ph.D.
Chief, Department of Research
Assessment and Training
New York State Psychiatric
Institute, New York

Anne H. Flitcraft, M.D.
Associate Professor of Medicine
University of Connecticut School
of Medicine, Farmington, CT

Edna P. Foa, Ph.D.
Professor of Psychiatry
Director, Center for the Treatment
and Study of Anxiety
Medical College of Pennsylvania
and Hahnemann University
Philadelphia

Ellen Frank, Ph.D.
Director, Prevention of Depression
and Manic Depression Program
Western Psychiatric Institute and
Clinic
Professor of Psychiatry and
Psychology
University of Pittsburgh School of
Medicine, Pittsburgh, PA

Ellen W. Freeman, Ph.D.
Director, PMS Program
University of Pennsylvania Hospital
Research Professor in Obstetrics,
Gynecology and Psychiatry
University of Pennsylvania School
of Medicine, Philadelphia

Anne Geller, M.D.
Chief, Smithers Addiction
Treatment and Training Center
St. Luke's-Roosevelt Hospital
New York
Associate Professor of Clinical
Medicine
Columbia College of Physicians
and Surgeons, New York

Judith Hammerling Gold, C.M.,
M.D.
Psychiatrist in private practice
Halifax, Nova Scotia, Canada
Chairperson, LLPDD Work
Group, *DSM-IV* Task Force

Marla Jean Gold, M.D.
Assistant Professor of Medicine
Medical College of Pennsylvania,
Philadelphia

Frederick K. Goodwin, M.D.
Professor of Psychiatry
Director, Center on Neuroscience,
Behavior and Society
George Washington University
Medical Center, Washington, D.C.

Marcia B. Greco, M.A., Education
and Human Development
Past Director of Education and
Outreach
Depression After Delivery
Morrisville, PA

Katherine A. Halmi, M.D.
Professor of Psychiatry
Cornell University Medical College
Director, Eating Disorder Program
New York Hospital–Cornell
Medical Center, Westchester
Division, White Plains, NY

Gloria Hamilton, Ph.D.
Associate Professor of Psychology
Middle Tennessee State University,
Murfreesboro, TN
Clinical Psychologist
Tara Treatment Center
Franklin, TN

Jean A. Hamilton, M.D.
Betty Cohen Professor of Women's
Health
Director of the Institute for
Women's Health
Medical College of Pennsylvania,
Philadelphia

Eric Hollander, M.D.
Professor of Psychiatry
Director, Anxiety, Compulsive and
Impulsive Disorders Program
Director of Clinical
Psychopharmacology
Mount Sinai School of Medicine,
New York

Luanne Holsinger
State Board Member, Virginia
Alliance for the Mentally Ill
Volunteer, National Alliance for
Research on Schizophrenia and
Depression (NARSAD)

Ann Jennings, Ph.D.
Director, Trauma Initiative
Maine Department of Mental
Health and Mental Retardation
Augusta, ME

Helen Singer Kaplan, M.D.
(deceased)
Former Director, Human Sexuality
Program
New York Hospital–Cornell
Medical Center, New York

Ira R. Katz, M.D., Ph.D.
Professor of Geriatric Psychiatry
University of Pennsylvania Medical
Center

Lisa Joan Kaylor, M.S.Ed., N.C.C.
Member, Board of Directors, and
Secretary
Obsessive-Compulsive Foundation,
Inc.
Member, Board of Directors, The
Trichotillomania Learning Center
Santa Cruz, CA

Jean Kirkpatrick, Ph.D.
Founder, Women for Sobriety
Quakertown, PA

Mary P. Koss, Ph.D.
Professor of Family and
Community Medicine, Psychology
and Psychiatry
University of Arizona, Tucson, AZ

Sue A. Kuba, Ph.D.
Associate Professor
Coordinator, Behavioral Medicine
and Health Psychology
California School of Professional
Psychology, Fresno

Ellen Leibenluft, M.D.
Chief, Unit on Rapid Cycling
Bipolar Disorder
Clinical Psychobiology Branch
National Institute of Mental
Health, Bethesda, MD

Henry Lesieur, Ph.D.
Professor of Criminal Justice
Illinois State University
Normal, IL

Freda C. Lewis-Hall, M.D.
Director, Lilly Center for Women's
Health
Eli Lilly and Company,
Indianapolis, IN

Charles Lieber, M.D.
Director, Alcohol Research and
Treatment Center
Bronx Veterans Affairs Medical
Center, Bronx, NY
Professor of Medicine and
Pathology, Mount Sinai School of
Medicine, New York

Carole Lieberman, M.D., M.P.H.
Assistant Clinical Professor of
Psychiatry
University of California, Los
Angeles (UCLA)

Michael R. Liebowitz, M.D.
Director, Anxiety Disorders Clinic
Columbia-Presbyterian Medical
Center–New York State Psychiatric
Institute, New York
Professor of Clinical Psychiatry
Columbia University College of
Physicians and Surgeons, New York

Nancy L. Marshall, Ed.D.
Senior Research Scientist
Center for Research on Women
Wellesley College, Wellesley, MA

Bonnie Maslin, Ph.D.
Psychotherapist, New York City
Author, *The Angry Marriage:
Overcoming the Rage, Reclaiming the
Love* (Hyperion), 1995

Caroline Adams Miller
Author, *My Name Is Caroline*
(Bantam Books), 1988

Laura J. Miller, M.D.
Assistant Professor
Department of Psychiatry
University of Illinois at Chicago

Robert B. Millman, M.D.
Director, Alcohol and Drug Abuse
Center
New York Hospital–Cornell
Medical Center

Carol C. Nadelson, M.D.
President, CEO and Editor in
Chief, American Psychiatric Press
Washington, D.C.
Clinical Professor of Psychiatry
Harvard Medical School,
Boston, MA

Mimi Nichter, Ph.D.
Department of Anthropology
University of Arizona, Tucson

Susan Nolen-Hoeksema, Ph.D.
Associate Professor of Psychology
University of Michigan
Ann Arbor, MI

Malkah T. Notman, M.D.
Clinical Professor of Psychiatry
The Cambridge Hospital and
Harvard Medical School
Cambridge, MA
Training and Supervising
Psychoanalyst
Boston Psychoanalytic Institute

Silvia W. Olarte, M.D.
Clinical Associate Professor of
Psychiatry,
New York Medical College
Valhalla, NY

John M. Oldham, M.D.
Director, New York State
Psychiatric Institute
Professor and Vice Chairman
Department of Psychiatry
Columbia University College of
Physicians and Surgeons
Coauthor, *The New Personality Self-
Portrait* (Bantam Books), 1995

Laszlo A. Papp, M.D.
Director, Biological Studies Unit
New York State
Psychiatric Institute, New York
Associate Professor of Psychiatry
Columbia University

Barbara L. Parry, M.D.
Associate Professor of Psychiatry
Associate Director, Consultation-
Liaison Psychiatry
University of California, San Diego
Medical Center

Holly G. Prigerson, Ph.D.
Assistant Professor of Psychiatry
University of Pittsburgh School of
Medicine
Department of Psychiatry, Western
Psychiatric Institute and Clinic

Valerie Raskin, M.D.
Assistant Professor of Psychiatry
University of Illinois College of
Medicine, Chicago

Gail Erlick Robinson, M.D.
Chair, APA Committee on Women
Professor of Psychiatry, Obstetrics
and Gynecology
University of Toronto

James C. Rosen, Ph.D.
Clinical Psychologist
Professor of Psychology
University of Vermont, Burlington

Jerilyn Ross, M.A., LICSW
President
Anxiety Disorders Association of
America, Rockville, MD

David R. Rubinow, M.D.
Clinical Director
National Institute of Mental Health

Mary V. Seeman, M.D.
Director, Schizophrenia Program
Clark Institute of Psychiatry
University of Toronto

Sally K. Severino, M.D.
Professor and Executive Vice Chair
Department of Psychiatry
University of New Mexico,
Albuquerque

Deborah A. Sichel, M.D.
Hestia Institute
Center for Women and Families
Wellesley, MA

Margaret Spinelli, M.D.
Director, Maternal Mental Health
Program
New York State Psychiatric
Institute, New York

Donna E. Stewart, M.D., D.PSCH.
Lillian Love Chair of Women's
Health, Toronto Hospital
Professor of Psychiatry, Obstetrics
and Gynecology, Anesthesia,
Surgery, Family and Community
Medicine
University of Toronto

Nada L. Stotland, M.D.
Associate Professor of Clinical
Psychiatry, Department of
Psychiatry and Obstetrics and
Gynecology
University of Chicago

Susan A. Toms, R.N.C., M.S.
Cofacilitator of the Perinatal
Bereavement Support Group
Montefiore Medical Center, Weiler
Division, Bronx, NY

Lynn Weber, Ph.D.
Founder and Director
Center for Research on Women
University of Memphis (Tennessee)

Myrna M. Weissman, Ph.D.
Professor of Epidemiology and
Psychiatry
Columbia University College of
Physicians and Surgeons, New York

Richard M. Wenzlaff, Ph.D.
Associate Professor of Psychology
Division of Behavioral and Cultural
Sciences
University of Texas, San Antonio

Sharon C. Wilsnack, Ph.D.
Chester Fritz Distinguished
Professor
Department of Neuroscience
University of North Dakota School
of Medicine, Grand Forks, ND

Katherine L. Wisner, M.D.
Associate Professor of Psychiatry
and Reproductive Medicine
Director, Women's Services
Mood Disorders Program
Case Western Reserve University
School of Medicine, Cleveland, OH

Paul Wood, Ph.D.
President
National Council on Alcoholism
and Drug Dependence, Inc.,
New York

Nancy Fugate Woods, Ph.D., R.N.,
F.A.A.N.
Professor of Nursing
Center for Women's Health
Research
Department of Family and Child
Nursing
University of Washington, Seattle

Kimberly A. Yonkers, M.D.
Assistant Professor
Departments of Psychiatry and
Obstetrics and Gynecology
University of Texas Southwestern
Medical Center, Dallas

Contents

A Note to the Reader:
What Is the *DSM-IV?*

In order to identify and treat mental illness, an accurate method of diagnosis is needed. Unlike other medical illnesses, such as diabetes or cancer, in mental disorders there are no blood tests or cellular pathology with which to confirm a diagnosis. Many symptoms of mental disorders can be vague and hard to sort out. So mental health professionals turn for help to the *Diagnostic and Statistical Manual of Mental Disorders*, published by the American Psychiatric Association.

The manual is currently in its fourth edition, published in 1994. The *DSM-IV* is the work of a twenty-seven-member task force; it took five years to complete and called upon more than one thousand mental health professionals and researchers to develop updated scientific criteria for 290 mental disorders. Diagnostic criteria for each disorder have been tested among more than seven thousand patients.

However, the *DSM-IV* has limits. Like its predecessors, it's an installment of a work in progress, reflecting ongoing changes in thinking and research. Some disorders that appeared in previous editions have been eliminated (such as *self-defeating personality disorder*), and others have been renamed (as with *late luteal phase dysphoric disorder, LLPDD,* now *premenstrual dysphoric disorder, PMDD*) and revised. While others are still considered unofficial, and are mentioned in the manual as meriting "further study."

While the current edition of the *DSM* takes gender, culture and ethnicity into account, much of the research on which diagnostic criteria are based was done largely in men. Moreover, there are ongoing controversies about many of the diagnostic categories, including PMDD (see page 202).

The diagnosis of mental illness is not always precise; men and women often display a "spectrum" of problematic behaviors, overlapping disorders, or symptoms that fail to meet diagnostic criteria, but which are nonetheless troubling and disabling.

The *DSM-IV* is neither the last word nor the only word on mental illness. But since it is the reference most widely used by mental health professionals (and by insurance companies for determining the bases for reimbursement), its diagnostic criteria will be used to provide a framework in which to discuss mental disorders in this book. The *DSM-IV* diagnostic criteria, adapted with the permission of the American Psychiatric Association, are offered solely as points of reference, not as a means of self-diagnosis.

Mental Wellness
for Women

Misunderstood: Women and Mental Illness

I felt like I was surrounded in darkness and sadness that never went away . . . even when something wonderful would happen, I was never truly happy. . . . If I could have lain down, gone to sleep and never woken up, it would have been perfectly okay with me. CAREN, AGE 35

Caren is *not* alone. As many as *half* of all American adults have experienced some form of mental illness at least once during their life. Perhaps a third suffer a mental disorder during any given year! Yet a major national survey found that fewer than half of those people received professional treatment for these disorders. Unfortunately, many of us still attach a stigma to mental illness, even though most people believe it can be treated.

But mental illness *is* a bona fide medical problem. More days are spent in bed as a result of major depression than as a consequence of any other disorder except heart disease. Depression alone costs Americans almost $44 billion a year in treatment and lost productivity—*more than* the tab for cardiovascular disease.

Although rates of mental illness are similar for men and women, certain disorders seem to be more common in women. Until fairly recently, these differences were not acknowledged or even studied, the result being large gaps in our knowledge about the diagnosis, treatment and course of mental illness in women. Only in 1994 were gender and cultural factors first taken into account in the most often used diagnostic tool, the *Diagnostic and Statistical Manual of Mental Disorders, Fourth Edition (DSM-IV)*.

HOW THIS BOOK CAN HELP YOU

The National Institute of Mental Health (NIMH) offers this definition of mental wellness:

> "Mentally healthy people understand they are not perfect nor can they be all things to all people. They experience a full range of emotions, including sadness, anger, and frustration as well as joy, love, and satisfaction. While they typically can handle life's challenges and changes, they can reach out for help if they are having difficulty dealing with major traumas and transitions—loss of loved ones, marriage difficulties, school or work problems, the prospect of retirement.

> "Unfortunately, many wrongly believe their symptoms are their own fault or are caused by personal weakness. They think that if they try hard enough they can overcome their problems by themselves and they suffer needlessly."

The goal of this book is to *prevent and reduce that needless suffering* and to help women maintain—or attain—mental wellness, as well as to become informed consumers of mental health services. We'll examine the current research into the origins, diagnoses and symptoms of mental disorders in women, and offer, where possible, advice on prevention.

We will look at how experiences in a woman's life cycle, from childhood, puberty, pregnancy and menopause to old age, can impact on her emotional well-being, as well as contribute to addictive behaviors, eating disorders, body-image distortion and major psychosocial problems such as violence and sexual abuse.

We'll discuss the different types of mental health professionals and the therapies they offer, as well as the medications used to treat mental disorders (and whether they affect women differently). We will look at racial and cultural issues, which may present barriers to mental health care for some women, and hear from women of different backgrounds describing their struggles and victories over mental illness.

Scientific data are changing all the time. Although some of the data we're going to explore have been published and peer-reviewed by the scientific community, other information is still very preliminary and under investigation. Everything, however, has been carefully reviewed by the experts who shared with us their cutting-edge research in the field. Each chapter has been prepared with the technical guidance of the Department of Psychiatry at New York University Medical Center, the NYU School of Medicine, and the NYU Women's Health Service.

However, before we explore these often explosive issues, there are things that should be stated.

- Differences in mental illness in men and women arise from a complex interaction among biological, genetic, behavioral and environmental factors, not gender itself.

- Gender differences in mental illnesses cannot be blamed solely on female hormones or on the societal roles, stresses and life experiences unique to women.

- Gender variances in mental health statistics cannot be viewed solely as a reflection of women's supposed tendency to visit doctors more often, and to report more symptoms.

- The increased incidence of certain mental disorders among women should not be interpreted with outmoded sex stereotypes: the "emotional" (weak and hysterical) woman, compared with the "stoic" (strong and capable) man.

- Apparent gender differences in certain brain structures do *not* indicate differences in mental *abilities* between the sexes. Nor have these gender differences been linked to mental disorders.

With that said, let's look at the statistics.

THE GENDER GAP: WHAT WE KNOW

Two major surveys—the National Institute of Mental Health (NIMH) Epidemiological Catchment Area (ECA) study of eighteen thousand people in five urban areas, and the NIMH-sponsored National Comorbidity Survey of over eight thousand households across the country—have found that men and women are *equally likely to suffer from mental disorders*. Where men and women part company is in the *patterns of mental disorders*. While seventeen million Americans suffer from major depression, women are affected twice as often as men. The National Comorbidity Survey, reported in the *Archives of General Psychiatry* in 1994, found that more than 21 percent of women had suffered an episode of major depression during their lifetime, compared with 12.7 percent of men.

Surveys by the NIMH indicate that of the more than four million Americans with panic disorder, women outnumber men two to one. Eating disorders are nine times more common among women than men. Women also suffer from *seasonal affective disorder (SAD)* and *somatization disorder* (emotional problems that produce physical complaints) four times more often than men. On the other hand, *antisocial personality disorder*, conduct disorders, alcoholism and drug addiction are almost five times more common in males.

Schizophrenia, characterized by delusions, hallucinations and withdrawal from society, affects some 2.5 million Americans, men and women equally. *Bipolar disorder*, or *manic depression* (wide mood swings from depression to manic euphoria), afflicts more than 3 million men and women, and 5 million people suffer from *obsessive-compulsive disorder (OCD)*. Incidence rates for these disorders are about the same for men and women, but there are some important gender differences.

Women develop schizophrenia between the ages of twenty-five and thirty, while men become ill much earlier, between the ages of sixteen and twenty-five. In bipolar disorder, women have more depressed episodes; women are also five to six times more likely than men to have "rapid cycling," where moods frequently switch back and forth between mania and depression, sometimes within hours.

Some disorders are unique to women's reproductive biology. A majority of women report some mood swings in the week or so before menstruation, with an estimated 3 to 7 percent suffering severe premenstrual depression and other symptoms now classified as *premenstrual dysphoric disorder (PMDD)*. Bipolar illness, schizophrenia and anxiety or panic disorders can also worsen premenstrually. After giving birth, between 10 to 15 percent of women experience *postpartum major depression* and around 1 in 1,000 women suffer a *postpartum psychosis*. Despite persistent myths, there is no clinical evidence that menopause triggers, or substantially increases, the risk of depression.

But older women are more vulnerable to *Alzheimer's disease*, which accounts for a majority of cases of *dementia*, progressive cognitive decline.

What accounts for these gender variances? Is it biology or psychology? brain structure or genes? hormones or environment? There is no one simple answer. There may never be. "A strong role for biology is supported by studies showing similar rates of depression and other mental illnesses in women across many cultures, the fact that sex differences in the rates of some disorders occur after puberty, as well as newly observed gender differences in the brain, and women's differing physiological responses to stress," observes Susan J. Blumenthal, M.D., M.P.A., U.S. assistant surgeon general and deputy assistant secretary for women's health in the Department of Health and Human Services.

Genes can also affect a person's predisposition to mental illness, Dr. Blumenthal notes. Sixty to 80 percent of people diagnosed with depression have a family history of the disease; half of all cases of schizophrenia may be influenced by genes.

Individual personality and the way we cope with stress also increase vulnerability to depression and other mental disorders. Dr. Blumenthal notes that the *interaction* of biological, genetic, psychological, environmental and social factors influences rates of mental disorders. "The adverse effects of inferior social status, impaired self-esteem, sexual abuse and sex discrimination, economic inequities and constricted educational and occupational opportunities, in part, may account for higher rates of some mental disorders such as depression among women," she adds.

BECOMING FEMALE

One thing is clear: Women's mental health is definitely not related to Sigmund Freud's notion of "penis envy." Freud, the inventor of psychoanalysis, believed that some of women's psychological problems stemmed from grief and shock as little girls when they discovered they didn't have a penis. He felt females devalued themselves and their bodies, forming dependent relationships with men as a sort of substitute for a phallus.

Freud was a product of the Victorian Age, when women had little power or status, and were expected to submit to men. Some of his ideas about women have become outmoded with our increased knowledge of human development and psychology. We now know that becoming "female" is a process that merges biology with behavior and environment, what experts call a *biopsychosocial model*.

Your *biological* sex is determined by which sex chromosomes you inherit at conception. Women inherit two "X" chromosomes; men inherit "X" and "Y" (a man's X chromosome is passed along from the mother). All embryos start out as female. During the early embryonic stages, these chromosomes trigger the formation of the primary sex organs (or *gonads*): testes in males, ovaries in females. The sex organs then produce the hormones responsible for development of the reproductive organs: the vagina, uterus and fallopian tubes in females and the penis, seminal vesicles and prostate in males. Sex hormones also influence structural brain development. At puberty, another surge of hormones triggers secondary sex characteristics, such as breasts or facial hair.

Behavioral scientists generally agree that our "core gender identity" is firmly established before eighteen months of age, and has a great deal to do with interactions with people early in life.

Even before a child is born, parents have differing expectations for each sex, formed by their own backgrounds and experiences. Many cultures value male children more highly, with special rituals surrounding the birth of a boy. Culture also dictates sex-coded dress, which establishes gender for all to see; newborn boys are wrapped in blue blankets in hospital nurseries, the girls in pink. Later on, many cultures impose rigid standards of "modest" dress for women. For example, under strict Islamic law, girls must wear head coverings and women must be veiled from head to toe; ultra-Orthodox Jewish women traditionally wear wigs after marriage.

Parents unconsciously relate to newborn daughters and sons differently. Studies show parents engaged in more motor activity with boys, and more nurturing play with girls. Inborn temperamental differences in male or female infants may prompt some of this behavior (see page 14), but some is due to culture. These different communication styles and signals are absorbed into a child's sense of self.

Then there's the development of "gender role," how women are expected to behave (the "social" component of the biopsychosocial model), according to culturally determined attitudes, expectations and behaviors considered "appropriate" for a female.

After an early *oedipal* phase where girls and boys express normal over-attachment to the opposite-sex parent, boys typically begin to identify with their fathers, girls with their mothers. For example, little girls absorb the idea that women have babies and cuddle their own baby dolls; boys imitate powerful male figures, like soldiers, superheroes or cowboys. Boys are encouraged to be competitive and aggressive toward their peers; girls are taught to be cooperative and compliant, and to think about the feelings of others, says Carol C. Nadelson, M.D., professor of psychiatry at Harvard University and editor in chief of the American Psychiatric Press. "The concept of being a 'good girl' exerts a powerful influence on girls growing up," she says.

Children develop distinct preferences in playthings, despite the best efforts of some parents to purchase "gender-neutral" toys. This may be due, in part, to television advertising (think Barbie and G.I. Joe) and to children's television programming, which still leans heavily on mostly male cartoon superheroes. But some of these preferences may be "prewired" at birth. Children begin to play separately; the boys in action-oriented play, the girls in quieter games and dress-up.

As they mature, girls and boys begin to adopt the social and cultural roles assigned to their sex. Most male cultural stereotypes emphasize power, aggression, confidence and nonemotionality; many female stereotypes emphasize passivity, dependence, emotionality and specific physical characteristics (such as slenderness). By puberty, a girl has formed a mental "ideal" of femininity that she will strive to achieve, and which may be at odds with her personality and desires.

How Your Brain Works

Fig. 1 (A, B, C): The Three Parts of the Brain

Source: National Institute of Neurological Disorders and Stroke, National Institutes of Health

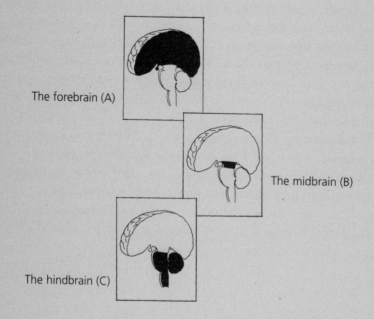

The forebrain (A)

The midbrain (B)

The hindbrain (C)

The brain is divided into three basic units, each having a specific function. The forebrain (A), primarily consisting of the *cerebrum* and structures hidden beneath it, is governed by conscious thought. It is the source of intellectual activities. It also holds your memories, allows you to plan and enables you to imagine and think.

The hindbrain includes the brain stem, the upper part of the spinal cord and a wrinkled ball of tissue called the *cerebellum* (C). The hindbrain controls vital functions such as respiration and heart rate. Above it lies the midbrain (B), which controls some reflex actions, and is also responsible for voluntary movements. The brain stem and cerebellum operate automatically, and control reactions to external stimuli.

These "higher" (thought) and "lower" (reflex) responses of the brain work in split-second concert. "For example, if you prick your finger with a needle, nerves in the finger transmit a signal to the brain stem, which sends a signal back to the finger, so you feel pain and recoil reflexively. But it is the cerebrum that recognizes the actual source of the pain as a needle, through sight and memory," explains Herman J. Weinreb, M.D., assistant professor of neurology at NYU Medical Center.

Fig. 2: The Structures of the Brain

Source: National Institute of Neurological Disorders and Stroke, National Institutes of Health

1. Cerebellum
2. Cerebrum
3. Frontal lobes
4. Motor area
5. Broca's area
6. Parietal lobes
7. Sensory areas
8. Occipital lobes
9. Temporal lobes

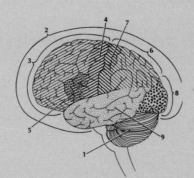

The cerebellum (1) is responsible for learned rote movements. When you play the piano or ride a bicycle, you're activating the cerebellum. The cerebrum (2) sits at the topmost part of the brain and is the source of intellectual activities.

The cerebrum is split into two halves, or *hemispheres,* by a deep fissure. The two hemispheres communicate through a thick tract of nerve fibers within this fissure, called the *corpus callosum.* The cerebral hemispheres are made up of an outer layer about the thickness of a stack of two or three dimes, called the *cerebral cortex* (so-called *gray matter*), and an inner layer (*white matter*). Most of the actual information processing in the brain occurs in the cerebral cortex, says Dr. Weinreb.

The cortex is gray because nerves in this area lack the insulation that make most other parts of the brain appear to be white. These structures are actually quite large, and are folded and creased to fit into the small space of the skull. The folds and creases add to the surface area of gray matter, increasing the quantity of information that can be processed.

The ability to form words seems to lie primarily in the left hemisphere, while the right hemisphere seems to control many abstract reasoning skills (and emotions). Each hemisphere primarily governs the opposite side of the body. When one side of the brain is damaged, the opposite side of the body is affected.

(continued)

The right and left hemispheres of the cerebrum are each divided into *lobes,* named for the main bones of the skull behind which they are located. The two *frontal lobes* (3) are associated with speech. In the rearmost portion of each frontal lobe is a *motor area* (4), which helps control voluntary movement, like moving the lips. Also in the left frontal lobe is *Broca's area* (5), which translates thoughts into words. The unique facets of our personality, the way we think, feel and create, are also controlled by the frontal lobes. The brain's *limbic system,* the seat of emotion, is also located within the frontal lobes.

Behind the frontal lobes are the *parietal lobes* (6). The forward parts of these lobes are the primary *sensory areas* (7), receiving information about temperature, taste, touch and movement from the rest of the body. Reading and arithmetic are also functions of each parietal lobe.

In the back of the brain, the *occipital lobes* (8) process images from the eyes and link that information with images stored in memory. Damage to these lobes can cause blindness.

Finally, there are the *temporal lobes* (9), which nest under the parietal and frontal lobes, near the ears. At the top of each temporal lobe is an area that receives input from the ears. The underside of each temporal lobe plays a crucial role in forming and retrieving memories (including those associated with music). Other parts of this lobe seem to integrate memories and sensations of taste, sound, sight and touch.

Fig. 3: Other Brain Structures

Source: National Institute of Neurological Disorders and Stroke, National Institutes of Health

10. Hypothalamus
11. Thalamus
12. Hippocampus

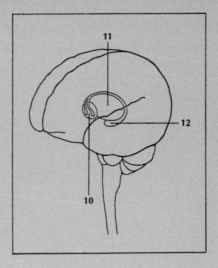

Deep within the brain lie other structures that function as "gatekeepers" between the spinal cord and the cerebral hemispheres. These structures determine our emotional state, modify our perceptions and responses accordingly and allow us to initiate movements without thinking about them. Like the lobes, these structures come in pairs, one in each half of the brain.

The *hypothalamus* (10) is only about the size of a pearl, but it is a powerhouse. It regulates functions like blood pressure and body temperature, sleep and waking and appetite and sexual behavior. The hypothalamus regulates the endocrine system, producing substances that trigger or block the release of key hormones, including sex hormones. It is also an important emotional center, controlling chemicals that make you feel exhilarated, angry or unhappy. Nearby is the *thalamus* (11), a key relay station linking the cerebral hemispheres to the other parts of the nervous system.

An arch of nerve cells links the hypothalamus and the thalamus to the *hippocampus* (12), a tiny nub that holds our memories and acts as a memory indexer, sending them to the appropriate part of the cerebral hemisphere for long-term storage and retrieving them when necessary.

(continued)

Also deep within the brain are the *basal ganglia,* clusters of nerve cells surrounding the thalamus that initiate and integrate movements; the *nucleus accumbens,* which controls feelings of pleasure; and the *pituitary gland* (a pea-sized extension of the brain located just behind the bridge of the nose), which produces a variety of hormones controlling sexual development, ovulation and metabolism (among other things).

Fig. 4: A Nerve Cell

Source: National Institute of Neurological Disorders and Stroke, National Institutes of Health

1. Cell body
2. Dendrites
3. Axon
4. Sheath
5. Sacs
6. Neurotransmitters
7. Synapse
8. Receptors

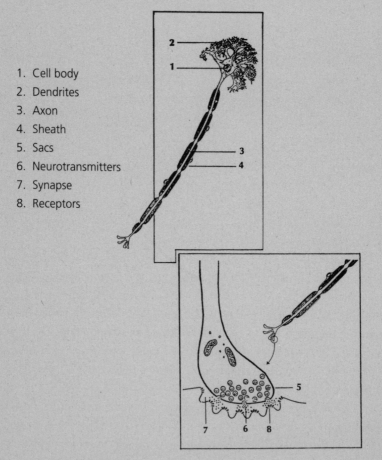

The brain could not perform any of these amazing functions without communication between nerve cells, or *neurons*. Neurons consist of three parts: the cell body (1), which contains the nucleus; *dendrites* (2), which extend outward from the cell body like branches of a tree and receive signals from other cells; and the *axon* (3), which connects it to other cells. Surrounding the axon is an insulating sheath (4), made of *myelin,* which helps nerve signals travel faster and farther.

Neurons "talk" to each other by transmitting electrical impulses through chemicals called *neurotransmitters* (6), sending the chemical from storage sacs (5) to receptor sites on other neurons. These neurochemicals are released from one nerve cell, travel into the synapse (7)—the space between the neurons—and attach to receptors on the next nerve cell (8). After the message has been transmitted, the neurotransmitter must then be removed from the receptor site. In some cases, the chemical travels back to the sending cell; this is called *reuptake*.

Scientists now believe disorders of mood, anxiety, personality, thought and even eating are caused by problems with reuptake, imbalances or breakdowns in neurotransmitter systems in specific areas of the brain, especially in the limbic system.

There are dozens of neurotransmitters, produced in different areas of the brain. Each performs a variety of functions according to which receptor they lock onto, in which part of the brain. Some neurotransmitters control movement and activity, others govern mood or appetite.

Neurotransmitters help the brain communicate with the body along a vast communications network, which includes the spinal cord, called the *central nervous system*. Within this network, the *autonomic nervous system* controls involuntary functions like breathing and heartbeat; sensory functions and muscle movement are controlled by the *somatic nervous system*.

Emotions also trigger reactions in the brain and body through the *sympathetic nervous system*. When we're under stress, for example, signals are sent to the brain that activate the sympathetic nervous system to produce stress hormones, which trigger increases in heart rate, blood pressure and breathing.

ARE THERE "MALE" AND "FEMALE" BRAINS?

We now have convincing evidence that there *are* differences in the brains of men and women, which affect the processing of information. And there are suggestions, mostly based on animal studies, that testosterone and estrogen may affect early development of the brain.

In both males and females, some 200 billion brain cells are formed within the first months of fetal life. Half of them die by the twentieth week of gestation. As the fetus develops, neurons form the basic structures of the brain, which in turn produce key brain chemicals and hormones. As more neurons grow, they move into place to create the specific brain areas described earlier, constructing networks among these regions, which allow information to be shared.

Estrogen and testosterone do not appear to affect the early formation or growth of human neurons, but animal studies suggest they can latch onto nerve cells that have hormonal receptors, potentially affecting the way neurons make connections.

Before age one, trillions of connections called *synapses* are made among brain cells. One neuron may have thousands of synapses. The brain produces more synapses than it needs and those which are not reinforced by stimulation from a baby's environment—sights, smells, sounds, touch—shrink and may die off. Experts say that a stimulating early environment may produce as much as 25 percent more brain connections.

"In animal studies, one can see gender-related differences in the structure of the brain, differences in the branching patterns of dendrites and axons, different synapse formation, differences in concentration of neuroregulators, different physiologic responses, and even differences in behavior," says David R. Rubinow, M.D., clinical director of the National Institute of Mental Health. "We do know that neurons act very differently in the presence of sex hormones."

Some scientists say that areas of the brain governing behavior like aggression may have more receptors for testosterone, the "male" hormone. However, it may not be that hormone by itself that produces such behavior, since much of the testosterone is converted in the brain to estrogen by the enzyme *aromatase*, notes Dr. Rubinow. So it may be the number of estrogen receptors on brain cells (and the way they function) that may differ in men and women.

"Many sex differences represent organizational effects. In animals, exposure to sex hormones during certain small 'windows' of development permanently alters brain structure and function," says Dr. Rubinow. For instance, scientists say, both hemispheres of the female brain develop evenly, so *both* can be used for verbal processing. Girls seem to acquire language skills earlier and faster than boys. In males, the right hemisphere appears to be more developed than the left, with more specialization for visual function and manipulating the environment. So boys may react more to visual stimuli as infants, and often appear to be better at tasks requiring spatial or mechanical skills.

Other differences: The corpus callosum in women is shaped differently than in men, which may help explain why women are able to use both sides of their brain for language. Women also appear to have more neurons in the cerebral cortex for processing language, vocal tones and music. Such findings could explain why women are better at deciphering both the meaning and the emotional content of words in another person's tone of voice.

These observations about humans were based largely on autopsy studies or psychological testing. Now there is growing evidence that men and women also *use* their brains differently, evidence that is emerging from studies using new brain imaging techniques that show the brain in the *act* of thinking (and feeling).

Thinking and sensory and motor activities alter blood flow and oxygen use in areas of the brain, producing signals that can be picked up on a *magnetic resonance imaging (MRI)* scanner. One 1995 study conducted at Yale University, utilizing a real-time MRI technique called *functional magnetic resonance imaging (FMRI)*, found that men and women use different areas of the brain when decoding words. Nineteen men and women were given pairs of nonsense words and asked to determine which pairs rhymed. All of the men used one small area in the *left frontal gyrus* located behind the eyebrow (long thought to be the location where speech is produced). Eleven of the nineteen women used this same region, *plus* a comparable area behind the *right* eyebrow.

Positron emission tomography (PET) scans also measure energy use within the brain. One PET study asked men and women to recognize sad or happy faces, and showed that men had to use more of their brain and work harder at it than women.

Many experts believe that this kind of brain *lateralization* may be one reason why boys have a higher incidence of developmental disorders affecting speech and language, such as autism. Neurologists have long observed that women recover more quickly than men from strokes in the left hemisphere of the brain, regaining language use more quickly, for example.

Other gender differences observed in infants may relate to brain lateralization: Baby girls react more to noise, touch and pain; baby boys are more sensitive to light. Boys tend to be more irritable and cry more; girls are generally calmer and more easily soothed. These differences may be one reason that parents react differently to baby boys and girls.

Sex-linked sensory differences persist throughout life. As adults, women seem to have a keener sense of taste and smell and have more sensitivity to noise than men. Visual acuity seems sharper in men, and male responses to visual stimuli are more pronounced. Women respond more strongly to verbal stimuli. On psychological tests, women score higher in areas linked to right hemisphere function, such as verbal skills, emotion and empathy; men score higher in abstract reasoning and spatial relations, areas associated with left hemisphere function.

In adulthood, sex hormones may affect levels of certain neurotransmitters. For example, low levels of, and reuptake problems with, the neurotransmitter *serotonin* (which affects mood and appetite), have been linked to depression, seasonal affective disorder and *premenstrual syndrome*.

Dr. Rubinow cautions against overinterpreting information about gender-related brain differences, noting that the exact effects of sex hormones in the human brain are still unclear.

MERGING BIOLOGY, BRAIN AND BEHAVIOR

Biological development, the alleged lateralization of brain function, the differing socialization of boys and girls and the environments we grow up in, all interact to make us who we are. These factors affect our development, our self-esteem, how we learn, our relationships, how we handle stress . . . and *perhaps* our risk of some forms of mental illness.

Some recent studies offer provocative suggestions of how these factors interact during a child's formative school years. In the early grades, boys are often more active and more inattentive than girls, who acquire earlier the social skills that enable them to sit still and the verbal skills to participate in class. Consequently, boys' fidgeting attracts more attention from teachers and they are often labeled as having behavioral or learning disabilities, such as hyperactivity or dyslexia (typically thought to be more common in boys).

However, a 1992 Yale University study of 445 children followed from kindergarten through third grade found that when children labeled by their teachers as dyslexic were independently tested, some boys thought to be dyslexic were not, and that the problem had gone unrecognized in some girls who did have dyslexia. In fact, the study showed that just as many girls as boys had learning problems, but that the boys' *behavior* attracted more notice from their teachers; girls with learning problems had to have significantly more disability, and show more distress, to get noticed in class.

Recent studies also show that at *all* grade levels, girls receive less attention in school; boys are called on more often and receive more one-on-one help from teachers. That hampers not only a girl's education, but also her self-esteem. One survey by the American Association of University Women found that girls generally start out on an equal footing with boys in science and math, but by junior high many may lag behind. Also lagging is girls' self-esteem; studies show that girls tend to be more self-critical than boys, rating themselves lower on their performance in many areas.

Combine all this with the emotional impact of making the transition to secondary school; the hormonal, physical and social changes of puberty; and a girl's attempts to achieve the feminine "ideal" she perceives as valued, and a pattern emerges. While rates of childhood depression are the same for both sexes, after puberty the rate rises for girls. Surveys show that girls aged fourteen to eighteen have consistently higher rates of depression than boys the same age, and report more symptoms of depression. While girls catch up and often surpass boys academically by high school and college, these gender differences in depression continue.

Studies show that boys tend to react to depression by misbehaving or fighting, girls by brooding and isolating themselves. Later in life, researchers have found, men are more likely to respond to stress with physical activity or aggression (as well as alcohol and drug abuse), while women internalize distress.

Effects of the "Female Experience"

Differing (and often conflicting) family, work and social roles, and victimization may also contribute to gender differences in the incidence and symptoms of some mental disorders, especially depression.

"Stress, poverty, violence, powerlessness, ethnic, racial and sexual orientation all intercede in a woman's life experience," comments Leah J. Dickstein, M.D., professor and director of the Division of Attitudinal and Behavioral Medicine in the Department of Psychiatry and Behavioral Sciences at the University of Louisville School of Medicine. "But until recently, there's been very little research about the differences in the incidence and diagnoses of psychiatric disorders in women, or in their treatment needs and responses."

New data show that major depression typically hits women in their mid to late twenties, a few years earlier than men, reemerging in the years preceding menopause. The American Psychological Association Task Force on Women and Depression notes that vulnerability to depressive symptoms is higher in mothers of young children and in women taking care of aging parents.

Depression is considered the most common disorder of older people (affecting about 20 percent of Americans over sixty-five). Women live longer than men and are more likely to be widowed and live alone in their old age, losing important social support networks.

The odds of having a mental disorder are twice as high for separated or divorced people, as they are for those who are married. But marriage is no panacea. Nearly half of women experiencing difficulties in their marriage may be clinically depressed.

More women than men live in poverty, often due to divorce or widowhood. Over one third of all American households are headed by women living below the poverty line. Studies show that people in the lowest socioeconomic groups are two and a half times more likely to suffer mental disorders than those in higher income groups.

African-American, Latina and Native American women suffer a disproportionate share of this nation's poverty, as well as other socioeconomic risk factors: poor education; low-status, high-stress jobs; having several young children at home; and single parenthood. Many bear the stress of discrimination, as do lesbians.

Women are more likely to be victims of abuse. One in every five girls may have suffered sexual abuse as a child; two million to four million women are physically battered each year by their partners; and one in every four women may be assaulted or raped. An estimated 50 to 70 percent of women hospitalized for psychiatric reasons have experienced abuse.

While a 1995 survey found that women contribute half to all family incomes, many women remain stuck in low-wage, low-mobility jobs, and earn less than seventy-five cents for every dollar paid to men. Sexual harassment on the job adds to stress. A recent survey by the Families and Work Institute found that a majority of women in two-paycheck families also work an extra twenty-one hours a week doing domestic chores and providing child care.

However, no direct, clinical cause-and-effect relationship has been established between mental disorders and any of these social factors, except for violence. We now know that women (and children) suffer *posttraumatic stress disorder (PTSD)* as a consequence of child abuse, battering or rape. Women may develop alcohol or drug dependency as a result of victimization, violence and PTSD. Other mental disorders have also been linked to a history of violence and abuse.

Many women have limited access to mental health care. Fifteen percent of American women aged eighteen to sixty-four lack health insurance, with African-American, Latina, Asian or other minorities even less likely to have coverage. Experts say, too, that many women are inadequately diagnosed and inappropriately treated, all too often prescribed mood-altering drugs.

Given these complex influences, it's easy to see why the relationship between gender and mental illness is a complicated, sensitive and often politically charged issue. However, it's about time we explored this issue objectively.

That's what this book will do.

Just as important, we will offer critical advice for women on dealing with the stresses of everyday living, to help them lead happier, and mentally healthier, lives.

CHAPTER 2

Mood Disorders

Depression is the most common mental disorder among American women. As many as seven million American women are thought to be suffering from a diagnosable depression.

Depression has many faces. Some women may feel like a dark cloud has followed them most of their lives, but they can still function. Others stop eating and sleeping, barely summoning the will to keep going. Still others ride an emotional roller coaster, soaring to euphoric highs, then plunging into despair.

According to the American Psychiatric Association's *Diagnostic and Statistical Manual of Mental Disorders, Fourth Edition (DSM-IV)*, the two major forms of *clinical depression* (that is, depression that can be diagnosed as a medical illness) are *unipolar* and *bipolar* (or *manic*) depression.

In full-blown manic depression, moods can swing from extreme elation to deep sadness. The moods are "polar" opposites, hence the term "bipolar." In major depression, there is one predominant mood, so it is referred to as "unipolar." People with unipolar depression have one or more periods during their lifetime where they feel sad, apathetic and hopeless. In bipolar depression, these "down" times are interspersed with bursts of excessive energy and feelings of euphoria called *mania*.

Unipolar depression can occur within a specific period as *major depression*, or in a milder, more chronic form called *dysthymia*. Other mood disorders include *postpartum depression*, major depression occurring after childbirth, and *seasonal affective disorder* (*SAD*).

We now know that major depression is a biological *and* psychological illness that affects thinking and emotion, and every aspect of our physical functioning. Many depressive episodes are triggered by stressful life events, such as the loss of a job or a loved one. Once that biological process is triggered, major depression can recur without provocation (see page 33).

Depression is a medical illness, not a personal weakness. Like other medical illnesses, *depression can be treated* with medication, but also with therapy or a combination of both. The symptoms and treatment of depression vary from individual to individual. But there are some common risk factors among women.

Quiz: Are You at Risk for Depression?

Sources: U.S. Department of Health and Human Services; the National Institute of Mental Health

Some women may have a biological vulnerability to depression, but life stresses can also trigger the disorder. Check the statements that apply to you.

- Do you have a family history of major depression or other mood disorders?
- Have you ever had an episode of major depression or been diagnosed with a personality disorder?
- Do you suffer from any other serious illnesses, like cancer or heart disease?
- Are you between the ages of twenty-five and forty-four (peak ages for major depression)?
- Do you feel stuck in a low-paying, low-status job with little control over your work?
- Are you having a hard time juggling societal and personal roles (e.g., being a wife, a mother and a working woman)?
- Are you married and not getting along with your husband?
- Are you at home with several small children?
- Have you had a recent loss or misfortune?
- Do you have the primary caretaking responsibility for an ailing parent?
- Do you have a problem with alcohol, cocaine or other addictive drugs?

❧ *Martha's Story* ❧

"When I had my first episode of depression back in 1960, far less was known about depression than we know today. . . . I was on the staff of a major university, and I noticed I began to lose interest in the things I used to enjoy, like reading a book on a cold winter evening. I experienced loss of appetite, weight loss, cried a lot. . . . one day in the office, I was trying to do some simple arithmetic and couldn't. Can you imagine what that was like for a former teacher? I was scared. Something was happening to me and I didn't know what it was. Because we didn't talk about depression in those days. . . .

"The treatment . . . back then was psychoanalysis. It's a long, arduous process where you analyze your thoughts, feelings and your behavior. . . . I went through that and I recovered. . . . I thought it would never happen again. But the depression reappeared. And . . . despite the fact that I had gotten my doctorate, had published papers in professional journals and given presentations at professional meetings, I felt inferior, inadequate and incompetent. Depression can wreak havoc with your self-esteem. . . . I had difficulty concentrating. I'd pick up one book and I'd try to read it, but I couldn't grasp it. . . . I was scared to death.

"Later, I saw a psychiatrist who had done research at the National Institute of Mental Health, and he said, 'Martha, this is a medical illness. Not a weakness.' Which was a relief. . . . Still, it was so hard for me to accept. I guess I wanted to think that I was in control . . . that if I just did something different, I wouldn't be depressed."

❧

MAJOR DEPRESSION

We often use the word "depression" to describe the sadness we feel after a loss or disappointment. But major depression is more than feeling sad. It is a biochemical illness with symptoms that affect the body as well as the mind, explains Bruce Rubenstein, M.D., director of Behavioral Health Programs at NYU Medical Center.

"The most typical symptoms of major depression include a persistent blue mood, a constant feeling of emotional pain and sadness, crying a great deal, as well as low energy, difficulty concentrating and, most tellingly, an inability to enjoy things you usually enjoy," explains Dr. Rubenstein. These symptoms may come on suddenly or gradually over a period of days or weeks, and persist for weeks or months. Major depression can affect memory, energy levels, motor function (movement and activity), appetite, sleep, sexual functioning and the immune system.

There may also be *psychomotor changes*, such as feeling so slowed down that when asked a question it may take more time than usual to answer. Some people have *agitated depression*—they're irritable and can't seem to sit still—while others are unable to eat or get out of bed, says Dr. Rubenstein. With severe depression, a person may feel worthless, that life isn't worth living, and may even have thoughts of death or suicide.

The key is that symptoms represent a sudden change and continue for two weeks or more, especially with a loss of interest in normally enjoyable activities, stresses Nada L. Stotland, M.D., an associate professor of clinical psychiatry at the University of Chicago and coeditor of *Psychological Aspects of Women's Health Care* (American Psychiatric Press, 1993).

"Symptoms can also vary with age. For example, a college-age woman who is depressed may have trouble falling asleep, or sleep too much. An older woman may have little trouble falling asleep, but may awaken before she wants to, and can't fall back asleep," Dr. Stotland notes. "Classic depression causes you to lose your appetite and lose weight. But younger people . . . may soothe themselves by eating too much and gain weight.

"Unfortunately, these are not symptoms which are likely to lead a woman to the doctor, because she may be sitting around feeling she's no good, telling herself it doesn't matter anyway, why waste energy seeing a doctor," she adds.

Most surveys find rates of depression among women of color somewhat lower than for their white counterparts. But experts say this may be due in part to differing symptomatology and less access to medical services. Data from the

National Lesbian Health Care Survey (a survey of almost two thousand women identifying themselves as lesbian), reported in 1994, showed that 37 percent of respondents had experienced a "long depression or sadness" at some point in the past, and 11 percent were currently experiencing depression (with a like number under treatment). Almost 50 percent of the women surveyed had sought counseling for depression at some time in their lives.

Depression can be triggered by (or coexist with) other mental problems, including eating disorders and anxiety disorders, as well as Alzheimer's disease. In older people depression may even be *mistaken* for Alzheimer's.

Substance abuse may cause depression (mania can be triggered by cocaine or other stimulants), as can some medications (such as drugs to control high blood pressure). Some 40 percent of women stop taking higher-dose oral contraceptives due to depressive symptoms. Major depression can result from medical conditions such as *hypothyroidism*, or underactive thyroid (see page 34), multiple sclerosis or pancreatic cancer. It can develop after a heart attack or in reaction to another serious illness.

"A complete medical evaluation should rule out substance abuse, the effects of medication or a medical condition, and take into account any recent bereavement and any family history of health problems before a diagnosis of major depression can be made," stresses Dr. Rubenstein.

Symptoms of Depression

Sources: *Diagnostic and Statistical Manual of Mental Disorders, Fourth Edition* 1994, American Psychiatric Association; National Institute of Mental Health; U.S. Department of Health and Human Services

Major Depression

A clinical diagnosis of *major* depression is based on having five (or more) of the symptoms listed below, nearly every day for more than two weeks, which represent a change from previous functioning and cause significant distress or impairment in work, family or personal relationships and other important areas of life. Major depression also may be diagnosed if the symptoms persist for longer than two months after a bereavement.

- Persistent sad or "empty" mood most of the day. Children and adolescents may appear irritable.

- Loss of interest or pleasure in ordinary activities, including sex.

- Decreased energy; feeling fatigued or "slowed down" nearly every day.

- Increased irritability, agitation or restlessness.

- Excessive crying.

- A decrease or increase in appetite; significant weight loss or gain. Children may fail to make expected weight gains.

- Trouble falling asleep, staying asleep or waking early; sleeping more than usual.

- Difficulty thinking, concentrating, remembering things or making decisions.

- Feelings of hopelessness, worthlessness or helplessness, or inappropriate guilt.

- Recurrent thoughts of death or suicide; suicide plans or attempts.

- Headaches, stomachaches, backaches or pains in joints or muscles not caused by disease and which do not respond to treatment.

Dysthymia

Dysthymia is characterized by a depressed mood most of the day accompanied by two or more of the following symptoms, for a period of at least two years (one year for children and adolescents), where a person is never without the symptoms for more than two months at a time.

- Poor appetite or overeating.

- Insomnia or hypersomnia (sleeping too much).

- Low energy or chronic fatigue.

- Poor concentration or difficulty making decisions.

- Feeling of hopelessness, despair or pessimism.

- Low self-esteem or self-confidence, or feelings of inadequacy.

Dysthymia is a milder, chronic form of major depression. It often begins in childhood or adolescence, and may be harder to recognize. "Some people may be naturally more moody or negative than others. To them the glass is always half-empty, rather than half-full," remarks Dr. Rubenstein. Some people blame themselves for their lingering sadness; others simply accept it as part of life, or as a facet of their personality. One form of dysthymia, *melancholic depression,* is characterized by negative thinking and intense feelings of personal inadequacy.

As many as 6 percent of Americans may develop dysthymia at some point during their lives. Perhaps 10 percent of dysthymic people may also suffer a concurrent episode of major depression (so-called double depression). Dysthymia can also occur with anxiety and panic disorders, and with substance abuse.

Some women perform so well on the job that even if things start to slide, it's hard to tell they're depressed. Warning signs of depression at work can include: decreased productivity, a sudden drop in morale, lack of concentration, accidents, and a rise in the number of sick days, or days taken off from work.

Many people with dysthymia consult a physician because they feel "unwell," but if no physical cause is found, their underlying depression goes undiagnosed. It's estimated that 25 percent of the population may have depressive symptoms which do not meet diagnostic criteria, and almost two thirds are women.

๑ Susan's Story ๑

"My battle with this illness [manic depression] goes back . . . to the confused third grader . . . with chronic and unbearable migraine headaches . . . through my junior and senior years of high school when my concentration was ruined and I was unable to sleep. . . . And I had to be tutored at home. . . .

"Can you imagine the pain of not knowing what to call what was happening to me? I spent fourteen years navigating a maze of doctors, procedures and diagnoses. I lost a big part of my life to a disease that had no name, and lost a big part of my digestive system, excised piece by piece in seven separate surgeries, to repair misdiagnosed, figmentary problems.

". . . Before I was diagnosed, I became a successful businesswoman, president of my own company by age twenty-seven. . . .

I was affluent, I had a closet full of clothes, I took luxurious vacations. But . . . I almost bankrupted my company when the manic phase of manic depression kicked in, as it inevitably does.

"In the manic phase of my illness, I made dozens of . . . trips to Los Angeles—thirty-two times in sixty days—spending tens of thousands of dollars, wasting money I didn't have, feeling invincible. . . . I hardly slept, I hardly ate. I talked a mile a minute, slurring my words, which is a typical symptom of mania. . . . Then, I started to lose touch with reality . . . that was a horrible out-of-control time . . . But it finally precipitated my diagnosis.

"For some women, the defining moments of their lives are their wedding day, the birth of their first child, their graduation from college. For me, it was commitment to a psychiatric ward at age twenty-seven, by my own husband of two months. It was an indescribable experience: the fear, the humiliation, the degradation, and confinement of a month-long hospitalization. But it was also a breakthrough . . . because at the end of it, my illness finally had a name. After twenty-eight days, after treatment with antipsychotic drugs and lithium, I was able to leave and start a new life."

Susan Dime-Meenan, C.B.A., is the executive director of the National Depressive and Manic Depressive Association. The above remarks are reprinted with her permission.

BIPOLAR DISORDER/MANIC DEPRESSION

Manic depression affects more than three million Americans, men and women in fairly equal numbers. However, the course of bipolar illness in women appears to be different, with more depressive episodes and fewer manic episodes.

Bipolar women are up to three times more likely than bipolar men to have "rapid cycling," where wide mood swings may occur within hours or days of each other, notes Ellen Leibenluft, M.D., chief of the unit on rapid cycling bipolar disorder at the National Institute of Mental Health.

"If female hormones play a role, it appears to be indirect," she says. "There's no evidence so far that rapid cycling is worse during different parts of the menstrual cycle, but women with bipolar illness are at very high risk for postpartum episodes. There is also some indication that sex hormones may affect the body's sleep-wake mechanism, which is disrupted in rapid cycling."

The *DSM-IV* lists two major types of bipolar disorder: *bipolar I*, where there has been at least one manic or mixed pattern (see below) as well as one or more periods of major depression, and *bipolar II*, in which major depression alternates with *hypomania*, a less extreme form of mania.

Bipolar disorder can occur in several patterns. In the *rapid-cycling* pattern, episodes of severe mood swings occur more than four times a year (in rare cases, from week to week). In the *mixed pattern*, symptoms of mania and depression may occur together (such as being agitated or irritable, as well as sad and suicidal) nearly every day for at least a week. A milder variant, *cyclothymia*, is marked by periods of hypomanic and depressive symptoms (but not severe, numerous or long enough to be diagnosed as hypomania or major depression) over a two-year period.

Before a diagnosis of bipolar illness can be made, medical illnesses such as *hyperthyroidism*, caused by an overactive thyroid, and the effects of medications or drug abuse should be ruled out, stresses Dr. Leibenluft. Hyperthyroidism can produce "hyperactive" symptoms akin to symptoms of mania.

A *manic episode* is defined as a period of abnormally euphoric or irritable mood, lasting at least one week, during which a person may have excessively "high" or euphoric feelings; inflated self-esteem or unrealistic, grandiose ideas about one's abilities or talents; increased energy or activity; restlessness; racing thoughts; increased talkativeness (or ceaseless, rapid talking); increased sexual drive; nonstop social activities; a decreased need for sleep and extreme distractibility.

A person may show uncharacteristically poor judgment, engaging in spending sprees, gambling or foolish business investments or promiscuous sexual behavior. Such symptoms must be sufficiently severe to cause marked impairment in occupational functioning, social activities and relationships, or to necessitate hospitalization to prevent harm to self or others.

A *hypomanic episode* is characterized by having only *three* of the above symptoms, within a period of extremely elevated mood or irritability lasting at least four days, but is not severe enough to cause marked impairment. In a "mixed" episode, every day during a one-week period, a person has symptoms of both a major depressive episode (see box, page 24) and shows symptoms like mania, often with depression predominating.

While bipolar disorders typically appear suddenly, the onset can also be gradual, beginning with hypomania. In women, the episodes of depression, lasting days, weeks or months, are usually longer and more frequent than periods of mania.

Cyclothymia generally begins gradually in late adolescence or early adulthood, with many people eventually developing more severe bipolar illness. Bipolar disorders can persist into old age, but little is understood about their course in older people.

Some experts believe that people in creative professions, such as artists and writers, seem especially prone to bipolar disorders and cyclothymia; in the hypomanic phase, they may be unusually creative and productive, doing some of their best work.

As with Susan Dime-Meenan, manic depression may take years to recognize and diagnose, even after someone first seeks help. A 1993 report by the National Depressive and Manic Depressive Association, surveying five hundred of its members, found that it took an average of eight years to get a correct diagnosis, with patients often seeing as many as three doctors.

Hypomania can be an early-warning sign of bipolar disorder, but it feels so good to the person experiencing it that they will often tell concerned friends and family that nothing is wrong. (A decreased need for sleep can be a key sign, Dr. Leibenluft points out.) The report noted that since symptoms first appear in adolescence, they may be dismissed as "teenage" emotional problems that will be outgrown, or may be misdiagnosed as depression. "Hypomania can be very subtle and it's not until the disorder reaches full-blown mania that it's often diagnosed," says Dr. Leibenluft. "People with hypomania can be quite functional, they can channel it and be very productive."

The side effects of bipolar illness can also be attributed to alcohol or drug abuse (which is common in people with bipolar illness), or as poor work or school performance.

SEASONAL AFFECTIVE DISORDER

Seasonal affective disorder, or *SAD*, is a form of depression apparently caused by seasonal shifts in daylight hours, which affect the body's twenty-four-hour sleep-wake cycle, or *circadian rhythm*. SAD can occur as arising during a particular major depression or bipolar disorder period of the year, over the course of two years. Other symptoms include lethargy, sleepiness and carbohydrate cravings. SAD affects as many as 20 percent of the population to varying degrees, four times as many women as men. A 1996 study of twins published in the *Archives of General Psychiatry* suggests that genetics may play a role in 29 percent of the cases of SAD.

The circadian rhythm in people with SAD undergoes a "phase disturbance" when the days grow shorter and nights grow longer in the late fall. They tend to awaken with the delayed dawn, rather than at their usual time. Their body clocks get out of sync, causing a chain reaction that results in depression. For some people with SAD, therapeutic doses of bright light in the morning can reset their body clock and help lift their depression.

SAD also seems to be related to disruptions in the release of a hormone called *melatonin*, a substance that signals the body when to go to sleep and when to awaken. Melatonin is produced in the darkness by the pea-sized *pineal gland*, located beneath the brain; production stops when daylight hits the retina of the eye. Recent studies suggest that people with SAD may secrete melatonin even in ordinary room light after dark, or that the retinas of people with SAD (especially women) may be less sensitive to light in the winter months.

Light therapy is currently the most effective treatment for SAD. However, experiments are under way using drugs that suppress melatonin, as well as using devices that produce an artificial "dawn" during sleep (light can penetrate the eyelid).

Medications that stimulate production of serotonin, a neurotransmitter that regulates mood and appetite, seem to help people with SAD. Studies show that a region in the brain thought to be a key part of the body clock displays seasonal variations in serotonin. Levels of serotonin are lower in winter for people with SAD, possibly indicating lower serotonergic function.

People with SAD have intense cravings for sweet and starchy carbohydrates (cookies, bread, pasta, potato chips), which stimulate production of serotonin. Normally, carbohydrates make us feel sleepy; people with SAD are energized by them. This may date back to caveman days when humans stocked up on food, then hibernated all winter. It is also perhaps one reason why some people (including those with SAD) tend to gain weight during the winter.

There is also very limited data, mostly from animal studies, indicating that sex hormones may regulate circadian rhythms. Estrogen appears to lengthen the sleep phase and advance the onset of sleep, notes Dr. Leibenluft. That may help explain, in part, why SAD and rapid-cycling bipolar disorder (both of which disrupt circadian rhythms) are more common in women than in men. It may also explain why women with major depression report more *hypersomnia*, sleeping more than usual, than do men. (Sleep disruption can also be a sign of an imminent bipolar episode.)

Some research has also shown that people with bipolar disorder suffer more mania during the summer months and more depression in winter, Dr. Leibenluft adds.

⮬ *Keshia's Story* ⮭

"I was only twenty-five, but I felt exhausted all the time. I didn't feel particularly sad. Just bone tired and dead inside. I had headaches. Stomach upsets. I went to a doctor, but she couldn't find anything physically wrong. . . . I didn't have the energy to call my friends. . . . It was all I could do to drag myself to the office in the morning. I wasn't even interested to watch TV or read the newspaper. Nothing was worth the effort. The best way to describe it is that I felt like I was slowly fading away, being erased. I just wanted to sleep and disappear. . . .

"This went on for weeks, then months. . . . I even thought about killing myself, and that really scared me. I was never that kind of person. I come from a family of strong black women. My mamma raised five children by herself after Daddy left. . . . She had shouldered so many heavier burdens, and here I was thinking my life was too hard to bear. I felt very guilty about that, like I was a weak person . . . unworthy of my heritage. . . .

"But when I found myself wandering around in a hardware store, looking at the bug killers, the weed killers . . . and wondering what kind of poison would be fastest, that's when I . . . I knew I couldn't carry *this* burden alone anymore."

DEPRESSION IN WOMEN OF COLOR

Symptoms of major depression can differ strikingly among cultures and among various ethnic and racial groups, not always fitting the standard diagnostic criteria.

A 1994 population study by the federal Centers for Disease Control and Prevention found rates of depression twice as high among African-American women, compared with white women. Studies show that women in nearly all Latino subgroups have more depressive symptomatology than men of similar backgrounds. But experts say that depression is underdiagnosed and undertreated in women of color.

According to Freda C. Lewis-Hall, M.D., former special Advisor to the Office for Special Populations at the National Institute of Mental Health, the number one symptom among African-American women is a change in appetite, rather than feeling sad or a drop in self-esteem. "African Americans . . . are more likely than white women to report somatic symptoms, primarily loss of appetite, dizziness, headache, gastrointestinal distress and chronic fatigue, and are less likely to connect them to depression," says Dr. Lewis-Hall, now director of the Lilly Center for Women's Health at Eli Lilly and Company.

Studies show that blacks also report greater irritability and fewer feelings of lethargy. Sleep disturbances in African Americans may take the form of *isolated sleep paralysis*, a stage between sleeping and awakening when one is paralyzed and actually dreaming while awake. This nonpathological phenomenon is more common among blacks than whites, and appears to be associated with hypertension and panic disorder, says Dr. Lewis-Hall. However, when a person describes the problem, it may be seen as hallucinations, sometimes leading to a misdiagnosis of psychosis, especially schizophrenia.

Lack of information about depression, limited access to medical care, suspicion of the (largely white) medical and mental health establishment and, as with Keshia, a woman's own belief that she must shoulder all burdens, may cause fewer African-American women (and other women of color) to report being depressed and seek help, says Dr. Lewis-Hall.

Recent studies show that 44 percent of Latino *medical* patients present symptoms of depression, says Silvia W. Olarte, M.D., an analyst and chair of the American Psychiatric Association's Committee of Hispanic Psychiatrists. "Latinas tend to somatize more than other groups, with more chronic abdominal pain reported by people with undetected depression," she observes. "Somatization is a very strong way of communicating their emotional anguish."

The *DSM-IV* notes that among Latino (and Mediterranean) cultures complaints of "nerves" (*ataques de nervios*) and headaches are frequent somatic symptoms of depression. Latinas are less likely to report being depressed because of cultural stigmas about mental illness and *marianismo*, the belief that women are supposed to endure suffering for the good of their family. They often lack insurance and access to mental health care.

According to the *DSM-IV*, among Chinese and other Asian cultures, physical symptoms of depression may be viewed as physical weakness or energy "imbalance." Asian groups may also believe that emotional distress results from a lapse in willpower, and people may not seek help out of a desire to avoid social stigma and shame (loss of face).

Of course, these are generalizations and don't apply to every African American, Latina or Asian American. But experts are now beginning to examine how depression and other mental disorders manifest themselves in different groups and cultures.

THE BIOCHEMISTRY OF MOOD DISORDERS

Two 1994 studies in the *Archives of General Psychiatry* suggest that, while stressful events can provoke an initial episode of depression, in people with a biological depression it may recur without any significant environmental stress, or may be triggered by smaller amounts of stress. One possible reason may be found in the brain-hormone system called the *hypothalamic-pituitary-adrenal axis* (*HPA axis*). The HPA axis involves activation of these three glands, and the regulation of the hormones they produce, including stress hormones.

Major depression has been linked to overarousal of the HPA axis and overproduction of stress hormones, including *cortisol*. Another HPA-axis hormone is *corticotropin-releasing hormone*, or *CRH*, which mediates our reactions to stress (increases in breathing, blood pressure and blood sugar, and the release of cortisol, all part of the body's "fight-or-flight" response).

"Under normal conditions, when stress subsides, the HPA axis returns to normal. But in some people, each time there's an episode of stress, there's a larger response by the HPA axis, or other neurochemical systems—until it takes very little stress to provoke that response. In some people, that response may eventually occur without any stimulus at all; the HPA axis becomes chronically overactive," explains Frederick K. Goodwin, M.D., former director of the National Institute of Mental Health, who now heads the Center on Neuroscience, Behavior and Society at George Washington University Medical Center. "This biological 'kindling' may help explain why major depression is a recurrent illness. Perhaps eighty percent of people who have one episode of unipolar depression will go on to have another."

Women have a larger response to stress in the HPA axis, with a two to three times greater outpouring of stress hormones than men, says Dr. Goodwin. Overactivity of CRH may also contribute to anorexia nervosa (since it suppresses appetite), panic disorder and obsessive-compulsive disorder.

Another gender difference is thyroid disorders. Thyroid hormones, which control metabolism as well as mood, are regulated by another brain-hormone system, the *hypothalamic-pituitary-thyroid axis* (*HPT axis*). Recent studies have linked major depression and bipolar disorder to underproduction of thyroid hormones, or *hypothyroidism*, which is more common in women.

Both the HPA and HPT axes also undergo major shifts during pregnancy (resulting in lower blood levels of thyroid hormone), which could be one possible trigger for postpartum depression.

For years, scientists have also believed that the neurotransmitter serotonin plays a major role in depression. Levels of serotonin, which can be measured in blood platelets, are lower in people with major depression; drugs that boost serotonin relieve symptoms of depression. But until recently, there was no direct evidence of serotonin's role.

Now scientists have actually *observed* impaired brain activity involving serotonin using neuroimaging. Neurologists can actually "see" some of the effects of depression by measuring electrical activity in the brain with an *electroencephalograph* (or *EEG*), or by *positron emission tomography* (*PET*) scans. Subjects are given injections of glucose containing minute amounts of radioactivity. Glucose is cell fuel, so active areas of the brain take in more blood containing glucose, and glow brightly on the scan.

Scientists at the New York State Psychiatric Institute, Columbia University and the University of Pittsburgh compared PET scans of six patients diagnosed with major depression with six normal controls, after giving them all a serotonin-boosting drug along with glucose. The researchers reported in 1996 in the *American Journal of Psychiatry* that the depressed patients showed a blunted response to serotonin release in certain areas of the brain, while the controls did not.

The first-ever imaging studies of serotonin synthesis in the brain, reported in 1997 by scientists at McGill University in Montreal, revealed that men's brains make 52 percent more serotonin than women's. This may be one of the biggest differences found in male and female brains unrelated to sex hormones. Some gender differences have also been found in the limbic system, considered the seat of emotion, with women showing more activity than men when asked to recall sad memories.

Other PET scan studies reveal *decreased* activity in people with depression in the rear portions of the brain's right hemisphere which helps regulate attention to a task. So, lessened activity in that region could explain why depressed people can't seem to concentrate. The right hemisphere also regulates the HPA axis and the release of stress hormones, affecting motor activity and reaction time, perhaps explaining why some depressed people feel "slowed down."

According to a report in a special 1993 issue of the *Journal of Affective Disorders*, some scientists believe that emotional stimuli may engage the right hemisphere of the brain in women more than in men. Studies have also shown that women tend to cope with depression with strategies like brooding, while men tend to distract themselves with work or sports. The report suggests that physical activity may stimulate the right hemisphere, which may "normalize" the HPA axis and help alleviate some of the symptoms of depression. Many therapists routinely recommend exercise as part of treatment.

Much of this research is still speculative, but it offers some tantalizing hints regarding differences between the genders in depression, and it may provide directions for treatments tailored to women.

Is It in Our Genes?

Depression also seems to be genetic, which is not surprising considering that 50 percent of our genes relate to the brain.

Children with one depressed parent are two to three times more likely to suffer from depression by the time they reach age eighteen than children of nondepressed parents; the risk doubles if both parents have had depression, says Dr. Goodwin. Such children also have an earlier age of onset, a longer recovery period and a higher recurrence rate. Recent studies of identical female twins (who have identical genes) show that if one twin has major depression, there's a 70 percent likelihood the other twin will have it, compared with 25 percent among nonidentical twins.

Rates of bipolar disorder are also higher when there's a family history of depression. Scientists at Thomas Jefferson University say they may have found a gene that predisposes people to manic depression but that research is still very preliminary.

ꙮ *Caren's Story, Continued* ꙮ

"My father had major depression, but we never talked about it. . . . Everyone said, 'Well, he has reason to be upset.' The year before his first admission to the hospital, he and my grandfather went in together on a big business venture. But it was a bad year, and not only did my father and mother lose a lot of money, but my mother's family lost everything, too. And my father felt responsible. So he probably had a depression related to a life event. But, probably, just as it did with me, it didn't go away.

"When I got my depression, I wanted all the information I could get about his history. When I finally read his medical records, it was a shock. He went through the exact same things I had. The panic attacks, the uncontrollable weeping at inappropriate times, the suicidal ideations, sleep disorder, the loss of interest in family, kids, work. . . . It was me. It was like reading myself on this piece of paper.

"I think my own depression really started when Daddy died. . . . We were expected to go back to school the day after we buried him and be perfectly normal. . . . I was crying, trying to figure things out. My mother couldn't deal with it. . . . She wasn't a bad mother, she just didn't know how to deal with my grief.

"For the rest of my family, it seemed so easy. Just pick yourself up by your bootstraps and go on with your life. But unfortunately, I had major depression, or at least the beginnings of it. My family couldn't deal with me."

The idea that female biology plays a role in depression is suggested by population studies from different parts of the world, which consistently show higher rates of depression and dysthymia in women across different races and cultures, notes Myrna M. Weissman, Ph.D., director of clinical and genetic epidemiology at the New York State Psychiatric Institute, and a professor of epidemiology and psychiatry at the Columbia University College of Physicians and Surgeons.

It was Dr. Weissman and the late Gerald L. Klerman, M.D., who in 1977 published the landmark study that first documented the twofold greater risk of depression in women. Drs. Weissman and Klerman also studied data from ten countries (places as diverse as Canada, Puerto Rico, Germany and Korea).

The fact that gender differences in the incidence of depression begin at puberty also lends credence to biological theories, says Dr. Weissman. Women have a slightly earlier age of onset for major depression (the mid twenties) compared with men (late twenties to early thirties). Between ages thirty and forty-four, the rates of depression are almost *three* times higher in women than in men!

New data from Dr. Weissman's multinational studies reveal some interesting patterns: a peak in depression among women in all cultures during their childbearing years (though not necessarily related to the birth of a child), and again during the *perimenopause*. "This may reflect an initial episode of depression which occurs during a woman's twenties, which recurs in the years just before menopause, rather than a 'menopausal' depression," she reported to the American Psychiatric Association's annual meeting in 1995.

PSYCHOSOCIAL FACTORS

There are many psychosocial theories as to why there are higher rates of depression among women. "Because of the prime importance of relationships in women's lives, they are more sensitive than men to losses, particularly losses of attachment, which may increase their vulnerability to depression," says Dr. Weissman.

Susan Nolen-Hoeksema, Ph.D., an associate professor of psychology at the University of Michigan and author of *Sex Differences in Depression* (Stanford University Press, 1990), disagrees. She points to studies showing equal rates of depression among men and women after divorce or widowhood. "Women may be more vulnerable to depression because of differences in coping styles. Men are conditioned from childhood to go into 'action' following a loss or disappointment, either trying to change the situation or distract themselves," argues Dr. Nolen-Hoeksema. "Women tend to focus inward on their feelings in a passive, non-problem-solving way. And this 'ruminative' response may increase their feelings of hopelessness and helplessness, intensifying and lengthening depressive episodes."

Women are socialized to be more sensitive to the feelings of others, which may add to the number of stressful life events they experience compared with those of men, suggests Ellen Frank, Ph.D., professor of psychiatry and psychology at the University of Pittsburgh, and director of the Prevention of Depression and Manic Depression Program at the Western Psychiatric Institute and Clinic. "We call it 'the cost of caring,'" she comments.

Recent research by Dr. Frank and her colleagues found that among 135 patients with recurrent depression, over half of the women had experienced a severely stressful life event prior to becoming depressed, compared with less than a third of the men.

Compounding increased life stresses may be women's psychological reaction to the devaluation of their roles in society, their lower status and pay in the workplace, as well as sexual or physical abuse. Factor in the element of low self-esteem and lack of control over one's life, and you have what's called "learned helplessness," says Helen A. DeRosis, M.D., clinical associate professor of psychiatry at NYU Medical Center and coauthor of *The Book of Hope: How Women Can Overcome Depression* (Macmillan).

"When women are unable to change things in their lives, or when they don't meet our own expectations, they feel like a failure, and despise their shortcomings," says Dr. DeRosis. "This sense of failure feeds the depression; one feels more helpless and trapped. When these feelings become overwhelming, they are unconsciously 'depressed' for the purpose of numbing the pain, shame and guilt."

The concept of "learned helplessness" actually evolved from animal experiments. When an animal is put into a situation where it is helpless, it first resists and tries to escape. But when the animal finds that nothing it does works, it slips from anxiety into withdrawal, similar to a shutdown phase of depression.

In some people, this same reaction may occur as a result of problems in their job or in their relationships, where they feel increasingly powerless to make changes, says Dr. DeRosis.

❧ Caren's Story, Continued ❧

"When I was at the height of my depression, there were people in my department who would walk into my office and find me cowered underneath my desk crying. . . . There were decisions to make. I didn't know how to make them. . . . I didn't know what to feel. I wasn't happy, I wasn't sad, I wasn't anything. . . .

"I was married for several years. It was not a good marriage from day one. In fact, I think I got married to try to escape the depression. I got married to be happy. But basically, I couldn't talk about how I felt, so I made everything okay. . . . I was supposed to be this wonderful wife, this happy person, very successful at work. And I pulled it off most of the time. I just lied about everything. I lied about how I felt, I lied about what I wanted to do. What everyone else said or wanted to do, I just agreed, because it was easier . . . than having to face what I really felt, which was I didn't want to do anything.

"I started to oversleep and miss work. . . . My suicidal thoughts really started with this sleep thing. I would think, I just want to stay under these covers and not have to get up, so then I won't have to make decisions that are wrong, I won't have to feel sad, I don't have to try to figure out why I'm sad.

"I was burglarized shortly after my divorce and after that I bought a gun, which I still have. I slept with it in bed. I can think of many, many a morning when I knew I had to get up to go to work and I'd look at it. A fleeting thought. I could never commit suicide, I know. But now, as a healthy person, I can look back and can still say shooting myself or swallowing a bottle of Valium would have been ten times easier than what I had to do to get healthy. But those suicidal thoughts are what made me finally get some help."

TREATING MOOD DISORDERS

Psychotherapy

Psychotherapy, or talk therapy, deals with the psychosocial aspects of depression, such as problems in relationships, adverse life events, personal losses, and emotional reactions that carry over from childhood and can affect thinking and behavior.

The 1990 *American Psychological Association National Task Force Report: Women and Depression Risk Factors and Treatment Issues* found that several forms of therapy that focus on active problem solving, rather than rumination, may be especially beneficial to women.

COGNITIVE THERAPY: Is designed to change the negative or distorted patterns of thinking, such as pessimism, self-devaluation and lack of self-esteem, that contribute to depression.

BEHAVIOR THERAPY: Does not explore thoughts or feelings, but rather tries to change depression-related behaviors, such as social withdrawal. Also may use a combination of *cognitive-behavioral therapy* (*CBT*).

INTERPERSONAL PSYCHOTHERAPY (IPT): A brief form of treatment that focuses on a woman's particular relationships and personal problems, and strives to teach women how to handle these more effectively.

SOCIAL SKILLS TRAINING: Aims at improving social interaction and communications skills.

PSYCHODYNAMIC THERAPY: A form of psychotherapy focusing on the underlying, often unconscious factors that determine how we behave and adjust to life experiences.

(For more detailed information on the different types of psychotherapy, see Chapter 12.)

Therapy may include exercise, which can biochemically reduce symptoms of depression, as well as reduce social isolation, and may improve self-image. Phototherapy (exposure to high-intensity light) may be used to treat *seasonal affective disorder* (SAD).

Pharmacotherapy

Psychotropic medications correct the chemical imbalances in the brain that cause symptoms of mood disorders. Long-term medication may be needed to prevent recurrent episodes of major depression and bipolar disorder. Antidepressants are not "uppers" or stimulants. They act chemically in the brain to eliminate or reduce the sadness and lethargy of depression, and help the depressed person feel the way she did before becoming depressed.

There are a wide variety of antidepressants which are not only effective in treating major depression, but can also be helpful in treating dysthymia, anxiety (which is present in many depressed people), phobias and other problems. However, it may take between one and three weeks (sometimes more) before an improvement is felt. Some symptoms lessen early on, others later.

"It's not clear why some people respond better to one medication than another. It may simply be a matter of their individual biochemistry," comments Norman Sussman, M.D., clinical associate professor of psychiatry and director of the Psychopharmacology Research and Consultation Service at NYU-Bellevue Hospital Center. "Several medications may need to be tried until an effective one is found."

There are five basic categories of antidepressants, and each affects chemical messengers in the brain differently.

SELECTIVE SEROTONIN REUPTAKE INHIBITORS (SSRIs): Block the reabsorption of the neurotransmitter serotonin in certain areas of the brain, prolonging its mood-lifting effects and eliminating symptoms of depression.

Since the first SSRI, *fluoxetine (Prozac)*, was approved by the Food and Drug Administration in late 1987, it has been used by more than seven million people in the United States. Newer SRRIs, like *sertraline (Zoloft)* and *paroxetine (Paxil)*, are also being prescribed extensively. These drugs have become popular partly because they have fewer side effects than tricyclic antidepressants, take effect quickly and are well tolerated by people who have trouble taking medications. "It's also virtually impossible to overdose on SSRIs. You do not get increasing effects, or any euphoria, from taking more of an SSRI. So they are much safer than tricyclic antidepressants," adds Dr. Sussman.

The major drawback to SSRIs is their sexual side effects; 40 percent of women report decreased sexual desire and others are unable to reach orgasm (or have delayed orgasms), says Dr. Sussman. Strategies for such sexual problems include stimulants like *yohimbine* (Yocon), giving lower doses of drugs or shorter-acting drugs like sertraline and allowing weekend "holidays." There is also a withdrawal syndrome with SSRIs, which can include crying jags, irritability and flu-like symptoms.

Another drawback to SSRIs (and other new antidepressants) is their high cost. A big-city pharmacy may charge upward of $150 for sixty tablets of the lowest dose of sertraline, compared with $8.50 for sixty tablets of the tricyclic *amitriptyline (Elavil)*.

MIXED REUPTAKE INHIBITORS: So-called fourth-generation antidepressants, including *nefazodone (Serzone)* and *venlafaxine (Effexor)*, block serotonin reuptake and inhibit reuptake of norepinephrine, another neurotransmitter involved in depression. Both drugs cause little or no sexual dysfunction or insomnia, but women can bruise very easily with venlafaxine, says Dr. Sussman. Effexor also causes some withdrawal symptoms.

ATYPICAL ANTIDEPRESSANTS: Include *bupropion (Wellbutrin)* and *trazodone (Desyrel)*, which are chemically unrelated to other antidepressants.

Bupropion appears to affect the neurotransmitter dopamine, a brain chemical involved in thought and movement disorders, while trazodone seems to increase serotonin levels.

The first in another new class of antidepressants, *mirtazapine (Remeron*), was approved in 1996. Mirtazapine stimulates release of serotonin and norepinephrine, and blocks two specific serotonin receptors in the brain. Its mechanism of action reduces the serotongeric side effects seen with some SSRIs, such as decreased sexual drive, nervousness and insomnia. Mirtazapine is designed to be used in people who suffer sleep disturbances and anxiety as part of their depression. It has not been shown to cause birth defects, but it should be used cautiously in pregnant women and during breast feeding.

TRICYCLIC ANTIDEPRESSANTS: Are so named for their three-ring molecular structure. They block the reuptake of norepinephrine and, to some extent, serotonin, relieving many of the emotional and physical symptoms of depression. Their major drawback is their unpleasant side effects, caused by their action on other neurotransmitters (see box, page 43). Tricyclics are very potent, and overdoses can be deadly, so most physicians will dispense only a week's worth at a time, and only for short periods of time.

"Tricyclics may be very effective for seriously depressed patients, especially those in inpatient settings, where their intake can be monitored," says Dr. Sussman. "We might also use tricyclics in patients who have taken them before successfully. And they may be prescribed when cost is a major consideration."

MONOAMINE OXIDASE INHIBITORS (MAOIS): Were the first antidepressants and have been in use since the 1950s. MAOIs suppress the enzyme *monoamine oxidase*, which breaks down neurotransmitters in the *synapse*, the space between two nerve cells. That allows the chemical messengers between neurons to remain active longer. MAO inhibitors affect dopamine, which is also implicated in depression.

MAOIs are most often used for "atypical" depressions marked by oversleeping, overeating, lethargy, anxiety and panic attacks, says Dr. Sussman. The major drawback is that they can have potentially dangerous interactions with certain foods and other medications (see page 45). New, safer MAOIs are on the way. "Some people consider MAOIs to be the most effective of the antidepressants," says Dr. Sussman. "MAOIs seem to work when other treatments have failed. Despite their drawbacks we may turn to MAOIs when patients don't do well with other medications."

Lithium is a mood stabilizer (see page 46), mostly used to treat bipolar disorder. It may be given as a maintenance treatment for recurrent depression (or added to drug therapy).

Other drugs used to enhance the effectiveness of antidepressants include thyroid hormones, certain stimulants, anticonvulsants and buspirone. Antidepressant treatment usually is given for a minimum of several months, and may last a year or more. Recent clinical trials have found that long-term treatment with antidepressants can reduce the frequency and severity of depressive episodes in people with recurrent depression.

Antidepressant Medications

Sources: Medical Economics, Inc., *Physicians' Desk Reference*, 1995; Harold I. Kaplan, M.D., and Benjamin J. Sadock, M.D., *The Pocket Handbook of Psychiatric Drug Treatment* (Williams and Wilkins, 1995); *The American Psychological Association National Task Force Report on Women and Depression*, 1990

Selective Serotonin Reuptake Inhibitors/SSRIs: fluoxetine (Prozac), sertraline (Zoloft), paroxetine (Paxil) and fluvoxamine (Luvox).

Potential Side Effects: Restlessness, insomnia, nausea, diarrhea and sexual dysfunction (in women, reduced sexual desire and delayed orgasm). Less common side effects can include forgetfulness, slowed movement, fatigue, lethargy, tremor, muscle twitches, difficulty with voluntary movements (*dyskinesia*) and worsening of existing Parkinson's disease.

Withdrawal symptoms can include irritability, nausea, dizziness, diarrhea and eye movement disturbances.

Warning: Studies suggest that fluoxetine can be used safely during the first trimester of pregnancy, but may carry an increased risk of miscarriage.

Mixed Reuptake Inhibitors: venlafaxine (Effexor) and nefazodone (Serzone).

Potential Side Effects: For venlafaxine: nausea, drowsiness, dizziness, dry mouth and constipation. For nefazodone: nausea, nervousness, sleep disturbances, constipation, weakness, sweating and, in higher doses, increased blood pressure.

Mirtazapine (Remeron): the first of a new class of antidepressants. It is taken in a single dose before sleep.

(continued)

Potential Side Effects: Excessive sleepiness, increased appetite, weight gain, dry mouth, dizziness, increases in cholesterol and triglycerides, impaired cognitive and motor function. Patients should not use alcohol while taking this medication.

Warning: Mirtazapine carries an increased risk of the potentially deadly disorder *agranulocytosis*, which depletes infection-fighting white blood cells. Patients should alert their physician if they develop fever, chills, sore throat or signs of infection. Clearance may be slowed in elderly patients, so it should be used cautiously. It can also worsen liver or kidney dysfunction. Because of potentially dangerous interactions, it should not be used with MAOIs.

Bupropion (Wellbutrin): a "monocyclic" antidepressant. (Unlike other antidepressants, which can be taken once a day, bupropion must be taken two or three times daily.)

Potential Side Effects: Dry mouth, constipation, weight loss, headache, insomnia, nausea, cough. Less commonly, restlessness, agitation and irritability may occur.

Warning: Bupropion may carry a slight risk of seizures in high doses (400–600 mg a day and over). Bupropion can interact with MAOIs, and should not be coadministered. It may also interact with the anticonvulsant carbamazepine (Tegretol), the ulcer drug cimetidine (Tagamet), the antiseizure medication phenytoin (Dilantin) and certain barbiturates.

Trazodone (Desyrel): an atypical antidepressant

Potential Side Effects: It is extremely sedating, and is often prescribed to help people with sleep problems and/or given as a sleep aid for people taking MAOIs. However, it can also help low desire and orgasmic dysfunction in women taking SSRIs.

Other side effects include dry mouth, dizziness, blurred vision, constipation and urinary retention. In people over age sixty trazodone may cause low blood pressure and dizziness when going from a prone to standing position (*postural hypotension*).

Tricyclic Antidepressants: include amitriptyline (Elavil), nortriptyline (Aventyl), amoxapine (Asendin), imipramine (Tofranil), trazodone (Desyrel) and clomipramine (Anafranil).

Potential Side Effects: Tricyclics lower levels of the neurotransmitter *acetylcholine* in a variety of nerves all over the body, resulting in *anticholinergic* symptoms, such as constipation, blurred vision and dry mouth. Side effects like drowsiness are produced by the effects of tricyclics on certain *histamine receptors*.

Other side effects include dizziness when changing position, increased sweating, urinary retention, rapid heartbeats (*tachycardia*), sedation, restlessness, headaches, changes in sexual desire, decrease in sexual ability, muscle twitches, fatigue, weakness and weight gain. Tricyclics may provoke manic episodes and worsen psychotic disorders.

Common Drug Interactions: Thyroid hormone, oral contraceptives and the ulcer medication *cimetidine* (*Tagamet*) may decrease plasma levels of tricyclics. Tricyclics may block the effects of the antihypertensives *propranolol* (*Inderal*) and *clonidine* (*Catapres*), and add to the sedating effects of antipsychotic drugs. Interaction with over-the-counter cold preparations and alcohol can depress the central nervous system.

Warning: Overdose requires immediate medical attention. Symptoms include rapid heartbeat, dilated pupils, flushed face and agitation progressing to confusion, loss of consciousness, seizures, irregular heartbeats, cardiorespiratory collapse and possibly death.

Tricyclics can cause problems in people with liver or kidney disease. Narrow-angle glaucoma can be aggravated by anticholinergic drugs; patients must use pilocarpine eye drops.

Monoamine Oxidase Inhibitors/MAOIs: include tranylcypromine (Parnate), phenelzine (Nardil), isocarboxazid (Marplan) and selegiline (Deprenyl).

Potential Side Effects: Low blood pressure, weight gain, fluid retention, sexual dysfunction and insomnia.

MAOIs can cause potentially life-threatening hypertensive reactions with foods rich in *tyramine,* a substance that acts similarly to adrenaline, causing dangerous surges in blood pressure. Tyramine-rich foods include: any aged cheese (such as Camembert, Edam or cheddar); cheese-containing foods; alcohol (especially Chianti, red wine, beer and ale); beef or chicken liver; pickled or smoked fish, poultry and meats; broad beans (fava); avocado; soy products (like tofu) and sour cream.

(continued)

Signs of a tyramine cross-reaction can include severe high blood pressure, headache, nausea, vomiting, rapid heartbeat, confusion, psychotic symptoms, seizures, stroke and coma. Patients should also be warned that bee stings can cause a hypertensive crisis. Such a hypertensive crisis can be treated with the calcium channel blocker *nifedipine* (*Procardia*).

Warning: Inhibition of the MAO enzyme can cause severe and possibly fatal interactions with other medications, including over-the-counter cold preparations, local anesthetics, amphetamines, antihistamines, insulin, narcotics and anti-Parkinsonian medications. Patients need to obtain a complete list of restricted medications, foods and drinks from their physician or pharmacist.

MAOIs should be avoided by people with cardiovascular or renal disease, hyperthyroidism and seizure disorders. MAOIs can also worsen symptoms of Parkinson's disease and provoke hypoglycemic reactions in people with diabetes.

Lithium: See chart on page 48.

Different types of medications are used for bipolar illness, chief among them, lithium.

LITHIUM: Lithium is a mineral salt present in certain rocks and in mineral springs. In the nineteenth century, people "took the waters" at these springs, by bathing in and drinking lithium-rich water.

It's not fully understood how lithium works. It is believed to inhibit the action of an enzyme found in brain cells, decreasing their response to various neurotransmitters. It is also believed to affect the movement of calcium and sodium in and out of cells, which influences nerve impulses along cells.

Lithium is most effective against mania. It can diminish symptoms in about five to fourteen days (especially if given early in a hypomanic episode). However, it may take days to months until mania is fully controlled. Antipsychotic medications (see page 102) or benzodiazepines may be used initially to control severe mania until the lithium begins to take effect. Antidepressants may be added in the depressive phase of bipolar disorder.

Lithium is widely used as a long-term preventive treatment for bipolar disorders. New studies indicate that it may also decrease the severity and frequency of recurrent unipolar depression.

About one in ten patients with bipolar disorder do not respond to lithium, and this problem is more common among women, says Dr. Ellen Leibenluft. Women are also more likely to be rapid cyclers, who also have a lesser response to lithium.

Bipolar illness can worsen in the postpartum period. Recent studies suggest that lithium given after delivery can help prevent postpartum affective psychosis. (Women are advised not to breast-feed while on lithium or other psychotropic medications. See page 284.)

Doses of lithium may vary over time. There's a fine line between an effective dose and a toxic dose. Blood tests are needed every few months to regulate lithium levels in the body.

Because of lithium's effects on sodium, anything that removes water from the body and lowers sodium levels—heavy sweating from prolonged exercise, fever, vomiting, diuretics (even weak ones like coffee and tea) or a low-salt diet—may cause a toxic buildup of the drug (see page 48). Adequate fluid and salt intake is essential.

As many as 75 percent of people who take lithium will experience side effects, especially during the first weeks of treatment, but that can be helped by adjusting the dose.

ANTICONVULSANTS: Anticonvulsant medications, used to treat epilepsy, can help curb manic episodes in patients who do not respond to lithium. One theory is that anticonvulsants dampen repeated electrical stimulation of certain areas of the brain similar to the stimulation that causes epilepsy. This repeated stimulation (possibly triggered by psychological stresses) may then transmit impulses through the nervous system that lead to manic behavior.

The anticonvulsants most widely used in treating bipolar disorder are *carbamazepine (Tegretol)*, *valproic acid*, *sodium valproate (Depakene)* and *divalproex sodium (Depakote)*. In 1995, the anticonvulsive Depakote was approved by the FDA for treating manic-depressive illness. Unlike lithium, these drugs are effective for rapid cyclers. Valproic acid has been found effective in treating both manic and depressive episodes. Some studies have also found that adding valproic acid to lithium can help a nonresponding patient respond to lithium.

Most side effects are mild, but carbamazepine can cause a potentially lethal blood disorder, so patients require weekly blood tests (see page 48), adding to the expense of the drug.

Antimanic Medications

Sources: Medical Economics, Inc., *Physicians' Desk Reference*, 1995; Harold I. Kaplan, M.D., and Benjamin J. Sadock, M.D. *The Pocket Handbook of Psychiatric Drug Treatment* (Williams and Wilkins; 1995)

Lithium: lithium carbonate (Lithane, Lithobid) and lithium citrate (Cabalith-S) are the most common forms of lithium.

Potential Side Effects: Slight nausea, stomach cramps, diarrhea, weight gain, fluid retention, muscle weakness and feelings of being tired, dazed or sleepy; patients may also develop hand tremors. Lithium may worsen Parkinson's disease. It can also cause kidney changes, accompanied by increased thirst and urination. Patients may also experience disturbed vision, perceptual distortions and memory impairment.

Lithium can also lower white blood cell counts, and requires periodic blood tests to monitor against the rare possibility of bone marrow depression. Long-term lithium treatment can worsen certain skin conditions, such as acne or psoriasis. Some 15 to 20 percent of patients may develop severe skin rashes.

Signs of lithium toxicity may include nausea, vomiting, drowsiness, mental dullness, slurred speech, confusion, dizziness, muscle twitching, irregular heartbeat and blurred vision. A lithium overdose can be life threatening and requires immediate medical attention.

Warning: Lithium may either not be recommended or may be given with caution when a person has existing thyroid, kidney or heart disorders or epilepsy. Patients need to be monitored for possible kidney problems. In patients with hypothyroidism, lithium may cause enlargement of the thyroid gland (goiter).

Anticonvulsants: valproic acid/sodium valproate (Depakene), divalproex sodium (Depakote), carbamazepine (Tegretol).

Potential Side Effects: For carbamazepine, nausea, vomiting, gastric distress, constipation or diarrhea, and loss of appetite. When used in combination with lithium, it can cause drowsiness, confusion, twitches, tremor and incoordination. Ten percent of patients may develop *leukopenia,* a drop in white blood cells.

In higher doses, carbamazepine can cause two potentially serious blood disorders: *agranulocytosis* and *aplastic anemia.* Signs include fever, sore throat, infections, mouth ulcers, easy bruising, pallor or weakness. Patients need blood tests every two weeks to monitor for these conditions, as well as tests for liver and kidney function.

The most common side effects of valproic acid are nausea, vomiting and sedation. These can be minimized by taking the drug with meals. Uncommon neurological side effects may include hand tremors, lack of coordination (*ataxia*), headache, anxiety and depression. Valproic acid has additive depressant effects when taken with alcohol. There can also be drug interactions with other anticonvulsants.

Warning: These anticonvulsants have been associated with neural tube defects, such as spina bifida, and should be avoided during pregnancy and breast-feeding.

ҽ *Marcia's Story* ҩ

"I was fortunate, I saw people going through ECT (electroconvulsive therapy) before I actually had it myself. And it is not horrible. . . . You're given a muscle relaxer and you're put to sleep for about ten minutes. You feel nothing and then you wake up. I remember it was seven o'clock and then I woke up and it was seven forty-five. You're a little groggy. After the first treatment, I had a severe headache. But after that, not much in the way of severe side effects.

"I had some short-term memory loss, but it all came back. It was stuff like I couldn't remember my phone number but I could punch it out on the phone. Or, I knew everybody's faces, but I couldn't remember their names. It was a little bit bothersome. But because I had seen other people go through ECT and I saw their memory come back, I was pretty confident. And even though I wasn't cured after the first time, I saw light at the end of the tunnel. In all, I had about eight treatments."

Marcia B. Greco is the past director of education and outreach for Depression After Delivery, National. The above remarks are published with her permission.

ELECTROCONVULSIVE THERAPY (ECT): In some cases, electroconvulsive therapy (or electroshock therapy) is used to treat severe bipolar disorder, or to help people with chronic major depression that has not responded to medication.

According to Bruce S. Klutchko, M.D., clinical assistant professor of psychiatry and director of the Electroshock Service at NYU Medical Center, the therapy involves delivering a mild electric current to both frontal lobes for two seconds or less, "firing" a large number of neurons. This produces a convulsion in the cerebral cortex of both hemispheres, lasting forty-five seconds to one minute. This induced convulsion is not violent, with few of the jerky muscle movements commonly associated with an epileptic seizure. During the procedure, a person is put to sleep with a mild anesthetic, and there is no pain. They awaken a few minutes later feeling tired and calmer, and can go home or to work.

"During the convulsion extra amounts of certain neurotransmitters are produced, including serotonin, flooding neuroreceptor sites, making them less sensitive to the particular brain chemical. This 'down-regulation' reduces the symptoms of mania or severe major depression," explains Dr. Klutchko.

A total of eight to ten treatments is needed and, in many cases, the normalized receptor sensitivity is permanent. Some patients experience memory loss, which is temporary.

Between 15 and 30 percent of patients may not respond to (or cannot tolerate) medication. Among those patients, 90 to 95 percent *will* respond to ECT. It's estimated that 50,000 to 100,000 people undergo ECT treatments every year in this country.

Which Treatment Works Best?

Many studies indicate that the best treatment for major depression may be a combination of psychotherapy *and* antidepressant medication. Guidelines for primary care physicians in diagnosing and treating major depression, issued in 1993 by the Federal Agency for Health Care Policy Research (AHCPR), note that a limited course of psychotherapy helps more than half of those with mild to moderate depression. But if psychotherapy produces no effect by six weeks, or does not result in a nearly full remission in three months, switching to medication is "highly recommended."

"We know that symptoms of depression are biologically mediated, so we need to address the biological aspects in order to treat it. If a person had an ulcer, you would use medication to relieve symptoms first, not focus on trying to talk them out of it, even though stress can cause ulcers," says Dr. Rubenstein.

About three fourths of people affected by depression have episodes that recur over a period of years. For those people, depression may become a chronic, lifelong problem, which may need long-term preventive medication.

Unfortunately, recent studies show that as many as 75 percent of women with clinical depression are *not* being treated at all. New evidence suggests one untreated episode of depression may increase the chances of a repeat episode. So if you are experiencing *any* signs of depression, don't hesitate to get help.

CHAPTER 3

Anxiety and Panic

Although the word "anxiety" is commonly used to mean stress, fear or worry, *anxiety disorders* are a cluster of specific, clinical illnesses, including panic disorder and phobias.

According to the National Institute of Mental Health, anxiety disorders are the most common mental health problem in this country, affecting more than twenty-three million Americans (almost 13 percent of the population), two to three times as many women as men.

Although anxiety disorders are highly treatable, as few as one fourth of those suffering from these disorders are under treatment. NIMH estimates that at least 70 percent of people suffering from anxiety disorders also have at least one other condition (such as substance abuse) that requires treatment. The cost of anxiety disorders is staggering: about $47 billion a year, much of it in reduced or lost productivity.

WHAT IS ANXIETY?

Most of us have felt anxious or fearful. Our stomach feels tied in knots, our hearts pound, our palms sweat. That is a natural physiological response to stress, whether it's being late for work or actually being in danger, such as driving in a bad storm. In this fight-or-flight response, the brain activates the sympathetic nervous system, which triggers production of stress hormones by the adrenal glands that sit atop the kidneys. These *adrenergic* hormones, *adrenaline* and *noradrenaline* (also known as *epinephrine* and *norepinephrine*), increase heart rate, blood pressure and breathing, pumping oxygen and fuel (glucose and simple fats) to our muscles. Once we perceive that we're out of danger, other hormones like *acetylcholine* counteract these physiological effects, and we calm down.

Back in prehistoric times, this response probably helped provide quick energy to attack or flee a charging saber-toothed tiger. In modern times, lesser threats trigger this same response: an angry boss or spouse, a screaming baby, having too much work to do, or sitting in a traffic jam. Tension and anxiety arise from normal life changes or stresses, such as the loss of a loved one or a divorce. Experts say that some anxiety is even healthy; it can spur us to work harder, or alert us to a problem that needs correcting, like an ongoing conflict at home or at work.

In anxiety disorders, however, sufferers have an *extreme* reaction to situations (or memories), and to real or perceived dangers, explains Michael R. Liebowitz, M.D., director of the Anxiety Disorders Clinic at the Columbia-Presbyterian Medical Center in New York City. "Mental symptoms of anxiety can include feelings of terror, dread or apprehension, uncertainty, nervousness, impatience, irritability, difficulty concentrating and feelings of unreality," says Dr. Liebowitz.

Physical symptoms include pounding or rapid heartbeat, chest pain, difficulty breathing and faintness, dizziness or sweating, all often mistaken for a heart attack. A woman can experience stomach upsets, cramps, nausea, constipation or diarrhea, and she may be diagnosed with *irritable bowel syndrome* (*IBS*). Anxiety can also provoke insomnia, fatigue, trembling or chills, frequent urination, muscle aches and dry mouth. When these symptoms are so severe that a woman cannot function or enjoy life, then they are considered a clinical anxiety disorder, says Dr. Liebowitz.

According to the *DSM-IV*, there are seven basic categories of anxiety disorders.

- GENERALIZED ANXIETY DISORDER (GAD): Excessive anxiety and worry out of proportion to a situation, persisting for six months or longer and which a person finds difficult to control.

- PANIC DISORDER: Repeated, unprovoked attacks of terror, with physical symptoms and worries about having another attack.

- PHOBIAS: Extreme, irrational and chronic fears of animals, places, objects or situations, which may provoke panic attacks.

- AGORAPHOBIA: A disabling fear of leaving home or of being in public places, where escape may be difficult. Agoraphobia can occur with or without panic disorder.

- OBSESSIVE-COMPULSIVE DISORDER (OCD): Recurrent anxiety-provoking thoughts, images, or impulses (such as a fear of being contaminated by germs) that cause a person to perform repetitive actions (like hand washing) to reduce anxiety.

- POSTTRAUMATIC STRESS DISORDER (PTSD): An extreme, long-lasting reaction to a traumatic event (such as a rape or mugging), which may cause the person to keep reliving the event with "flashbacks" or nightmares, retreating into emotional numbness.

- ACUTE STRESS DISORDER: The development of symptoms similar to those of PTSD, within one month after a traumatic event. In contrast to PTSD, however, symptoms last a maximum of one month.

It's estimated that over 30 percent of women have experienced an anxiety disorder sometime during their life. Seven percent of women have suffered agoraphobia, 5 percent of women have had panic attacks and almost 16 percent have had phobias. Anxiety disorders can occur in clusters, such as panic attacks with agoraphobia. About half of panic disorder patients have had an episode of major depression. A third may abuse alcohol or other addictive substances.

Anxiety can be triggered by medical problems including endocrine disorders such as hyperthyroidism, low blood pressure or irregular heart rhythms and respiratory conditions such as asthma. Certain medications, including high blood pressure drugs, digitalis, thyroid hormones, bronchodilators, antidepressants, decongestants, over-the-counter diet pills and steroid nasal sprays, can cause anxiety symptoms.

Caffeine can cause nervousness and irritability, as can substance abuse, particularly severe alcohol withdrawal, or use of stimulants such as cocaine and amphetamines.

Quiz: Are You at Risk for Anxiety?

We all worry. And we are all afraid from time to time. But some women find themselves caught up in a disabling cycle of anxiety and fear. Check the statements that apply to you. (Adapted from: *DSM-IV*; Understanding Panic Disorder, National Institute of Mental Health, 1993)

- Do you experience sensations of overwhelming anxiety, fear or terror for no apparent reason?

- Do you experience episodes of overwhelming fear coupled with rapid or pounding heartbeats, chest pain, rapid breathing, smothering or choking sensations, sweating, trembling or faintness?

- Do you feel extremely anxious in social situations or in certain places?

- Are you afraid of having embarrassing problems (such as fainting or diarrhea) in certain places or situations, and not being able to escape?

- Are you terrified of specific things like animals, insects or being in an elevator?

- Do you avoid social events, specific situations, places or even objects because of your anxiety or recurrent fears?

- Are you terribly afraid or worried about being embarrassed, or about people observing or criticizing you?

- Do you worry constantly about normal events or occurrences?

- Do you have difficulty sleeping or concentrating because of worry?

- Do you feel extremely irritable or tense because of worry?

- Do you engage in repetitive behaviors that temporarily seem to ease anxiety?

- Do these odd repetitive behaviors or repeated anxious thoughts seem to take on a life of their own?

✒ *Evelyn's Story* ✑

"My agoraphobia began as panic attacks when I was fourteen. . . . I would be sitting in the classroom and my heart would start pounding, and I would have this overpowering feeling that I had to get out at all costs. That my life depended on it. . . .

"My legs would feel all rubbery. . . . I'd have this choking sensation, a feeling of being disoriented. People's voices would sound funny, as if they were coming from very far away. . . . I saw a psychiatrist for ten years, but that did not help. . . . I had every test imaginable, but there was nothing physically wrong with me.

"I chose a college that was fairly near my home. I even managed to graduate, which took a lot of effort on my part. By that time the panic attacks began to take over my life. At first I could go on buses, but then I couldn't make myself get on a bus. So I switched to the subway. . . . But you cannot get off a train in a tunnel. If I took a taxi, I might get caught in traffic and if I had to get out, I would be frightened because I wouldn't know how to get home.

"I knew I could not take on a job . . . unless it was on the first floor, so I would not have to take an elevator. I began avoiding certain places. Once you have an attack in a particular place, that place becomes contaminated and you don't want it to happen again, so you avoid that particular situation or that place. So, little by little, it began to narrow down to where I virtually couldn't leave the house at all.

"I married a man who was very understanding about my fears; we lived in the suburbs where life was less crowded and, for me, less fearful. But after my son was born, I really wanted to get out and enjoy more of life. That's when I finally got help."

PHOBIAS

The most common of anxiety disorders are phobias, affecting more than twenty million Americans (about 11 percent of the population). More women experience phobias than men, and women suffer more intense symptoms.

A phobia is a persistent, excessive fear of a specific object or situation, prompted by the presence or anticipation of the phobic stimulus. Exposure provokes an immediate anxiety response, with symptoms such as rapid heartbeat, trembling, sweating, dizziness, shortness of breath, nausea or abdominal distress or a panic attack.

People either avoid or endure contact with the feared object or situation with intense anxiety or distress (or suffer anxious anticipation of the contact), which interferes significantly with the person's normal routine, occupational or academic functioning or social relationships.

There are three broad categories of phobias:

SIMPLE PHOBIAS: Exaggerated, unreasonable terror of objects such as animals, insects, blood or water; of environments (heights, storms, etc.); or of situations, like receiving an injection or being in an elevator or a plane. The National Comorbidity Study found that the lifetime prevalence of simple phobias is over 11 percent, affecting more than twice as many women as men. It's estimated that twenty-five million Americans are afraid of flying. Fear of high places is called *acrophobia*; fear of closed spaces (like elevators) is *claustrophobia*.

SOCIAL PHOBIA: (or *Social Anxiety Disorder*) is an excessive fear of failure or ridicule associated with any public activity, including eating in restaurants, attending parties, using public lavatories or making speeches or presentations. Social phobias are different from the occasional anxiety we may feel encountering new situations or meeting new people. A woman fears she will act in a way that will be embarrassing or display physical symptoms of anxiety, says Dr. Liebowitz. She may become convinced that everyone will notice her sweaty palms, for example, and this only makes her anxiety worse. She knows her fear is exaggerated, but cannot do anything about it, and may even restrict her activities, hampering advancement on the job or progress in school.

Social phobias appear to affect about 13 percent of the population, men and women in fairly equal numbers, often first appearing during adolescence. However, many people don't usually seek treatment until their mid-twenties.

AGORAPHOBIA: Is a crippling terror of being alone in public places, or suffering a panic attack (or other physical problem) in a place where escape might be difficult. The term is Greek, literally meaning "fear of the marketplace." Agoraphobia affects almost 7 percent of the population; an estimated 75 to 86 percent of those affected are women, many of them aged fifteen to thirty-four.

Agoraphobic fears typically include: being out of the home alone; being in a crowd; standing in line; being on a bridge; traveling in a bus, train or car; or fearing that one may have an attack of dizziness or diarrhea in public. People react to their fears by severely restricting activities or not going out at all.

Agoraphobics typically develop their first symptoms in their mid-twenties, but may not seek help until ten years later.

↜ *Faye's Story* ↝

"My first panic attack happened live on the air, while I was anchoring the late weekend news ... about six years ago. . . . I hadn't been feeling well for a while, but I didn't know what was wrong.

"I was two thirds of the way through the newscast, and just got this overwhelming feeling that I was going to faint . . . I just couldn't draw a breath. . . . I had numbness in my hands, numbness in my face, I was sweating, I was hyperventilating . . . my peripheral vision seemed to fade to black. . . . I figured I was either having a heart attack, or I was having a stroke. . . .

"I looked right into the camera and said, 'We'll be right back.' And the director said into my earpiece, 'Faye, you have more to read,' but I just shook my head and they went to commercial. Fortunately, the weather segment was next . . . and the weatherman signed off. So it really wasn't that apparent on the air. But when they cut away, I literally fell off the chair. . . .

"They called an ambulance, but the EMTs . . . did absolutely the worst thing you can do for a person who's having a panic attack. They gave me oxygen . . . which just prolonged the attack, sent it into overdrive. . . . I had all of these tests, a CAT scan, brain scans, heart tests. I was healthy as a horse. Finally, they said I'd had a panic attack and I needed to talk to my own doctor and maybe think about seeing a therapist.

"I was under a lot of pressure at the time. I was renegotiating my contract, I had two young children at home. I was supposed to be working part-time, but . . . I was working much more than that. . . . After the first attack, I was having panic attacks three and four and five times a day . . . but I kept dragging myself in to work, because I didn't want people at work to know. But I was a wreck."

PANIC DISORDER

It's estimated that more than two million Americans have panic disorder, attacks of terror accompanied by physical and emotional distress that, like Faye's, seem to come from nowhere.

Panic attacks themselves are defined in the *DSM-IV* as periods of intense fear accompanied by physical symptoms. Attacks can last between five and twenty minutes, and are usually accompanied by physical symptoms such as rapid heartbeat, chest pain, sweating, chills or hot flushes, trembling, choking or smothering, nausea and rapid breathing known as *hyperventilation*. The person may feel a sense of unreality, an overwhelming sensation of impending doom and a desire to escape, or terror that one is dying or having a heart attack. They are often rushed to an emergency room, but no physical problem can be found. Then the same thing happens again a few days or weeks later.

Panic attacks usually start when people are in their twenties, often occurring during a time of transition, stress or crisis, for example, a divorce or when leaving home to go to college.

Up to 7 percent of Americans have suffered a panic attack at some point, but when four or more attacks occur within a month, it is considered to be panic disorder. Often people feel a constant *anticipatory anxiety* about the next attack. This may escalate to the point where a woman becomes afraid to leave home, drive, or perform any activity associated with the panic attack. The resulting *agoraphobia* can be severe and disabling, with one quarter to one half of people suffering major depression.

GENERALIZED ANXIETY DISORDER (GAD)

Generalized anxiety disorder affects more than 5 percent of Americans aged fifteen to forty-five, and twice as many women as men. Risk factors include being separated, widowed, divorced, unemployed and being a homemaker.

Contrary to traditional thinking, GAD can greatly interfere with a person's life.

Women who suffer from generalized anxiety disorder often describe it as being followed by a perpetual "cloud of doom" that doesn't seem related to anything specific. That anxiety ranges from mild tension and nervousness to uncontrollable feelings of dread, lasting at least six months.

Depression can produce anxiety attacks and vice versa. However, anxiety disorders generally do not produce the same amount of lethargy as depression. Moreover, anxious people have trouble falling asleep, while depressed people often wake up early. Unlike depression, a woman with anxiety can enjoy things and can be cheered up.

People with GAD may experience occasional physical symptoms, such as a pounding heart, sweating and a sinking feeling in the stomach. Untreated, GAD can produce chronic headaches, insomnia and extreme fatigue. Many women turn to alcohol or tranquilizers for relief. The physical symptoms combined with concern over alcohol or drug abuse often finally prompt a woman to seek help.

OBSESSIVE-COMPULSIVE DISORDER (OCD)

As many as five million Americans may suffer from obsessive-compulsive disorder (OCD): endless cycles of repetitive thoughts and actions taken to calm anxiety or prevent a perceived danger.

We've all worried whether we locked the front door or left the stove turned on. After checking once or twice, most of us forget about it. But people with OCD check repeatedly, fearful that danger lurks outside, or that a fire is starting in the kitchen, explains Eric Hollander, M.D., professor of psychiatry and director of the Anxiety, Compulsive and Impulsive Disorders Program at the Mount Sinai School of Medicine in New York.

OCD is characterized by *obsessions*, repetitive, intrusive thoughts, impulses, or images that provoke anxiety. These in turn provoke repetitive behaviors called *compulsions*, which are designed to reduce anxiety. "These compulsions become rituals which make the person with OCD feel safe, that they are magically warding off harm to themselves or others," says Dr. Hollander.

One common obsession is fear of contracting germs from other people or objects, then compulsively washing the hands (even to the point of skin becoming raw). Another common obsession involves fear of harming another person, so that someone may repeatedly retrace an automobile route where they hit a bump, just to make sure their car did not strike a pedestrian.

Common compulsions include repeated counting or rearranging of objects (trying to keep them in perfect order or alignment), or mental acts, such as endlessly praying silently. People with OCD may perform these rituals for hours every day, deriving only temporary relief from their anxiety.

"Initially, people with OCD struggle to suppress their obsessive thoughts and compulsive behaviors, which they know are silly, keeping them secret. In fact, many people are able to keep their symptoms under control during working or school hours," says Dr. Hollander. "But over time, this control may weaken and obsessive-compulsive habits may take over the person's life, making it impossible to live normally."

People with OCD may not seek professional help until they can no longer manage their symptoms. A recent Gallup survey, commissioned by the Obsessive-Compulsive Foundation, found that over half of people with OCD have considered suicide as the only way to stop their obsessive and compulsive behaviors.

Men and women are affected with OCD fairly equally. The symptoms typically begin during the teenage years or early adulthood. The illness can first appear (or worsen) during pregnancy. OCD is generally a chronic disease, lasting for years. There may be intervals when the symptoms are mild, but OCD does not go away without some form of treatment.

It is now generally accepted that OCD has a biological basis (see page 65); it is no longer attributed to attitudes learned in childhood (such as an inordinate emphasis on cleanliness). Two thirds of people with OCD have also suffered a bout with major depression at some point in their lives.

The National Institute of Mental Health cautions that people with OCD should not be confused with people who are sometimes called "compulsive" because they hold themselves to a high standard of performance at work or at play. However, compulsive gambling and compulsive hair-pulling (see page 63) *may* be related to OCD, since they involve uncontrollable, impulsive behaviors that relieve anxiety or bring gratification.

Other problems that may be related to OCD are *body dysmorphic disorder*, an obsessive preoccupation with a minor or imagined body defect, and *hypochondriasis*, obsessive fears of having a serious disease (see Somatoform Disorders, page 106).

"The eating disorder *anorexia* may also be related to OCD, since girls are obsessed with being fat, even after they have compulsively starved themselves," says Dr. Hollander.

⊱ *Joan's Story* ⊰

"I started pulling my hair when I was eleven. . . . The hair pulling became very severe between the ages of fifteen and thirty, to the point where I was about forty percent bald. I wore wigs and scarves, but I continued to pull. It was an irresistible urge.

". . . Human beings enjoy nibbling, picking, preening, just like our animal forebears. But in trichotillomania, the impulse becomes so strong that the person isn't satisfied with simple nibbling or preening. The hair pulling becomes destructive and addictive. . . . It doesn't hurt, it feels good.

"I no longer pull my scalp hair, but I pull hairs on my face and other parts of my body. . . . I also pick at my face and skin, and cuticles when I am very nervous.

"I was diagnosed when I was sixteen by a psychiatrist. He told me the technical name, trichotillomania. . . . I did psychotherapy, but that really had no effect. . . . I was finally able to get help when I was thirty-six, after reading a book about obsessive-compulsive disorder, *The Boy Who Couldn't Stop Washing*; I saw myself in Chapter Twenty-two, 'Jackie P., the Hair-Pulling Woman.'

"In the support group I founded, I learned I was not alone. I learned to take my recovery one day at a time, sometimes one minute at a time. . . . It's the same with an alcoholic and having one drink. I know if I pull one hair, I will pull more. . . . maybe it's genetic, or a chemical imbalance, or low self-esteem, or . . . stressors in a person's life. It all contributes.

"I became active in the Obsessive-Compulsive Foundation and started a support group for other people with trichotillomania. In doing that I feel that I have transformed the negative, destructive energy and negative feelings about myself into something positive. Once I started doing positive things, helping others, my self-image improved and I was able to control my pulling/picking behaviors. Today my pulling is in remission, and my picking is under control!"

Joan Kaylor, M.S.Ed., N.C.C., is a member of the board of directors of the Obsessive-Compulsive Foundation, based in Milford, Connecticut, and a member of the board of directors of the Trichotillomania Learning Center in Santa Cruz, California. The above remarks are printed with her permission.

—◦◦—

TRICHOTILLOMANIA

Compulsive hair pulling, or *trichotillomania*, is regarded by some experts as a subtype of obsessive-compulsive disorder, and people with the disorder often show symptoms of OCD. Like OCD, trichotillomania also tends to run in families. It is thought to be up to three times more common among women.

Although it is officially classified in the *DSM-IV* as an impulse control disorder, people with trichotillomania often pull their hair to relieve anxiety, says Dr. Hollander. One of the symptoms is an increasing sense of tension before pulling out the hair and a sense or relief, pleasure or gratification afterward. "That gratification may also turn the impulsive act of pulling hair into compulsive behavior," he says.

As with Joan, compulsive hair pulling often starts in the early teens (it can also begin in early childhood or even infancy). People may spend minutes to hours a day engaged in hair pulling, targeting just about any area where hair grows.

Some people with trichotillomania have experienced sexual or physical abuse or multiple early losses. Other associated symptoms include chronic nail or cuticle biting, thumb sucking, compulsive scratching or head banging. Some medications for OCD can be helpful in treating trichotillomania, says Dr. Hollander. Sometimes the effect may wear off with time, and combined drug and behavioral therapy is needed. (However, it's believed the disorder may stem from a different biochemical problem.)

POSTTRAUMATIC STRESS DISORDER (PTSD)

Posttraumatic stress disorder (PTSD) was first formally recognized in soldiers returning from the Vietnam War, and was included in the *DSM* in 1980. During the Civil War, such problems stemming from battle were called "neurasthenia" (a term later expanded to include anyone suffering from chronic fatigue and malaise). In World War I, symptoms like flashbacks, nightmares, depression and survivor guilt were termed "shell shock"; in World War II, the term was "battle fatigue."

PTSD is now known to occur in as many as one in every twelve adults (as well as in children) who have experienced or witnessed violent or traumatic events that pose the threat of death, serious injury or physical violation to themselves or others, including sexual abuse during childhood, rape, battering, violent crime or a natural disaster.

A major national survey of more than six thousand men and women aged fifteen to fifty-four found that PTSD occurred *twice* as often in women as men after a trauma. Experts speculate that some traumas that occur more often in women, such as rape, are more likely to trigger PTSD. According to the survey, published in the *Archives of General Psychiatry* in 1995, more women than men reported an incident of rape, sexual molestation, and childhood abuse. Other studies estimate that five million American women who have experienced abuse have suffered PTSD.

The most common initial (or *acute*) response to a trauma can include intense fear, helplessness, horror, a feeling of being dazed or even temporary amnesia (in children, reactions can include agitation, withdrawal or disorganized behavior). "In women who are victims of domestic violence or rape, the acute reaction may be 'hypervigilance,' characterized by fear, anxiety and panic," observes Anne H. Flitcraft, M.D., an associate professor of medicine at the University of Connecticut School of Medicine, and a noted expert on violence against women.

Later, the memory of the trauma is reexperienced in unpredictable, but recurring, ways. "The smallest and most tangential reminder brings a rush and flood of the experience back," Dr. Flitcraft explains. "In the next stage, the victim may begin to experience a numbness that represents a dissociation of the emotions from the memory of the experience. This split between the emotions and the memory becomes the basis for subsequent depression."

For a formal diagnosis of PTSD, the traumatic experience must manifest itself in at least one of the following ways.

- Recurrent and intrusive, distressing memories of the event, including thoughts, or flashes of images or perceptions.

- Recurring nightmares or daydreams involving the event.

- Feeling as if the event were happening again, with a sense of reliving the trauma with "flashbacks" or hallucinations. Children may reenact the trauma in play.

- Intense distress when exposed to objects, people, places or other "cues" that symbolize or resemble an aspect of the trauma. The patient tries to avoid activities, places, conversations, objects or people that recall the trauma; feels "numb" or detached emotionally; has a diminished interest in activities and cannot function in important areas of living. A person with PTSD may also suffer sleep disturbances, experience outbursts of anger, startle easily, have difficulty concentrating, experience sexual dysfunction, abuse drugs or alcohol or attempt suicide and will continue to be fearful and hypervigilant, says Dr. Flitcraft.

Symptoms can be immediate or delayed, lasting for months. The *Archives* survey found that in more than a third of cases, symptoms of PTSD lasted at least ten years after the trauma. In acute stress disorder, the same symptoms last a minimum of two days and a maximum of four weeks.

Until recently, treatment of PTSD was based on experience with male combat veterans. But that is changing, as more women serve in the military. In 1992, the first inpatient treatment facility for women veterans with PTSD was established at the Veterans Administration National Center for Posttraumatic Stress Disorder in Menlo Park, California. Many shelters for battered women offer specialized treatment for PTSD. (For more on women, violence and PTSD treatment, see Chapter 9.)

THE BIOLOGY OF ANXIETY DISORDERS

While posttraumatic stress disorder and the shorter-lived acute stress disorder have their primary origin in a specific experience, there is emerging evidence that anxiety disorders have biological underpinnings. It's theorized that people with some anxiety disorders may have an imbalance in certain neurochemicals, such as norepinephrine or serotonin, or that the brain is unable to regulate their reuptake. In panic attacks, certain areas of the brain are thought to be overactive.

Supporting evidence has emerged from experiments in which scientists induce panic attacks and other anxiety symptoms in a controlled laboratory environment. One chemical used to provoke panic attacks is carbon dioxide. Carbon dioxide is produced when we exhale after taking in oxygen. Many panic patients "hyperventilate," take very rapid, shallow breaths during attacks and even show chaotic breathing patterns at rest.

According to Laszlo A. Papp, M.D., director of the Biological Studies Unit at the New York State Psychiatric Institute, hyperventilation may also be caused by the imbalance of neurochemicals in the brain. For instance, carbon dioxide stimulates an area of the brain stem called the *locus ceruleus*, which secretes norepinephrine. "When patients with panic disorder inhale carbon dioxide, we find that they increase their breathing at a higher rate than normal controls, a condition we call carbon dioxide hypersensitivity. They seem to need to take in more oxygen," he explains. It's still unclear, he adds, whether hyperventilation *causes* panic attacks.

Recent research has also linked anxiety disorders to imbalances in the neurotransmitter serotonin. "Our research suggests that those individuals whose serotonin system is unusually sensitive have a greater sense of harm, that something bad may happen to them. And this is associated with a greater amount of OCD symptoms, particularly harm-avoidant behaviors," says Dr. Eric Hollander. "Over half of our OCD patients seem to have overly sensitive serotonin systems, and when we stimulate those receptors, we can actually provoke obsessive thoughts and compulsive behavior in the laboratory."

PET scan studies at Harvard, done while patients' phobias were stimulated in the lab, found heightened activity in the *paralimbic belt*, the so-called worry circuit, as well as the locus ceruleus. (A small 1996 Harvard study found physical brain abnormalities in women with OCD.)

More than fifteen years of animal studies also indicate that norepinephrine and epinephrine (adrenaline), which are activated during stressful or frightening events, enhance memories of those events; this process may be *another* pathway to certain anxiety disorders. A small 1994 study of nineteen women and seventeen men at the University of California at Irvine seemed to prove that theory in humans. The group listened to either of two recorded stories, one of which was designed to be emotionally disturbing. An hour before hearing the stories, half were given a placebo and half received *propranolol*, a drug known as a "beta blocker," which blocks the effects of stress hormones and is used to control high blood pressure. When participants took a memory test a week later, those who had received the placebo remembered more details of the emotional story than those who took the beta blocker; both groups remembered the emotionally neutral story equally well.

"Hormonal reinforcement may be why frightening memories stay so vivid. It's possible that each time a person retrieves the memory, this stimulation takes place, further reinforcing the memory. If the system is driven too hard, it may result in phobias or posttraumatic stress disorder," speculates Larry Cahill, Ph.D., lead author of the study and a research neurobiologist at the Center for the Neurobiology of Learning and Memory at U.C. Irvine.

Genetics is also under study. About half of all panic patients have at least one affected relative. Identical twins are four times more likely to have GAD than fraternal twins. OCD runs in families and is more common in identical twins, even those separated at birth and raised by different families.

There is *no* evidence to link anxiety with sex hormones. But some women report their first panic attacks postpartum, while others report fewer symptoms while they are pregnant.

THE PSYCHOSOCIAL ROOTS OF ANXIETY DISORDERS

A growing number of experts believe that personality traits make some people vulnerable to anxiety disorders.

For example, panic disorder (and agoraphobia) may be linked to acute separation anxiety in childhood. Separation anxiety may be one facet of an inborn "overreactive" temperament (stemming perhaps from a genetic glitch in brain wiring) that emerges in childhood, heightening a person's reactions to stress, increasing their vulnerability to anxiety disorders, says Dr. Michael Liebowitz. One recent study found that up to 50 percent of adults diagnosed with panic disorder and agoraphobia recalled experiencing severe anxiety whenever they were separated from their parents as children, with many refusing to go to school.

"This trait, a tendency to be shy, inhibited and fearful in reaction to unfamiliar people or places, is often apparent before age two, and appears to be more common in children whose parents have agoraphobia and panic disorder," Dr. Liebowitz points out.

Researchers at Harvard have been following groups of such children from around age two onward. One study found that children identified as "behaviorally inhibited" as toddlers reported a variety of phobic symptoms at age eight, including fear of strangers, crowds, speaking in front of class, being called on in class as well as fears of elevators, airplane travel, going outside or being in a room or staying home alone.

Other researchers are investigating links between anxiety and personality disorders. People with social phobias display personalities high in "harm-avoidance," as do individuals with *avoidant personality disorder*, a pattern of social inhibition fueled by feelings of inadequacy and hypersensitivity to any kind of criticism.

"About two thirds of OCD patients . . . overestimate the probability of harm associated with their behaviors; they are particularly harm-avoidant and are very reluctant to take risks," says Dr. Hollander. Some experts believe that women may have more harm-avoidant and reward-dependent traits than men, which may explain the higher incidence in women of some anxiety disorders.

"These disorders can be seen in 'spectrums' that encompass different kinds of behaviors relating to both anxiety and personality disorders," adds Dr. Liebowitz. The panic spectrum may include agoraphobia as well as dependent personality and, perhaps, secondary substance abuse. The obsessive-compulsive spectrum can incorporate sexual obsessions, compulsive behavior, lack of impulse control, hypochondriasis, distorted views of body imperfections (known as *body dysmorphic disorder*, *BDD*) and trichotillomania. The social phobia spectrum can include a wide range of inhibited, fearful behaviors and social hypersensitivity.

"However, it's often difficult to tell whether what we're seeing is a manifestation of anxiety or depression, or whether it is a long-standing personality trait," comments Eric D. Peselow, M.D., a research professor of psychiatry at the NYU School of Medicine. "People who are dependent, avoidant and compulsive may actually have a form of anxiety or depression, rather than a specific personality disorder or style."

ᙓ Faye's Story, Continued ᙣ

"The medication helped to prevent the panic attacks when I had them all the time, but I have been mostly off of it for two years. . . . I've only had a couple of full-blown attacks. . . . But if I start to have symptoms again, I know they're not going to kill me. . . . I've learned a couple of little exercises to break an attack, so I don't always have to take medication. . . . When you feel you're starting to hyperventilate, you take a deep breath, hold it for twenty seconds and breathe out very slowly. That will stop the palpitations and heavy breathing. I've also learned some imaging to calm myself down. . . .

"I also give myself 'time-outs.' When I'm in a situation that's making me upset, I remove myself from the situation, do some deep breathing, and I go through this mental checklist: Nothing's happening, I'm okay, the kids are okay, my husband's okay. Whatever the situation is isn't going to kill me. . . . It's only going to last so long, then I'll be home and I'll be okay. I'm happy to say that I'm back at work part-time, and I can handle anything that comes my way."

Treatment of Anxiety Disorders

Anxiety disorders may be treated with medications, behavior therapy or, in many cases, a combination of the two.

Pharmacotherapy

BENZODIAZEPINES: Are the medications most often used to treat anxiety. The molecular shape of these drugs fits into specific brain receptors for *gamma-aminobutyric acid* (or *GABA*) like a key fits into a lock. Benzodiazepines increase the activity of GABA, which blocks the too-rapid release of norepinephrine (and other stress hormones) associated with symptoms of anxiety and panic. *Alprazolam* (*Xanax*) is the only benzodiazepine approved for the treatment of panic attacks.

In smaller doses, benzodiazepines act as *tranquilizers*, reducing nervousness and overexcitement. In moderate doses, they act as *anxiolytics*, turning off anxiety symptoms (such as racing pulse, rapid heartbeat and difficult breathing). In higher doses they act as *hypnotics*, producing drowsiness when anxious thoughts prevent sleep. Benzodiazepines take effect within hours.

Some individuals may remain on medication for as long as six months, which can have the potential for dependency (and abuse), as well as withdrawal problems. A withdrawal reaction may be mistaken for a return of the anxiety, since many of the symptoms are similar. To avoid or minimize withdrawal, doses are gradually tapered off. Because of their potential for dependence and abuse, benzodiazepines are usually prescribed for very brief periods (perhaps days or weeks), or sometimes occasionally for stressful situations or recurrent anxiety attacks.

BUSPIRONE (BUSPAR): A nonbenzodiazepine, buspirone has been approved for the short-term treatment of generalized anxiety. "Buspirone has none of the sedative effects of benzodiazepines, or their potential for abuse, and there are no withdrawal symptoms," explains NYU psychopharmacologist Dr. Norman Sussman. However, buspirone does not take effect as quickly as benzodiazepines, and a full clinical response may take two to four weeks.

BETA BLOCKERS: Help treat social phobias. Beta blockers like *propranolol* (*Inderal*) are normally used for high blood pressure; they slow heart rate and reduce flushing and other signs of anxiety.

MONOAMINE OXIDASE INHIBITORS: May be used to treat social phobias and panic. A number of clinical trials show that the MAOI *phenelzine* (*Nardil*), which blocks anxiety symptoms, has a response rate of 60 to 70 percent in treating social phobias. Other MAOIs may be used for their antidepressant effects in treating panic disorder.

ANTIDEPRESSANTS: Are used to treat a number of anxiety disorders. Paroxetine (paxil), a selective serotonin reuptake inhibitor (SSRI), was approved in 1996 for treating panic disorder. In PTSD, cognitive-behavioral therapy is used along with certain tricyclic antidepressants, which can also relieve anxiety symptoms. The tricyclic *clomipramine* (*Anafranil*) and the selective serotonin reuptake inhibitors *fluoxetine* (*Prozac*) and *fluvoxamine* (*Luvox*) have been approved for treating OCD. They are thought to reduce obsessions and compulsions by blocking reuptake of serotonin and decreasing activity in the frontal lobes, says Dr. Hollander. Large-scale studies of *clomipramine* show that half of patients have a 35 percent reduction in symptoms; smaller studies of SSRIs show symptom reductions in up to 70 percent of patients.

Unfortunately, most OCD patients relapse unless given long-term medication. Recent research indicates that psychotherapy combined with short-term medication may provide more lasting results.

Other drugs that may occasionally be prescribed for anxiety disorders include antipsychotic medications, barbiturates such as *phenobarbital*, and sedatives like *meprobamate* (*Equanil*).

Anxiety Medications

Sources: Medical Economics, Inc.; *Physicians' Desk Reference,* 1995; Harold I. Kaplan, M.D., and Benjamin J. Sadock, M.D., *The Pocket Handbook of Psychiatric Drug Treatment* (Williams and Wilkins, 1995)

Benzodiazepines: diazepam (Valium); alprazolam (Xanax); chlordiazepoxide (Librium, Librax, Libritabs); clonazepam (Klonopin); lorazepam (Activan); triazolam (Halcion).

Potential Side Effects: About 10 percent of patients experience drowsiness. Other side effects include dizziness, *ataxia* (incoordination of muscles involved in voluntary movement) and, rarely, cognitive deficits. Driving or operating machinery should be avoided while taking benzodiazepines.

Some medications increase blood levels of benzodiazepines including: *cimetidine* (*Tagamet*); the alcoholism treatment drug *disulfiram* (*Antabuse*); the tuberculosis drug *isoniazid* (*Nydrazid*); and oral estrogens. Benzodiazepines may raise blood levels of the heart drug *digoxin* (*Lanoxin*) and the anticonvulsive *phenytoin* (*Dilantin*). Over-the-counter antacids may also decrease absorption of benzodiazepines, and should be avoided.

Warning: Benzodiazepines carry a potential for physical and psychological dependence. If taken with alcohol (or other sedatives), marked drowsiness, disinhibition and even respiratory depression can occur. If taken with alcohol, antidepressants or antipsychotics it can result in seizures, coma or death. Signs of overdose include slurred speech, sedation, confusion, respiratory depression and memory problems. Immediate treatment is required.

Buspirone (BuSpar): a nonbenzodiazepine anxiolytic.

Potential Side Effects: Headache, nausea, dizziness, mild restlessness and, in rare cases, insomnia.

Warning: Buspirone may adversely affect patients with liver or kidney disease. It is unknown whether it passes into breast milk, and should be used cautiously (if at all) in nursing mothers.

Tricyclic Antidepressants: imipramine (Tofranil); trazodone (Desyrel); clomipramine (Anafranil); used to treat OCD.

(*continued*)

Potential Side Effects: Grogginess, headaches and constipation. Side effects of clomipramine include dry mouth and drowsiness and, in rare cases, seizures.

Selective Serotonin Reuptake Inhibitors (SSRIs): fluoxetine (Prozac), and fluvoxamine (Luvox); used to treat OCD.

Potential Side Effects: Nausea, diarrhea and sexual dysfunction.

Monoamine Oxidase Inhibitors (MAOIs): tranylcypromine (Parnate); isocarboxazid (Marplan); phenelzine (Nardil) is used to treat social phobias.

Potential Side Effects: Can include dizziness, fatigue, constipation and dangerous interactions with certain foods and medications.

Beta Blockers: propranolol (Inderal, Inderide); metoprolol (Lopressor); labetalol (Normodyne).

Potential Side Effects: Sluggishness, depression; some women report they have difficulty achieving orgasm. Beta blockers may worsen asthma and congestive heart failure and can interact with anticlotting or cholesterol-lowering drugs.

Warning: In very rare instances beta blockers can impair electrical rhythms in the heart, called "heart block." Doses of beta blockers need to be carefully regulated and anyone taking these drugs must be monitored by her physician.

Psychotherapy

Different forms of psychotherapy are often used in conjunction with medications for treating anxiety disorders.

COGNITIVE-BEHAVIORAL THERAPY: Combines cognitive therapy, which modifies or eliminates fear-inducing thought patterns, and behavioral therapy, aimed at changing destructive behaviors. Some experts believe that people with panic disorder have distortions in their thinking that give rise to an escalating cycle of fear.

Cognitive therapy helps patients to recognize events and thoughts that trigger anxiety, and to modify their response. For example, replacing alarmist thoughts like "I am having a heart attack, I'm going to die" with more moderate ones: "It's just a little dizziness, I can handle it." OCD patients are taught to label compulsions as part of a medical condition; they learn to resist them, eventually lessening their frequency. Cognitive therapy can produce lasting benefits in 80 percent of patients.

Incredibly, scientists have found that cognitive therapy may actually help "rewire" the abnormal brain activity that leads to OCD. A 1996 report in the *Archives of General Psychiatry* found that after ten weeks of cognitive therapy, PET scans of patients showed that abnormally increased activity was reduced in brain structures associated with OCD, a reaction previously seen only with the SSRI fluoxetine.

DESENSITIZATION: Is a form of behavioral therapy in which a patient is exposed to feared objects, places or circumstances (such as a bridge or elevator), for gradually increasing amounts of time, in an effort to "desensitize" the patient to what she fears.

To treat agoraphobia, a therapist might begin therapy at the patient's home but gradually take her on excursions to shopping malls or other places she has avoided. The therapy usually lasts eight to twelve weeks (or longer, depending on the patient).

Patients may also be taught breathing exercises. "People who have panic disorder have a tendency to breathe from the chest rather than from the abdomen, so training focuses on teaching them to breathe properly," explains Dr. Laszlo Papp.

SOCIAL SKILLS TRAINING: May be combined with desensitization to help people with social phobias. Behavioral techniques are used to help them become more confident in social situations, practicing conversational skills, giving talks or mingling with people at "parties" with the therapist or therapy group.

EXPOSURE/RESPONSE THERAPY: Is used in combination with drug therapy and behavior therapy to help people with OCD. The patient is deliberately exposed to the feared object or idea, either directly or by imagery, and stopped from carrying out her usual compulsive response.

The goal is to help the patient experience less anxiety from obsessive thoughts, and become able to refrain from compulsive actions, explains Edna B. Foa, Ph.D., professor of psychiatry and director of the Center for the Treatment and Study of Anxiety at the Medical College of Pennsylvania, who developed a number of exposure therapy programs. Dr. Foa says 75 percent of patients show lasting significant improvement with this therapy.

RELAXATION TRAINING: Teaches people to progressively relax different sets of muscles to eliminate tension and anxiety, while imagining anxious or threatening situations. Patients then use the exercises in stressful situations.

EMOTION-FOCUSED TREATMENT (EFT): Is a new brief therapy developed at the Western Psychiatric Institute in Pittsburgh for treating panic. In EFT, patients learn about panic disorders and their emotional responses to anxiety-provoking situations. The National Institute of Mental Health is conducting a study comparing EFT with cognitive-behavioral therapy.

Some individuals may require a combination of several types of therapy, as well as short-term medication to eliminate the debilitating symptoms of anxiety.

VIRTUAL REALITY: May take the treatment of high anxiety into the realm of high tech in the very near future. In this new therapy a patient "experiences" feared situations simulated by a computer, displayed visually inside the eyepiece of a special helmet.

The virtual reality (VR) visual display may include flight simulation (for people afraid of flying), the inside of an elevator (for people with claustrophobia) or a precipice at the edge of a tall building (for acrophobia). Scientists at Emory University, Georgia Tech and Clark University in Atlanta reported some success in 1995 in a small group of students who were afraid of heights. During the seven weekly sessions of VR therapy, the students stood at a railing during the simulation; it felt so *real* that some even experienced vertigo and vomiting.

Among those testing virtual reality as an anxiety/phobia therapy are the National Institutes of Health, the U.S. Army and a major California HMO, which views VR as a potentially cost-saving therapy of the future.

CHAPTER 4

Personality Disorders

[ach of us has our own distinct personality, predominant character traits that make us unique. But some people have what's known as "maladaptive" personalities: traits that put them in conflict with others, impulsive behaviors that sabotage their success. Extreme cases, which psychiatrists term *personality disorders*, involve distorted and inflexible thoughts and behaviors that make it impossible for that person to live a productive life or establish fulfilling relationships.

"There is considerable debate over whether one can diagnose maladaptive personality traits as an illness, which personality traits are, in fact, 'abnormal' and whether it is possible to treat severe personality problems," says Robert Cancro, M.D., Med.D.Sc., chairman of the Department of Psychiatry at NYU Medical Center. "Our personalities are shaped by genes, life experience and environmental factors. And you cannot separate personality from the nervous system. For instance, if you have a stroke or a head injury, your personality can change.

"A certain amount of maladaptive personality traits may well be inborn, and may not be as easily correctable in the way we can treat illnesses such as major depression," he adds.

The area of personality disorders is among the most controversial in psychiatry. In this chapter, we'll take a look at current thinking about the roots of personality, and ways personality disorders might be treated.

WHAT CONSTITUTES A PERSONALITY DISORDER?

It was only in 1980 that criteria attempting to *define* personality disorders were first included in the *DSM*. Since then, the criteria have undergone major revisions, and the process of defining personality disorders is still on-going.

"The question of when one's personality style becomes a problem is not something that easily lends itself to medical characterization," concedes John M. Oldham, M.D., director of the New York State Psychiatric Institute, and a member of the advisory committee on personality disorders for the *DSM-IV*.

"Acute disorders, such as major depression or panic disorder, have dramatic symptoms which flare up periodically. They are more easily diagnosed and often have a powerful biological component and can be treated with medication," says Dr. Oldham. "On the other hand, personality disorders are long-term patterns of behavior that are inflexible and maladaptive, that may only become apparent over time, and can last a lifetime unless they are treated in some way."

Instead of *symptoms*, psychiatrists assess personal *style* and behaviors, using measurement tools, such as the Personality Disorder Examination (PDE), to determine if personality traits have become abnormal (deviant), or pathologic (diseased).

The current diagnostic manual lists ten maladaptive personality patterns and suggests two others for further study:

- PARANOID PERSONALITY DISORDER: Characterized by extreme distrust and suspicion of others, interpreting everyday incidents or remarks as a personal attack or deliberate deception.

- SCHIZOID PERSONALITY DISORDER: Refers to people who neither want nor enjoy companionship or close relationships, and have a severely restricted range of emotions.

- SCHIZOTYPAL PERSONALITY DISORDER: Describes individuals who suffer extreme discomfort in close relationships, distortions in thinking and who display radical eccentricities of behavior.

- ANTISOCIAL PERSONALITY DISORDER: Applied to people with a disregard for the rights of others, who are always in trouble with the law.

- BORDERLINE PERSONALITY DISORDER: Describes a pattern of unstable self-image, personal relationships and moods and impulsiveness.

- HISTRIONIC PERSONALITY DISORDER: Refers to a person who is excessively emotional and attention seeking, often acting inappropriately sexually provocative.

- NARCISSISTIC PERSONALITY DISORDER: Describes a pattern of grandiose thinking, a need for constant admiration, coupled with a lack of empathy for others.

- AVOIDANT PERSONALITY DISORDER: Refers to someone who suffers extreme social inhibition and feelings of inadequacy and is hypersensitive to any form of criticism.

- DEPENDENT PERSONALITY DISORDER: Applied to an individual who is extremely submissive and clinging and displays an excessive need to be taken care of.

- OBSESSIVE-COMPULSIVE PERSONALITY DISORDER: Describes a person obsessively preoccupied with work, perfection and control.

   Other personality traits not formally classified as disorders include *depressive personality disorder* (characterized by chronic feelings of gloom) and *passive-aggressive personality disorder* (a pattern of negative attitudes and passive resistance to social and job responsibilities).

WHEN DO TRAITS TURN INTO TROUBLE?

All of us probably display some of these characteristics, to a certain degree, at one time or another. So how do you make the distinction, for example, between a person who is extremely egotistical and a person with a narcissistic personality disorder? Experts are wrestling with that very question.

   "In some people, personality traits or temperaments can become extreme or distorted," explains NYU's Dr. Eric D. Peselow. "In general, that distortion in personality is considered to be deviant when it is long-standing, interferes with a person's individual, interpersonal, or vocational functioning, or deviates from accepted social norms."

Another way of looking at it is that personality styles form a "spectrum," one end being normal, the other end being maladaptive. Dr. Oldham likens this spectrum to blood pressure: "A certain level is healthy, but when you turn the pressure up beyond a certain point, you become dysfunctional."

For example, he says, if a person is highly conscientious, organized and work oriented, it can be very useful in their career. "But if those same behaviors become too extreme, you can be disabled by them. You can become rigid, perfectionistic, and unresponsive—an obsessive-compulsive personality."

Personality traits may also reflect an individual's ethnic, social and cultural background, as well as recent stresses, losses or substance abuse. Some experts argue that borderline personality disorder stems from a history of childhood sex abuse and may actually be a form of posttraumatic stress (page 63).

Biological predisposition may be a factor. For example, schizotypal disorder is more common among people with close relatives with schizophrenia.

The first partial link between genetics and personality was uncovered early in 1996. Two teams of scientists reported in the journal *Nature Genetics* that people high in "novelty seeking" behavior share a variant of a gene that may cause the brain to respond more powerfully to dopamine, the neurotransmitter most strongly linked to pleasure- and sensation-seeking behavior.

Other recent research suggests that some features shared by depression, anxiety and personality disorders, such as anger and impulsivity, may have similar biochemical bases. For example, abnormalities in serotonin may be related to impulsivity.

Dr. Peselow is investigating whether some personality disorders may be manifestations of depression, anxiety or psychosis. "You may treat a person for depression and find that what you thought was a personality trait goes away when the depression does. Deviant personality traits remain stable over time."

People with possible personality disorders will usually not acknowledge maladaptive personality traits, says Dr. Peselow. So, the physician asks family members or other people to assess the individual. But what other observers report often varies widely. All of which can make a diagnosis difficult.

Experts say the only personality traits that can truly be labeled "disorders," based on current knowledge, are those which are inflexible and maladaptive. According to the *DSM-IV*, such a person must also display a pattern of behavior and inner experience that "deviates markedly from the expectations of an individual's culture." This includes distortions in thinking, in seeing oneself and others, and in emotional responses; difficulties in relationships and impulse control displayed in a broad range of situations. Clinicians must decide how well a person matches the prototype for each disorder.

A diagnosis should only be made when traits are present *outside* of another mental disorder, and are typical of a person's *long-term functioning*, says Dr. Peselow. However, there's a huge overlap between personality disorder and other problems. For instance, a person with borderline personality may be vulnerable to substance abuse or depression. An individual may be diagnosed as having several personality disorders, in varying degrees; or may be seen as having an "unspecified" personality disorder, one that is maladaptive but doesn't clearly fit one diagnostic criterion.

WHAT'S AN "ABNORMAL" PERSONALITY?

The *DSM-IV* clusters personality disorders based on behavioral similarities. Cluster A covers the odd-eccentric disorders (paranoid, schizoid and schizotypal); Cluster B encompasses the dramatic-emotional disorders (borderline, histrionic, narcissistic and antisocial); Cluster C, the anxious-fearful disorders (avoidant, dependent and obsessive-compulsive). While the "cluster" system isn't used for diagnosis, it provides a framework or model for looking at this scope of behaviors.

One such "dimensional" model looks at the traits of reward-dependence, novelty-seeking and harm-avoidance seen in anxiety. For example, the same harm-avoidant traits that may predispose a person to phobias and panic may *also* play a role in Cluster C personality disorders characterized by avoidant or fearful behavior. In fact, one recent study found that between 42 and 93 percent of people diagnosed with borderline, histrionic, dependent and avoidant personality disorders had a "comorbidity" (coexisting problem) with panic disorder.

Another approach looks at *character* as well as personality traits. The "Seven Factor Model of Personality," developed by C. Robert Cloninger, a professor of psychology and genetics at Washington University in St. Louis, adds three character traits—self-directedness (commitment to goals), cooperativeness and self-transcendence—and the temperamental trait of persistence, to the dependent/avoidant/novelty-seeking model.

"People who are mature and well adjusted tend to be high in self-directedness, they accept responsibility for what they do, know what they want to accomplish in life, are resourceful and self-disciplined. They are cooperative, socially tolerant, compassionate and principled," he says. "Someone who is immature and maladjusted, low in self-directedness, is blaming of others, doesn't feel that they have any direction in life, feels helpless, wants to be perfect and is not accepting of both their strengths and weaknesses. They are uncooperative, intolerant, insensitive to other people, revengeful and opportunistic. That immaturity is the core of all personality disorders."

Dr. Cloninger proposes that a "personality profile" be constructed using rating scales or detailed questionnaires, given to both patients and family members, and that a diagnosis (based on disorders listed in the *DSM*) be made depending on which temperamental qualities are maladaptive. Use of such dimensional models in conjunction with the *DSM-IV* is being studied.

Quiz: Personality or Problem?

Adapted from *Diagnostic and Statistical Manual of Mental Disorders, Fourth Edition* (*DSM-IV*), 1994, American Psychiatric Association

The following are characteristics of some of the major personality disorders. Check off those you think may apply to you, then give the list to someone close to you. Do others see you differently than you see yourself?

Borderline Personality

- I don't know who I am or what I want out of life.

- My close relationships always seem so stormy; one minute we're inseparable, the next minute I can't stand the person.

- I fall in love quickly and take a long time to get over it.

- I get angry over little things and can't control my temper.

- Sometimes I feel so empty or uncertain, I want to kill myself.

- When I sense a person I'm involved with may leave me, I'll try to do anything to make them stay.

- I can be reckless or indulgent: spending too much, eating too much, drinking too much or driving recklessly.

Narcissistic Personality

- People say I'm self-centered and always looking for attention.

- I often daydream about having a storybook love affair with a perfect man; reality never measures up.

- I get angry and impatient if I have to wait for something I want, even standing on line.

- I believe that the end always justifies the means.

- To make it in life you must be tough, even if it means stepping on or using others.

- I'm special; I only associate with others of high status.

- I often daydream about being successful, powerful or famous.

- I can't understand why people get upset with me.

Histrionic Personality

- People often tell me I act overly dramatic or theatrical.

- I always get very emotional about little things.

- I'm very conscious of how I look.

- I want to be as attractive as I can, and I'd undergo plastic surgery to achieve perfection.

- If I don't get my way, I often get angry or behave childishly.

- I like being the center of everyone's attention.

- People tell me I'm always fishing for compliments.

(continued)

Dependent Personality

- I have trouble making decisions without asking everyone I know for advice or reassurance.

- I prefer to let other people take the lead; I can't seem to get started on anything by myself.

- I allow others to make important decisions for me.

- I often agree with people, even when I think they're wrong, because I want them to like me.

- I'm easily influenced by other people.

- I'm afraid to be alone.

- I need someone to take care of me.

- I'm afraid of being rejected by others.

- I'm easily hurt when people criticize me.

WOMEN AND PERSONALITY DISORDERS

Some personality styles have been thought to be more common in women, dating back to the notion of the "hysterical female" ruled by hormones. But many experts contend that personality problems may stem from social conflict.

"Women's attempts to react to their sociocultural situation are often misdiagnosed as personality disorders," observes Leah J. Dickstein, M.D., director of the Division of Attitudinal and Behavioral Medicine at the University of Louisville School of Medicine. "Studies show that women with social problems are more likely to be given a psychiatric diagnosis and psychotropic drugs."

Some experts believe that histrionic personality disorder is more common in women, but the expression (and consequently the diagnosis) of the disorder may be influenced by sex roles and how we view them. Which personality do you think might be seen as histrionic: a man who dresses and behaves in an excessively "macho" style and boasts of his athletic prowess or sexual exploits, or a woman who dresses or behaves in an overly seductive way, and who brags that her boss is secretly attracted to her? The *DSM-IV* says that *either* could be diagnosed as histrionic.

In fact, personality disorders do not fit stereotypical gender patterns. Contrary to the myth that women are dependent and emotional, the rates of avoidant, dependent and histrionic personality disorders are about equal in both sexes. Between 50 and 75 percent of people with narcissistic personality disorder are *men*, while three quarters of those diagnosed with borderline personality disorder are women. Antisocial personality disorder is more common in men, as is obsessive-compulsive personality disorder. Rates of schizoid, schizotypal, and paranoid disorders are only slightly higher in men than in women.

⎯ *Danice's Story* ⎯

"My life . . . didn't match what everyone told me I should be, and I had no idea what it was I wanted or even what I wanted to be. So I started making up stories . . . small things at first, that I had done this thing or that. And people listened to me for the first time. . . . Then the stories got bigger and bigger. More dramatic. . . . I would say I had taken a vacation to Hawaii, and met this guy and he proposed and he had bought me all these wonderful things. . . . I even started to almost believe the stories myself. . . . And I found myself at twenty-four years old, not even knowing who I was. Everyone who knew me, knew this person that I had made up. . . .

"I picked relationships that I knew were going to end badly . . . but I would always be devastated when they ended. I would call the guy or write him. . . . I'd say I was pregnant, or that I was going to kill myself. . . . I didn't mean it, of course. . . .

"Even when the good stuff happened, there was still this feeling of nonfulfillment. . . . Finally I hit bottom. . . . I just felt, why not just kill myself, that's the only way I can get out of this. . . . I realized that I didn't want to live my life this way anymore. Somehow in all that anguish I had the sense to find a therapist. . . . That really turned my life around."

The Major Personality Disorders

BORDERLINE PERSONALITY DISORDER (BPD): Of all the personality disorders, none is more controversial than borderline personality disorder. Some experts argue that it is overdiagnosed in women (about 75 percent of those diagnosed with BPD are women). Others claim that such women may, in fact, be showing a reaction to sexual abuse or some other trauma in childhood.

Researchers at the University of Michigan at Ann Arbor found that 75 percent of inpatients in the Personality Disorders Program reported a history of childhood sexual abuse, and that sexual abuse itself was a strong predictor of the disorder. The researchers believe that while abuse may not actually cause BPD, it can lead to "abnormal interpersonal development that may harden into character pathology."

People with borderline personality disorder have difficulty establishing interpersonal relationships, usually having a string of relationships that swing from extreme involvement to cold indifference, from overidealization to vicious rejection. They fall "in love" at first sight, often making frantic efforts to avoid imagined abandonment. They may try to manipulate or "punish" others with suicide threats or self-injury. They may feel "empty," or show inappropriately intense anger.

Some experts describe BPD as a major "identity crisis," characterized by extreme uncertainty about many life issues, including career choices, long-term goals, choices in friends or lovers, questions of values and even sexual orientation.

People with borderline personality disorder may experience temporary, stress-related paranoid ideas or even detachment from reality. There can also be a destructive impulsiveness, including shopping or gambling sprees, casual sex, binge eating, shoplifting, promiscuity, substance abuse and reckless driving.

The disorder usually emerges during young adulthood; some people gain greater stability in their relationships and at work during their thirties and forties, and may improve over time. BPD often occurs along with mood disorders but, again, may be hard to distinguish from acute symptomatology, says Dr. Peselow.

HISTRIONIC PERSONALITY DISORDER: This disorder also begins in early adulthood. In clinical settings, histrionic personality disorder is diagnosed more frequently in women, but the actual population prevalence rates may be similar for both sexes.

People diagnosed with histrionic personality disorder are overly dramatic, emotional, erratic and attention seeking. They constantly seek praise or reassurance, are very impressionable and are overly concerned about physical attractiveness. Happiest when they are the center of attention, they may act or dress with an inappropriate seductiveness. In friendships or romance they become clingy and manipulative and may construct romantic fantasies about the object of their desire. They are easily influenced by others, especially strong authority figures who, they think, can provide magical solutions to their problems.

They may frequently complain of headaches, physical illness or poor health. But if these complaints predominate, the diagnosis may be somatization disorder (see page 106).

DEPENDENT PERSONALITY DISORDER: This is among the personality disorders most frequently reported in mental health clinics. In that setting it (as with histrionic disorder) is more common in women.

However, the *DSM-IV* cautions that dependent behavior should be considered pathological *only* when it is "clearly in excess of cultural norms or reflects unrealistic concerns." Some societies may foster passivity, over-politeness and deferential treatment of others. Many older women were raised to be dependent on, and submissive to, men, notes Dr. Dickstein.

In this disorder, dependent and submissive behavior must pervade every aspect of life. Women with this disorder are incapable of making everyday decisions by themselves, and obsessively seek advice and reassurance from others. A married woman may leave all major decisions to her spouse. She may be pessimistic, belittle her abilities and refer to herself as "stupid." Such people often volunteer for a task no one else wants in a bid to gain support from others. They hate being alone and feel incapable of taking care of themselves. They have a deep-seated fear of abandonment, and become heartbroken when a close relationship ends. There is also an increased risk of mood and anxiety disorders with dependent personality disorder.

AVOIDANT PERSONALITY DISORDER: This is a disorder equally common in men and women. The person who is afflicted with this disorder is an individual who feels so socially inhibited or inferior that he or she avoids any activity or social contact that may lead to criticism or rejection. These people yearn for social acceptance and are often upset by their inability to relate to others. They rarely have any close friends outside their immediate family, and are quiet in social situations for fear of saying something that would be thought silly or inappropriate.

Such individuals like to stick to their accustomed routines and may exaggerate risks involved in doing something new. For example, they may decline an invitation to attend a party in a strange neighborhood, fearing that they might become hopelessly lost.

The Other Personality Disorders

Although less commonly diagnosed in women, these personality disorders are not unknown among women.

PARANOID PERSONALITY DISORDER: This disorder is characterized by someone who harbors grudges for long periods, and who never forgets (or forgives) a real or imagined insult or slight. Such people are also "pathologically" jealous, questioning without good reason the trustworthiness and fidelity of their friends, lovers or spouses. They are rigid, unwilling to compromise, and often argumentative and critical of others, counterattacking when criticized, or when they feel threatened. As a result, they have major problems in the workplace, and may be seen by coworkers as devious, secretive and scheming.

NARCISSISTIC PERSONALITY DISORDER: This diagnosis describes a person with grandiose ideas about their own power, importance, talents or attractiveness, and who expects special recognition or treatment, whether or not they merit it. A majority are men.

But this exaggerated narcissism hides a fragile sense of self-esteem. Others' opinions are extremely important to them and they react with rage, shame or humiliation when criticized. They require constant attention and often fish for compliments.

These individuals are preoccupied with fantasies of success, power, beauty, brilliance or ideal love, and are chronically envious of anyone they perceive as more successful than they are. They lack empathy for others, and may take advantage of people or choose friends to achieve their own ends. Romantic partners are often treated as objects to bolster self-esteem.

OBSESSIVE-COMPULSIVE PERSONALITY DISORDER: This disorder is characterized by an intense need for control, and is seen twice as often in men. Such people are often perfectionists, preoccupied with cleanliness, order and personal control.

Often described as "workaholics," they rarely relax or take vacations and expect the same of others. They are stingy with their time and money, as well as with their emotions. These individuals may be so afraid of making a mistake that they avoid making decisions or completing tasks. They are equally indecisive about throwing anything away, and are often dubbed "pack rats."

"For the most part, these are not symptoms which make the person uncomfortable, but may drive the people around them crazy. They don't necessarily want to change until they get in trouble at work," comments Dr. Eric Hollander, of the Mount Sinai School of Medicine, an expert in obsessive-compulsive behavior.

SCHIZOID PERSONALITY DISORDER: This describes people who can be extreme loners. They usually have no close relationships, even with family members, and express little or no desire for sexual experiences. Men with this disorder rarely date or marry, but women may passively accept courtship and eventually marry. They may appear cold and aloof, rarely smiling. They often claim to have rarely experienced any strong emotions.

The schizoid personality is indifferent to the praise or criticism of others. Functioning on the job may be impaired, except in occupations where such people can work on their own. (However, experts caution that people of high intelligence with this disorder seem to function well, and their symptoms may be more subtle.) They may seem indecisive and even absent-minded. Some may have both schizoid and schizotypal personality disorder.

SCHIZOTYPAL PERSONALITY DISORDER: This disorder is characterized by eccentric behavior, ideas or beliefs, or extreme superstitiousness or "magical thinking," for example, the belief that others can read their mind. Schizotypal personalities may harbor bizarre fantasies or delusions, such as perceiving "evil forces" or seeing ghosts. (The *DSM-IV* is careful to separate such ideas from culturally held or religious beliefs.)

These people may have unusual patterns of speech or seem incoherent, often talking to themselves. Unlike schizophrenia, however, these people do not hallucinate or hear voices, and their behavior is not as extreme. They often appear unkempt, with strange mannerisms, appearing oblivious to behavioral norms. Not surprisingly, such people are impaired socially and at work; they may also be suspicious of others and live very isolated lives.

This disorder is more common among first-degree relatives such as a mother or sister, of people with schizophrenia. Symptoms typically begin in early adulthood. "It may well be that schizotypal, schizoid and paranoid personality disorders are a 'soft' form of psychotic illness," speculates Dr. Peselow.

ANTISOCIAL PERSONALITY DISORDER: This is the most common of the personality disorders among men, but some experts say it may be underrecognized in women. Quite simply, these are individuals who are unwilling to abide by society's rules and represent an extreme danger to others around them. They are often labeled "sociopaths" or "psychopaths."

They display a pattern of behavior, typically beginning in childhood or early adolescence, involving lying, stealing, fighting, truancy, vandalism and physical cruelty. As adults, they are unable to become responsible, independent and self-supporting; they cannot function in an organized way on the job or as a parent; and they may turn to illegal activities. They are often repeat offenders of crimes and are more likely to die a violent death than normal people. They may neglect or abuse their children or spouse, without guilt or remorse for their actions. They frequently lie, squander their money and cannot seem to maintain a monogamous relationship for more than a year.

Fantasies and "Fatal Attraction"

People with personality disorders often believe that relationships are more intimate than they actually are, and may be consumed by romantic fantasies. The extreme form of romantic delusion is called *erotomania*.

Although the idea of obsessive love has been around for centuries, erotomania was first described in clinical detail by a French psychiatrist, Gaetan De Clerambault, in 1921. The *DSM-IV* lists it as a delusional disorder in which the person believes someone, usually of higher status (a superior at work or a celebrity), is in love with them but is prevented from showing it.

"Erotomania can occur in any mental illness, including schizophrenia," explains Park Dietz, M.D., a forensic psychiatrist in Newport Beach, California, who wrote the definition of erotomania for the *DSM-IV*. "But when romantic delusions occur without other signs of mental illness, that's pure erotomania."

Those susceptible to erotomania are usually people from modest backgrounds, living quiet, lonely lives with few friendships or sexual relationships. Many spend their days toiling in low-level jobs. Since love is the ultimate form of approval, delusions of a love affair with someone rich and famous provide gratification when life fails to do so. The major clue that a person suffers from erotomania is the person's *total* belief in their delusion. No amount of "reality checking" by a therapist or friends can shake the conviction of a true eroto-manic, explains Dr. Dietz.

Erotomanics single out celebrities, or someone equally unattainable, be-cause their delusion usually involves highly idealized romantic love rather than sex. Many will write letters, send anonymous gifts or stalk their love object, says Dr. Dietz. "While 15 percent of people who write letters to celebrities do phys-ically approach them, violence is relatively rare," adds Dr. Dietz.

In the 1987 movie *Fatal Attraction,* Glenn Close played a woman obsessed with a married man with whom she'd had a casual affair. After he tries to break it off, she harasses him, slashes her wrists and even attempts to murder his wife. In reality, violence by women is rare; most women turn their rage inward.

"Glenn Close portrayed a 'borderline personality' type, someone with ex-treme mood swings, very impulsive and unstable, and who may also be pro-miscuous," explains Carole Lieberman, M.D., M.P.H., an assistant clinical professor of psychiatry at the University of California at Los Angeles. "This kind of person feels empty and bored and tries to fill the void with obsessive romantic relationships, feels intense anger at rejection and may try to hurt herself."

Women who need romantic delusions may have felt unloved as a child, says Dr. Lieberman. "The woman tries to heal the wound later on in life by having this grandiose fantasy of this wonderful man being madly in love with her. The more severe the wound, the deeper the need and the deeper the delusion."

Unlike erotomanics, women enmeshed in romantic fantasies know the man of their dreams doesn't love them. "It's not a delusion, it's denial. They are neurotic, not psychotic. They just can't give up their wishful thinking," she says.

In some cases, psychiatrists use antipsychotic drugs to help reduce the intensity of the delusion. Antidepressants may help when a romantic delusion is part of a mood disorder.

TREATING PERSONALITY DISORDERS

Unlike depression, personality disorders do not appear as a single episode or episodes. These are ingrained, lifetime patterns of thinking and behaving, which can be hard to change. Unlike most people suffering from phobias or anxiety, individuals with personality disorders often can't see or admit how their behaviors disrupt their lives. They're more likely to blame others, or "fate," rather than look to change themselves.

They usually seek help because of depression or anxiety, not because of their behavior, says Dr. Peselow. Sometimes people may be brought in by family members or referred by other physicians.

There are four basic approaches to treatment, depending on the disorder: psychotherapy, cognitive-behavioral therapy, marital, family or group therapy, and/or pharmacologic therapy.

PSYCHOTHERAPY: Is usually long-term. Psychoanalysis and psychodynamic therapy (see Chapter 12) are the preferred treatments for personality disorders, since they are aimed at "restructuring" personality.

Some studies have found that borderline patients take three to five times longer to show improvement than do people suffering from depression or anxiety (partly because they may take longer to establish a working relationship with their psychotherapist).

COGNITIVE-BEHAVIORAL THERAPY: Seeks to identify maladaptive thinking and behavior patterns, and then, step by step, tries to change them. For example, a woman diagnosed with dependent personality believes she is incapable of taking care of herself. The cognitive therapist would try to challenge this belief, showing the woman the ways in which she is capable, and helping her develop competence in other areas. Behavioral therapy would teach the person how to manage stress and improve interpersonal skills. This type of therapy is usually short-term.

MARITAL, FAMILY OR GROUP THERAPY: Personality disorders affect not only the individual, but their families and partners. Marital and family therapy is aimed at changing the way people interact with one another. In group therapy, people share their problems, getting feedback from each other and the group leader.

PHARMACOLOGIC THERAPY: Medications are usually given in conjunction with psychotherapy and are designed to relieve symptoms of depression, anxiety, agitation, panic attacks, impulsiveness, moods swings or disassociation. Medications used include antidepressants, antianxiety drugs, antipsychotics (in small doses), anticonvulsants and, in some cases, lithium.

Recent research into the biological underpinnings of anxiety and personality disorders suggests that serotonin abnormalities may play a role in certain personality disorders characterized by impulsivity and aggression.

The selective serotonin reuptake inhibitor (SSRI) *fenfluramine* (see page 43) was found to reduce such symptoms. Research at the National Institute of Mental Health also found that the MAOI *tranylcypromine* (*Parnate*) (page 45) helped some borderline patients regain mood stability, and the anticonvulsant *carbamazepine* (*Tegretol*) (page 47) could help them regain control over their impulsiveness.

CHAPTER 5

Thought and Perception

Just as mental illness can affect our moods and our personalities, it can also affect the way we think, and the way we perceive the world around us.

Thought disorders are characterized by disorganized, illogical thinking and speech, distorted emotionality and reactions, delusions (false beliefs with no basis in reality), hallucinations (seeing, hearing or even smelling things that do not exist) and a state known as "psychosis." A "psychotic" has difficulty separating real from unreal experiences, fantasies or thoughts. Thought disorders are equally common in men and women; a majority involve schizophrenia and its subtypes, as well as other psychotic and delusional disorders.

SCHIZOPHRENIA

Schizophrenia is the most chronic and disabling of the major mental illnesses. It is also vastly misunderstood.

The term comes from the Greek word *schizo*, which means "split." However, schizophrenia is *not* the same as "split personality," as many people mistakenly believe. Multiple personality is a different, and quite rare, disorder. The term *schizophrenia* was coined in the early part of this century by a Swiss psychiatrist, Dr. Eugen Bleuler, to describe the splitting, or shattering, of coherent thought, what he saw as the most prominent feature of the disorder.

In reality, schizophrenia may be more than one disorder, with different causes. It is extraordinarily complex, and experts caution that the official diagnostic criteria should only be seen as an attempt to summarize its major, outward signs. Although it is hard to make generalizations that can apply to all people diagnosed as having schizophrenia, we will try to provide a basic understanding of this illness.

❧ *Luanne's Story* ❧

"I started having problems when I was twenty-two years old. . . . It took about six years before I was correctly diagnosed. . . . By then I had a bad breakdown and I was delusional and hallucinating. . . .

"I had my first breakdown at college. I was sitting in a classroom and suddenly my vision seemed to narrow. . . . I was also paralyzed for about thirty seconds; I couldn't move anything but my eyes. I know my anxiety level had been very high for about nine months previously. So I just think my central nervous system went into some kind of shock.

"I saw a doctor, but he couldn't find anything physically wrong. He told me to go see a social worker. About a week and a half later, I ended up in a psychiatric hospital, where they put me on a small dose of a neuroleptic. I seemed to recover so well they thought it was just major depression. They gave me antidepressants, which alleviated some of the symptoms, but I still wasn't functioning. . . . I was hospitalized about seven times for about a month each, almost every year after that. During the last two breakdowns I was very delusional. And that's when the evidence of the schizophrenia really came out. . . .

"My delusions were about religion. I believed I was an angel . . . and I had to do certain things to save the world. . . . I felt like God was talking to me, and people who had died were talking to me. And I actually could hear a voice. It's like having a nightmare and not being able to wake up; you're living a dream, a bad dream. I also had what are called 'olfactory hallucinations.' One time I was in my bedroom and I smelled green beans, but nobody was cooking green beans. . . . Another time, I was walking in a field and I smelled gasoline. . . . It wasn't until they finally got me on the right medication that I was able to . . . see that it was a psychotic experience.

"I continued to work in between my breakdowns, and now I believe the stress of trying to hold down a full-time job helped to bring them on. I would become so lethargic, depressed . . . I would end up in a hospital for about a month. Each time . . . I would rest, they would adjust my medicine a little. Then I would go out and try working again. . . . Over time, my jobs would get less and less complicated; it got to the point I was doing a sorting job all day. I could not function in the world and that was extremely distressing to me."

Luanne Holsinger is a volunteer with NARSAD, the National Alliance for Research on Schizophrenia and Depression, and a member of the state board of the Virginia Alliance for the Mentally Ill. The above remarks are printed with her permission.

The *DSM-IV* lists several subtypes of schizophrenia.

- PARANOID SCHIZOPHRENIA: Is characterized by delusions or hallucinations of being persecuted, or of having extraordinary powers. This subtype usually occurs without disorganized thinking or behavior, or social and emotional withdrawal, but can feature anger and suicidal behavior.

- DISORGANIZED SCHIZOPHRENIA: Has as its main symptoms disorganized speech, eccentric behavior, and flat and inappropriate moods and emotions. Delusions or hallucinations may occur, but they are not prominent.

- CATATONIC SCHIZOPHRENIA: Is the most severe subtype, where a person becomes rigid and immobile, seemingly in a trance, not moving or speaking. Or, there can also be extreme, seemingly senseless, motor activity. In severe cases, a person may need supervision to avoid harming themselves or others.

There are also two related disorders:

- SCHIZOPHRENIFORM DISORDER: In this the symptoms are identical to those of schizophrenia, but last between one and six months, usually without impaired social or occupational functioning.

- SCHIZOAFFECTIVE DISORDER: Is diagnosed when a manic or major depressive episode occurs during the course of schizophrenia, or when the illness is characterized by major disturbances of mood.

Symptoms are characterized either as "positive," relating to disorganized thinking and speech, delusions and hallucinations, or "negative," relating to flat mood or emotions, social withdrawal and inability to feel pleasure. More subtle symptoms—such as social isolation; unusual speech, thinking or behavior; loss of interest in schoolwork or jobs; and deterioration in hygiene or grooming—may precede actual psychotic episodes. Symptoms can appear gradually, over a period of years, or have a sudden onset, known as *acute schizophrenia*.

One to two out of every one hundred people may develop schizophrenia during their lives; 2.5 million Americans currently suffer from the disorder. Although it affects men and women fairly equally, there are some important gender differences.

The first psychotic symptoms appear in women during their early twenties or thirties; symptoms emerge in men during the teens or twenties. Late-onset schizophrenia, after age forty-five, is also more common in women. This overall delay in psychotic symptoms in women may allow them to mature psychologically, socially, educationally and vocationally and thus "cushions" them during the early course of schizophrenia, suggests Mary V. Seeman, M.D., who heads the Schizophrenia Program at the Clark Institute of Psychiatry at the University of Toronto.

Women appear to have milder forms of the disease in the first ten years, with more mood symptoms than in psychoses. A recent small study at Harvard indicates that women may retain better cognitive skills, especially in language, than men. Women also seem to be more responsive to antipsychotic medication, so the initial prognosis is often better than for men with schizophrenia.

All of these differences may well be due to the effects of estrogen. "Studies show that during the phase of the menstrual cycle where estrogen levels are relatively high, the level of psychotic symptoms is lower, whereas during the phase where estrogen is relatively lower, severity of symptoms increase," Dr. Seeman told the annual scientific meeting of the American Psychiatric Association in 1995.

Women also seem to suffer fewer psychotic symptoms during pregnancy, whereas during the postpartum period they are more likely to have an increase in symptoms, or their first episode of psychosis. Many women worsen after menopause, and Dr. Seeman is now studying the effects of estrogen-replacement therapy.

Some people may have only a single psychotic episode; others suffer many episodes over their lifetime, but are able to lead relatively normal lives between episodes. The individual with chronic (continuous or recurring) schizophrenia often does not fully recover normal functioning and typically requires long-term treatment, usually medication, to control the symptoms.

Since psychotic symptoms can be triggered by underlying medical conditions, substance abuse, medications and head injury, a complete medical evaluation is needed to rule out other causes.

Through a Distorted Glass, Darkly

People with schizophrenia see the world as if through a distorted, fun house mirror. Normal brain systems that help us distinguish between what's real and what's imaginary do not seem to function well in these people, says schizophrenia researcher Arnold J. Friedhoff, M.D., the Menas S. Gregory Professor of Psychiatry at the NYU School of Medicine, and director of the Margaret S. Millhauser Laboratory for Research in Psychiatry and the Behavioral Sciences at NYU.

"For example, you're in the shower and think you hear the phone ringing, or you're walking on a dark street and imagine a shadowy figure lurking in the bushes. At some point, your senses and perception make you realize that you just imagined things. But for people with schizophrenia it's hard to tell the difference between what's in their head and what's really happening," explains Dr. Friedhoff. He compares this to a reverse LSD "trip"; instead of drugs producing hallucinations, in schizophrenia the brain *itself* triggers the hallucination. "It doesn't happen all the time, but when it does, it can be frightening. Imagine hearing voices telling you what to do, or believing that the people sitting next to you on the bus are plotting to kill you."

Delusions in schizophrenia commonly involve themes of persecution or grandeur, or that one is being cheated, harassed, poisoned, persecuted or conspired against. More bizarre delusions include someone believing that they receive radio signals from outer space through their dental fillings, or that a neighbor is controlling their thoughts. A person with schizophrenia may believe that they are God, the devil, or even the President.

To a person with schizophrenia, the world can seem baffling and changeable, without any of the landmarks we use to anchor ourselves to reality. This makes them feel anxious, confused and easily distracted. They may jump from thought to thought, topic to topic, in a jumble of words. People with schizophrenia may show "inappropriate affect," bursts of emotion in sharp contrast to what they are saying or thinking. Others are likely to become uncomfortable by this and tend to leave that person alone.

In "deficit" schizophrenia, a person displays "blunted" or "flat" emotional reactivity; they may talk in a monotonous tone of voice and never smile or frown. Some patients may sit as rigidly as a stone, not moving for hours and not uttering a sound. Or they may move around constantly, always occupied, wide awake, hypervigilant. Such people may not speak or interact with others and may feel little sense of purpose in life. One in four people with schizophrenia may attempt suicide.

Contrary to common beliefs, most schizophrenics are not violent and do not usually commit violent crimes. Instead, they tend to withdraw from social contacts, preferring to be left alone (in fact, many are homeless individuals).

The Biology of Schizophrenia

No one knows what causes this schism with reality. No specific gene has yet been found, no one biochemical defect has been proven totally responsible, and no stressful event alone seems sufficient to produce schizophrenia.

A growing number of scientists believe that schizophrenia may stem from glitches in brain development that occur midway through pregnancy, when neurons begin to finalize brain structure organization. Recent research suggests that these brain abnormalities may be caused by viral infections (especially influenza) during pregnancy, as well as by prenatal problems or birth difficulties. Some studies also suggest that women may be more vulnerable to such virus exposure in utero, while males may be more susceptible to developmental brain abnormalities and brain damage (especially during delivery).

New scientific research has pinpointed different areas of the brain that may produce the distorted thoughts and scrambled language of schizophrenia. Scientists at Johns Hopkins University have linked these symptoms to abnormal changes in the *planum temporale* (or *PT*) located behind either temple. Normally, structures related to language and thought tend to be larger on the left side of the brain; the Hopkins study found that the left PT of schizophrenic patients is abnormally small.

Other research points to damage or shrinkage of the left temporal lobe, an area crucial to hearing and speech; as well as to loss of tissue in and around the limbic system, key for emotion and memory. A 1995 University of Pennsylvania study found that the greater the decrease in the left temporal lobe volume, the more severe the negative symptoms. Greater decreases in right frontal lobe volume were associated with longer-term illness.

Abnormal activity in *specific* areas of the brain may produce hallucinations. Neuroscientists at New York Hospital–Cornell Medical Center and the Hammersmith Hospital and Institute of Neurology in London used new imaging techniques to capture fleeting patterns of brain activity *while* schizophrenic patients were having hallucinations. In patients with auditory hallucinations, abnormal activity was seen in the hippocampus and other areas deep within the brain. Patients with visual and auditory hallucinations had increased activity in surface areas of the brain responsible for complex vision and hearing. When the whole network was active, the brain created its own "reality."

These same abnormal neural circuits have also been identified with imbalances in certain neurotransmitters. For example, overactivity of the brain chemical dopamine has been linked to hallucinations, distorted thinking and agitation.

"Dopamine modulates the information that's being transmitted to the brain, modulating thought processes so that when adverse or extremely disruptive events occur, your thinking doesn't get confused," explains Dr. Friedhoff. "In a situation of extreme stress, such as in combat, the dopaminergic system seems to turn itself down. Your thinking becomes more focused, but you are less emotionally responsive. In patients with positive symptom schizophrenia, there may be a defect in the dopaminergic system so it can't turn itself down, and thinking becomes disturbed.

"Female hormones are mildly 'antidopaminergic,' which may account for the lesser severity of psychotic symptoms of schizophrenia in women," he adds.

Other scientists speculate that estrogen may act during critical developmental periods to protect women from increased dopamine activity, and that women who develop schizophrenia may be more susceptible to disruptions in the dopamine system. Recent research also suggests that an excess of serotonin produces the "negative" symptoms of schizophrenia.

Genes may play a major role. Children who have a schizophrenic parent have about a 10 percent chance of developing the disorder. Recent studies of twins have found that identical twins have more than a 50 percent rate of "concordance" (where both twins develop schizophrenia), whereas fraternal twins have the same concordance as nontwin siblings. "However, in almost every case where one twin is sick and the other is well, the twin with schizophrenia had a lower birth weight, supporting the theory of some developmental problem in utero," Dr. Friedhoff notes.

A unique study of such identical "discordant" twins led by Dr. Friedhoff at NYU has identified ten genes that appear to be inactive in twins who suffer from schizophrenia, but not in identical twins who do not have the disease. "One of the genes is normally active in a portion of the brain involved in hearing. The twin with schizophrenia had persistent auditory hallucinations, which raises the possibility that inactivation of this gene may be linked to this symptom," he says.

However, Dr. Friedhoff and other scientists stress that genes *alone* would not directly cause schizophrenia. While a person may inherit a predisposition to schizophrenia, the disease may only emerge when other factors are present (such as exposure to a virus during pregnancy).

❧ Luanne's Story, Continued ❧

"With the medicine I take every day, I rarely have any hallucinations from my schizophrenia. . . . If I do, it's just minor auditory hallucinations, usually at bedtime, which my doctor says is a period where your brain is relaxed and is more vulnerable to such things. I am on small doses of a neuroleptic and an antianxiety medication to help with my nerves. . . .

"I wouldn't be surprised if they don't find that those of us who are recovering from a serious psychiatric illness almost go through a posttraumatic stress syndrome. Because I still have nightmares that I'm going to get ill again. . . . But I realize that as long as I take my medicine, the chances are very slim.

"I do have to live with some limitations. . . . I have to limit my driving to two hours a day; concentrating on the road for a long period of time stresses me out. . . .

"But it is amazing to think that medication can restore what's been taken away in an illness like this. . . . that you can think and reason, and really be the person you were before the schizophrenia took over. . . . I am so grateful for that."

-—ᘐᘓ-—

Treating Schizophrenia

Unlike most psychiatric disorders, schizophrenia is best treated with medication, principally antipsychotic medications (also called *neuroleptics*), which can turn off the "voices" heard by some people with psychotic illnesses (such as schizophrenia), and help them to perceive reality more accurately. These medications cannot cure schizophrenia, but they eliminate many of the symptoms or make them milder. In some cases, medications can even shorten the course of the illness, says Dr. Friedhoff.

STANDARD ANTIPSYCHOTICS: Relieve the "positive" symptoms of schizophrenia, such as hallucinations, agitation, confusion and delusions. They are believed to work mainly by blocking receptor sites for dopamine in the brain. They can also reduce severity and frequency of schizophrenic episodes.

The most widely prescribed standard antipsychotic is *haloperidol* (*Haldol*). The major drawbacks to these drugs are their side effects, including movement problems and tremors.

ATYPICAL ANTIPSYCHOTICS: These are a new class of drugs that act on dopamine, serotonin and other neurotransmitters, affecting both the "positive" and "negative" symptoms of schizophrenia.

Clozapine (*Clozaril*) was considered a major breakthrough when it was approved by the U.S. Food and Drug Administration in 1990. Clozapine has a response rate of 60 percent, reducing symptoms in many patients who do not respond to standard antipsychotics, says Dr. Friedhoff. It acts on dopamine as well as other neurotransmitters, including serotonin, dampening the "positive" and "negative" symptoms of schizophrenia. Clozapine produces fewer movement and muscle problems, while easing both "negative" and "positive" symptoms. However, clozapine can cause a potentially lethal blood disorder, so patients need weekly blood tests (see page 102), adding to its already high expense (pills plus tests can cost up to $9,000 a year).

Another new atypical antipsychotic, *risperidone* (*Risperdal*), approved in

1994, appears to be even more effective than clozapine, with less severe side effects. It is an antagonist for both serotonin and dopamine. Because it is so new, risperidone is also expensive, costing around $2,000 a year.

Other new schizophrenia medications (including *sertindole* and *alanzapine*) are being tested at NYU Medical Center and elsewhere and should be approved shortly. Preliminary tests at Harvard of the drug *D-cycloserine*, used to treat tuberculosis, showed that it helped the "negative" symptoms of schizophrenia and improved cognitive function.

Responses to antipsychotic medications vary, with some symptoms diminishing in days, while others take weeks or months. Most patients experience substantial improvement in six weeks.

Antipsychotic medications are not addictive. Even though some patients experience sedation, these drugs are not "chemical straitjackets." (Daytime sedation can be reduced by taking the medication just before bedtime.) About 30 percent of schizophrenic patients do not respond to standard antipsychotics. However, women, particularly younger women, seem to be *more* responsive.

Three other drugs—lithium, the antiseizure medication *carbamazepine* (*Tegretol*) and benzodiazepines (such as *alprazolam*) may be helpful when taken with antipsychotics. Antidepressants can help treat depression occurring in schizophrenia.

One major problem is that, just as in other chronic illnesses, some patients may discontinue taking drugs because they start to feel better, says Dr. Friedhoff. Family members may wrongly believe that the person no longer needs medication, or that the drugs may be harmful. However, stopping medication increases the risk of relapse. Moreover, because of the nature of the illness, some patients are unreliable in taking medication, so new, long-acting injectable antipsychotics may be useful.

With continued drug treatment, about 40 percent of recovered patients will suffer relapses within two years of discharge from a hospital. That compares with an 80 percent relapse rate when medication is discontinued.

Drugs Used to Treat Schizophrenia

Sources: Medical Economics, Inc., *Physicians' Desk Reference,* 1995; Harold I. Kaplan, M.D., and Benjamin J. Sadock, M.D., *The Pocket Handbook of Psychiatric Drug Treatment* (Williams and Wilkins, 1995); Department of Health and Human Services, *Medications for the Treatment of Schizophrenia: Questions and Answers,* 1993

Standard Antipsychotics: Reduce "positive" symptoms of schizophrenia. They are classified as high-, intermediate-, or low-potency. High-potency antipsychotics require smaller doses to be effective. They include haloperidol (Haldol), fluphenazine (Prolixin, Permitil), trifluoperazine (Stelazine), pimozide (Orap) and thiothixene (Navane). Low-potency drugs include chlorpromazine (Thorazine), chlorprothixene (Taractan), thioridazine (Mellaril) and mesoridazine (Serentil). These drugs require higher doses to relieve symptoms. Intermediate-potency antipsychotics include perphenazine (Trilafon), loxapine (Loxitane) and molindone (Moban).

Potential Side Effects: Lower-potency antipsychotic agents are more likely to produce sedation, dry mouth, episodic low blood pressure and dizziness.

High-dose agents are more likely to produce several types of muscle problems (called *extrapyramidal* symptoms). These include *dystonia,* involuntary spasms in a muscle or group of muscles; *akathisia,* a feeling of restlessness that may result in continual leg movements and pacing; and *pseudoparkinsonism,* slowed or stiff movements resembling Parkinson's disease. Both dystonia and akathisia are reversible when doses are lowered or stopped; both can be treated with a variety of medications.

The most serious extrapyramidal side effect is *tardive dyskinesia (TD),* an irreversible neurological condition causing involuntary twitching of the lips, tongue, jaw, fingers, trunk, arms or legs. While TD doesn't interfere with mental functioning, it can hamper daily tasks like eating and walking. Patients must receive follow-up exams after three months of use, then every six months thereafter. Other side effects can include constipation, drooling, skin rashes, sun sensitivity, cholestatic jaundice (slowing of bile flow in the liver) and weight gain.

Clozapine (Clozaril): Reduces "positive" and "negative" symptoms.

Potential Side Effects: Drowsiness, dizziness, rapid heartbeat, constipation, headache and disturbed sleep. Less commonly, there is muscle rigidity, tremors, body shakes, weight gain and drooling, and a risk of tardive dyskinesia. Clozapine does not increase prolactin (which can cause problems with ovulation).

Warning: Clozapine carries a 1 to 3 percent risk of the potentially deadly blood disorder *agranulocytosis,* a depletion of infection-fighting white blood cells. If not diagnosed and treated immediately, agranulocytosis can lead to death. Patients using the drug are required to undergo weekly blood tests to monitor for the disease.

Risperidone (Risperdal): Reduces "positive" and "negative" symptoms.

Potential Side Effects: During the initial period after starting risperidone, it may induce *orthostatic hypotension,* a form of low blood pressure that can result in fainting after standing for long periods. It can also produce some extrapyramidal symptoms, as well as insomnia, agitation, headache, anxiety and rhinitis. Risperidone does not cause agranulocytosis, but it requires weekly blood tests.

๛ Luanne's Story, Continued ๛

"After I was diagnosed, I was put on disability, which has helped me tremendously. It has taken away the need to push each day, and taken away a lot of my stress. . . . I could also adjust my schedule. If I was having a bad day, I could take a day off, if I needed to rest. . . . My medication helps a great deal, also. . . .

"I personally feel like I'm now dealing with reality in my life and in the volunteer work I do for NARSAD. . . . One of my friends says I'm back to being the same person that I was when I was twenty-two. It's great to feel that way. Because this is a really tragic illness, where you lose your self when you're ill. . . .

"Like anyone else with a serious illness, I know I have to live with some limitations. But I'm willing to accept that. I'm just happy that I don't have breakdowns anymore. . . . The researchers with NARSAD are really changing the world for people like me, and it's great to be a part of that."

Social Help for People with Schizophrenia

Even if medication helps with the symptoms of schizophrenia, many patients still have extreme difficulty establishing and maintaining relationships. In addition, because so many schizophrenics frequently become ill during their college and career-building years, they are less likely to acquire the training required for skilled work. As a result, many people not only suffer thinking and emotional problems, but also lack social and work skills. Rehabilitation programs that emphasize social and vocational training may be able to help patients and former patients overcome such difficulties.

A 1994 study conducted at the University of Wisconsin followed 122 men and women over seven years, assigning half to intensive, community-based services, including medication, twenty-four-hour crisis counseling, help in finding jobs and housing, as well as coaching in everyday skills such as shopping, doing laundry and managing money. Those patients in the program spent only five days a year in the hospital or on the street, compared with fifteen days for people who were not in the program.

Psychotherapy may help schizophrenic patients understand their illness, enabling them to distinguish what's real and what's not. Family therapy and self-help groups can also provide resources for patients, caregivers and family members. The largest network of family help groups is run by the National Alliance for the Mentally Ill (NAMI, see Appendix II).

Community-based residential care or outpatient treatment facilities have become alternatives to long-term hospitalization for many chronically ill patients. However, such approaches appear to have limited value for acutely psychotic patients (those who are out of touch with reality or have prominent hallucinations or delusions), who may require long-term hospitalization.

DELUSIONAL DISORDERS

In contrast to schizophrenia, delusional disorders are characterized by delusions involving situations that *can* occur in real life, but still do not exist in reality. For example, a person may believe that their spouse is being unfaithful, or that a celebrity or powerful person is in love with them, when there is absolutely no evidence to support the idea.

Delusional disorders appear to affect men and women equally, occurring in middle or late adult life. They can be chronic, or clear up within a few months, never to recur. A few studies have found delusional disorders to be more common among relatives of people with schizophrenia. Types of delusions include:

- EROTOMANIC TYPE: Delusions that another person, usually of higher status, is in love with them from a distance.

- GRANDIOSE TYPE: Delusions of inflated power, worth, knowledge or a special relationship to a famous person or deity.

- JEALOUS TYPE: Delusions that a partner is unfaithful.

- PERSECUTORY TYPE: Delusions that a person is being persecuted, marked for murder, poisoned or badly treated.

- SOMATIC TYPE: Delusions that a person has a physical defect, body odor or disease.

A delusional person may believe that random, everyday events have a special significance which supports the theme of their delusion. A person with jealous delusions may display anger and violence; a person suffering from erotomania may stalk the object of their affections; a person with delusions of persecution may engage in lawsuits or write hundreds of letters to authorities.

In contrast to schizophrenia, the delusion is the *only* odd thing about the person and, apart from the impact of their delusion, social functioning is not terribly impaired. In contrast to normal fantasies, the person *acts* on their belief.

DISSOCIATIVE DISORDERS

In dissociative disorders, a person breaks away not only from reality, but from themselves, sometimes creating separate "personalities." This can occur suddenly or gradually, and may be a fleeting experience or a chronic problem. Dissociative disorders, once rare, have increased in incidence in recent years, and are thought by some experts to be a protective mechanism for dealing with trauma, such as early childhood sexual abuse (for more, see Chapter 9). In fact, dissociative symptoms are included in the descriptions of posttraumatic stress disorder and acute stress disorder, both of which can be triggered by abuse and victimization. Dissociative disorders include:

- DISSOCIATIVE AMNESIA: Is an inability to recall personal information, usually of a traumatic and stressful nature.

- DISSOCIATIVE IDENTITY DISORDER: Was formerly known as multiple personality disorder, where a person creates different identities or personalities, which can control their behavior. (Women seem to create more separate personalities than men, sometimes as many as fifteen.)

- DEPERSONALIZATION DISORDER: This disorder is characterized by a feeling of being detached from one's body or mental processes (as if the person is observing herself).

SOMATOFORM DISORDERS

Soma is a Greek word meaning "body." In "somatization," psychological distress is converted into bodily distress. Somatization disorders are usually characterized by having physical symptoms without an underlying medical condition.

Other somatoform disorders include *hypochondriasis*, in which a person believes or fears they have a serious illness, based on misinterpretation of physical symptoms or bodily functions, and *body dysmorphic disorder* (*BDD*), an obsession with imagined (or exaggerated) defects in personal appearance.

Somatic delusions or hallucinations (such as seeing and feeling insects on one's body) can occur in schizophrenia. Hallucinations and dissociative symptoms (such as amnesia) also occur in somatoform disorders. In fact, somatoform disorders were once classified as a variant of delusional disorders. What used to be referred to as "hysterical" blindness or paralysis is now known as a *conversion disorder*.

Somatization mostly occurs in women, especially those with little education or low socioeconomic status. BDD and hypochondriasis are equally common in men and women (hypochondria affects 4 to 9 percent of the population).

Not surprisingly, body dysmorphic disorder is linked with eating disorders (see Chapter 7). And recent studies also suggest it may be related to obsessive-compulsive disorder (with perhaps a third of people with OCD also having BDD). "These people are obsessed with the idea that something doesn't look right; half may also have delusions where they actually 'see' defects. They also display ritualistic or compulsive behaviors, like constantly putting on makeup to try to conceal imagined defects, undergoing plastic surgery over and over again, never feeling the defect has been corrected," explains OCD expert Dr. Eric Hollander of New York's Mount Sinai Medical Center.

However, unlike people with OCD, these people do not get relief from their behaviors; repeatedly checking themselves in the mirror only reinforces their belief. And, in contrast with people with OCD who know their thoughts and behaviors are silly but are driven to do them, many people with body dysmorphic disorder are convinced that their body defects are real.

Some medications that reduce symptoms of OCD have also proven helpful in treating people with body dysmorphic disorder.

CHAPTER 6

Women and Addiction

Many things can be considered "addictions": substance abuse—of alcohol, prescribed medications or illegal drugs—as well as self-destructive behaviors such as compulsive gambling, shopping, eating or even sex. While statistics show that fewer women than men abuse alcohol or hard drugs, women are no less vulnerable to addictions.

Addictive substances and behaviors have one thing in common: They change a person's mood, produce euphoria or relaxation, provide relief from stress or emotional pain.

The cycle of addiction is insidious and progressive. A person uses a substance to produce a mood change, then begins to need the drug more often and in bigger amounts to achieve that same effect—a state called "dependence," explains Marc A. Galanter, M.D., professor of psychiatry and director of the Division of Alcoholism and Drug Abuse at NYU Medical Center.

"When the dependent person tries to taper off or stop, they suffer physical or mental 'withdrawal' symptoms, and resume taking the substance to avoid those unpleasant symptoms," says Dr. Galanter. "Eventually, a person is unable to control their addiction, no matter what the consequences may be to themselves, their families, their finances or careers."

Addicted people can't control their intake or behavior (for instance, getting drunk when they intended to take only one or two drinks). They often express a desire to stop, or have made repeated, unsuccessful tries. They may spend a great deal of time trying to obtain the substance (especially if it's a restricted prescription or an illegal drug) and recovering from its effects.

Addicts also ignore important social, occupational or recreational activities because of substance abuse and may become impaired both socially and on the job, says Dr. Galanter. Addiction can lead to social and legal problems, loss of a job, divorce, injury or illness (including psychotic episodes, delirium, hallucinations, sexual dysfunction and sleep disorders), accidents and even arrest.

Addictive substances include alcohol, stimulants (like amphetamines), tranquilizers, marijuana, cocaine, hallucinogens, inhalants (such as amyl nitrate), nicotine, opioids (like heroin) and sedatives. Their addictive properties vary. One recent study found that nine out of ten people who try cigarettes become hooked. Studies show that 15 percent of those who try heroin become addicted, while only about 10 percent of drinkers develop problems with alcohol. Research indicates that women become addicted quickly to drugs like crack cocaine, even after experimental or casual use.

Behaviors are not officially classified as addictions. For example, the *DSM-IV* calls compulsive gambling an *impulse control disorder*. But it shares many of the same symptoms as substance abuse, such as the need to gamble to produce excitement (just as taking a drug produces a "high"), the need for increasing amounts of gambling to produce the effect, the failure of efforts to cut back and "withdrawal" symptoms. Other self-destructive "addictive" behaviors such as compulsive spending and promiscuity are also among the symptoms of borderline personality disorder (page 84), mania and hypomania (page 28).

According to a 1996 report, "Substance Abuse and the American Woman" by the Center on Addiction and Substance Abuse (CASA) at Columbia University analyzing data from hundreds of scientific articles, surveys and government reports, 4.5 million women are alcoholics or alcohol abusers, 3.1 million women regularly use illicit drugs such as cocaine, heroin or marijuana, 3.5 million misuse prescription drugs and 21.5 percent smoke.

Substance use and abuse have been reported to be more prevalent among lesbians and bisexual women. Surveys have found alcohol use among lesbian women as high as 31 percent, with similar rates for drug use; as many as 10 percent of lesbians consider their alcohol or drug use a problem.

Substance abuse often begins in adolescence. Recent surveys showing alcohol and illicit drug use rising among junior high, high school and college students. One recent study found that by the time they reach the eighth grade, 70 percent of American youngsters will have tried alcohol, 44 percent will have smoked cigarettes, 10 percent will have tried marijuana and 2 percent will have used cocaine!

Up to 3 percent of the population may be compulsive gamblers; one in three are women. And the numbers are rising as more states approve legalized gambling. About 6 percent of the population could be considered compulsive spenders, perhaps 60 percent of them women.

Millions of women could be helped by treatment for substance abuse and other addictions, but the CASA report says that less than 14 percent of women who need treatment are receiving it. The report says many physicians do not know the risk factors and symptoms of female substance abuse and many treatment programs are geared toward men (lacking key components like child care).

IS THERE AN "ADDICTIVE PERSONALITY"?

Despite the popular notion of an "addictive personality," there is no evidence such a thing exists.

"People who develop addictions to drugs or various behaviors have many problems in common, but there is no single predisposing personality trait," says Sheila Blume, M.D., medical director of Alcoholism, Chemical Dependency and Compulsive Gambling Programs at South Oaks Hospital in Amityville, New York.

"The difference between an alcoholic and a person who likes to drink is the loss of control. A healthy person stops on their own and can set limits if needed. The addict cannot. Her behavior becomes obsessive, destructive. Addicts lose the ability to take care of themselves," explains Dr. Blume.

Among the potential "triggers" for addictive behavior are hidden psychological problems. As many as 40 percent of addicts may have coexisting psychiatric disorders, including clinical depression, manic depression, anxiety, panic and attention deficit/hyperactivity. Those disorders may contribute to, result from or be worsened by drug abuse in as many as 70 percent of cases, says Dr. Galanter.

"A common thread among women who become chemically dependent is a history of abuse, either physical child abuse, sex abuse, rape or battering," says Machelle Allen, M.D., director of the Substance Abuse and Domestic Abuse Service at the NYU-Bellevue Hospital Center. "A lot of these women are suffering from posttraumatic stress syndrome, and are numbing themselves with drugs or alcohol." Nearly 70 percent of female substance abusers in treatment were sexually abused as children.

Many women who are chemically dependent also have coexisting problems not found among men, such as eating disorders and sleep disorders, says Dr. Allen. Women with an alcoholic or drug-abusing parent (or partner) are also at increased risk.

While alcoholism tends to run in families, a specific "alcoholism gene" has not yet been found. But studies have found that young adult sons and daughters of alcoholics appear to have less sensitivity to alcohol than children of nonalcoholics. So the offspring of alcoholics may have to drink more just to feel the effects of alcohol, leading to heavy drinking.

In addition, researchers at NYU Medical Center, the University of California, Los Angeles, and elsewhere, have found a gene that they believe may be linked not only to alcoholism, but also to drug abuse, nicotine addiction, compulsive eating and pathological gambling. The defective gene regulates the release of dopamine, which triggers feelings of pleasure in the brain. This chemical "reward" system does not appear to work in some people with addictions, producing anxiety and anger instead. Alcohol, cocaine and nicotine all are known to cause release of dopamine; people may use these substances to relieve unpleasant feelings, and therefore become addicted. The defective *D-2 dopamine receptor gene* has been found among people with severe alcohol problems. Recent PET scan studies of people in the throes of addiction also show heightened metabolic activity in areas of the brain which form a "pleasure pathway" known as the *mesolimbic dopamine system.*

A person's cultural background may also play a role. Some religious groups, including Muslims and Jehovah's Witnesses, forbid alcohol consumption, while drinking is regarded as a sign of sociability among some ethnic groups.

Age is no deterrent to addiction; as many as 4.1 percent of women over age 60 may be heavy drinkers. Other research indicates that social factors, like dropping out of high school (which predisposes to lower socioeconomic status), increase the risk of alcohol or drug abuse later in life.

However, the most important thing to understand is that substance abuse is not a character defect or a moral weakness, but a *medical illness,* just like diabetes or depression.

☙ *Ruth's Story* ☙

"I've been addicted to one thing or another my entire life. I never liked myself. My first drug of choice was books. I was a compulsive student. When that didn't work, I turned to food. I became a compulsive eater in the eighth grade. I was fat in high school and that just reinforced my low self-esteem.

"I was the oldest of seven kids. . . . My dad was a workaholic. . . . My mother is an alcoholic, but has never confronted it. . . . My brothers and sisters grew up out of control and all of them had alcohol problems. . . . So I do believe I was predisposed to it. But I don't blame my family anymore.

"I went to all-girl Catholic schools. When I started college at age sixteen, I had to start interacting with boys. I discovered that beer made me more outgoing and likable when I was with men. I progressed from beer to wine to vodka.

"When I went to law school, I used diet pills to stay awake so I could study. I passed the bar . . . but I never filled out the papers to get admitted until I was sober. . . . I worked at low-level clerical jobs . . . and stayed drunk.

"I got up in the morning and my whole goal was oblivion. . . . The more screwed-up things I did . . . like getting drunk . . . the more I hated myself. . . . One night, coming home in a stupor, I was almost raped in the lobby of my building. For me, that was the bottom. . . . I did not go back to work; I rarely got out of bed. Here I was, this great person with this law degree, this great background. I had one good dress, nowhere to go, no job, no friends. Nothing to do but get high, and when the money ran out, I couldn't even do that. I was one step away from the street, from being a dead person. Shortly after that, at twenty-five, I put myself in an in-hospital alcoholism program.

"Stopping drinking didn't solve all my problems, but it cleared a path for me to work on them. The mainstay of my recovery has been AA. . . . Now I'm practicing law. I'm lucky. I've been given more than a second chance, I've been given a million chances. I like myself now, I'm proud of myself. But believe me, sobriety is a constant struggle. I've fallen on my face hundreds of times in sobriety. But I always get up. And I keep on going."

---oc---

The Female Factor

Many women like Ruth have a history that includes unhappy childhoods, sexual abuse, violent spouses, failed marriages and unsuccessful careers. All of which can lead to depression, which can be both a cause and consequence of alcohol abuse.

A 1996 update of a major longitudinal study of women's drinking, conducted by neuroscience professor Sharon C. Wilsnack, Ph.D., at the University of North Dakota School of Medicine, found that over 20 percent of women with a history of childhood sexual abuse reported problem drinking and use of other drugs, and more than one third reported using illicit drugs. The study, which has followed more than one thousand women since 1981, also found that alcohol abuse makes women more vulnerable to sexual assault and rape.

Women have different patterns of alcohol addiction than men, suffering more cross dependencies, especially problems with prescription drug abuse (see page 118). A survey by Alcoholics Anonymous found that 40 percent of its female members were addicted to another drug; the number jumped to 64 percent for women under thirty.

One contributing factor may be that doctors tend to prescribe tranquilizers for symptoms of nervousness or anxiety that may actually be related to hidden alcohol abuse in women, says Nicholas A. Pace, M.D., an assistant professor of clinical medicine at the NYU School of Medicine, and a member of the board of directors of the National Council on Alcoholism and Drug Dependence (NCADD). "Women will go to a doctor for some of the secondary symptoms of alcoholism, such as sleep disturbances or nervousness, and not tell the doctor they're drinking. The doctor prescribes sleeping pills or tranquilizers, not realizing the woman has an alcohol problem, unknowingly fostering her cross addiction," says Dr. Pace.

"A woman may operate under societal constraints, saying it isn't proper to drink until evening," adds Dr. Blume. "So while a male alcoholic may take his first drink in the morning, a woman might take a Valium, and not have her first drink until later."

ALCOHOL *IS* A WOMAN'S PROBLEM

Most studies of alcoholism prior to the 1970s were done among men, leading experts to believe that alcoholism was rare among women. Today we know that this is not true; at least one third of alcoholics in the United States are women, and the numbers may be rising.

Many people like to "unwind" with a drink or two after work, and make alcohol part of every social occasion. The National Institute on Alcohol Abuse and Alcoholism found that a little over half of women who drink alcohol are light drinkers (less than four drinks per week), 29 percent are moderate drinkers (four to thirteen drinks per week) and 7 percent are heavy drinkers (more than fourteen drinks per week). Dr. Wilsnack's 1991 survey data found slightly lower numbers in each category.

One quarter of girls aged twelve to seventeen use alcohol. Adolescents most prone to problem drinking often have behavior or school problems. A 1995 survey by the Minnesota-based Hazeldon Foundation found that almost 67 percent drank (or used drugs) to "help forget their problems," rather than because of peer pressure.

While "binge" drinking in high school is almost twice as common among boys, some studies show a more than threefold increase in heavy drinking among college women. Women aged twenty-one to thirty-four report higher rates of problems like drunk driving, drinking-related job problems and conflicts with friends or family.

"Alcohol abuse is becoming more frequent among women at a younger age," comments Anne Geller, M.D., chief of the Smithers Addiction Treatment and Training Center in New York City, and past president of the American Society of Addiction Medicine. "In fact, one study shows that the risk of alcoholism for women in the current generation is equal to that of men in their fathers' generation. So, sadly, we are catching up with the men."

In the 1970s, it was assumed that women who were juggling multiple roles were at greater risk for alcohol abuse. But ten-year data from Dr. Wilsnack's study found that *lack* of social roles is a major risk factor. The CASA report found that 7.2 percent of unemployed women drink heavily, compared to 1.7 percent of working women and 0.9 percent of homemakers.

"Women who do not have fulfilling work, who are not in a meaningful relationship or who have no children turned out to be at higher risk. Women aged twenty-one to thirty-four, who were unmarried and unemployed (or working part-time) were at the highest risk," reports Dr. Wilsnack. "Women who had multiple social roles were actually at lower risk. It may well be that multiple roles provide more sources of self-worth and more social support."

For working women, alcohol and drug abuse may be fostered by low job status, job stress and sexual harassment. Studies show that women in occupations traditionally dominated by men are at increased risk of problem drinking. Also at risk are widows, women living with men outside of marriage and women whose partners are heavy drinkers.

Recent surveys on lesbian health indicate that 27 to 35 percent are either alcohol abusers or alcoholics, compared with a rate of 10 to 12 percent for women in the general population. "The social structure for this culture has for a long time been in an underground bar situation, where the habits used for people to communicate include alcohol and cigarettes," observes Marla Jean Gold, M.D., an assistant professor of medicine at the Medical College of Pennsylvania and a member of the advisory board of the Lesbian Health Fund. "We think that alcohol may be used to cope with internalized homophobia. And that alcohol may be used to ease the 'coming out' process, which can be stressful." Lesbian women in abusive relationships are also at increased risk.

Women aged thirty-five to forty-nine have the highest rates of chronic alcohol abuse problems, reports Dr. Wilsnack. Among the major risk factors: lack of employment, divorce or separation and heavy drinking by a spouse. Many middle-aged and older women may drink in the isolation of their homes.

African-American women are half as likely as white women to drink alcohol. However, black women who do drink are twice as likely to have an alcohol problem and up to six times more likely to develop cirrhosis. Hispanic culture discourages drinking among females, so Latina women are more likely than white or black women to be abstainers. But the more assimilated they become, the more likely they are to drink.

Problem drinking among Native American men has long been acknowledged as a major health problem, but alcohol abuse among Native American women has not been widely studied. One study found that the death rate from alcoholism among Native American women aged twenty-five to forty-five was *ten times higher* than for all other women in the United States. Deaths from alcohol-related illnesses are also high among Pacific Islander women; little is known about alcohol use among Asian-American women.

Three times more men than women meet the diagnostic criteria for alcohol abuse and dependence. However, says Dr. Geller, "women become alcohol dependent and suffer impairment at much lower doses and after a much shorter duration than men do. Women also develop end-organ damage at significantly lower rates of drinking than men do." For example, women can suffer liver damage on as little as 1.5 drinks per day, compared with 4 drinks a day for men with liver disease.

Fig. 5: What's in a Drink?
Comparison of Alcohol Content of Average
Servings of Beverages

Source: National Institute on Alcohol Abuse and Alcoholism

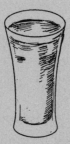 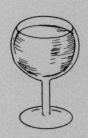

12 oz. Beer   5 oz. Table Wine   1 oz. Distilled Spirits
4.5% Alcohol   12% Alcohol   40% Alcohol (80 proof)

While women drink less than men do, they are more likely to consume spirits or wine, which have three to ten times more ethanol content per drink than beer. Federal dietary guidelines recommend that women consume no more than one alcoholic drink per day.

Why are women more sensitive to the effects of alcohol? For one thing, women have a higher percentage of body fat and less body water than men. Since alcohol dissolves more easily in water than in fat, alcohol becomes more concentrated in a woman's body. Women are also more sensitive to the effects of alcohol during certain times in the menstrual cycle, leading to higher blood concentrations of ethanol.

"Women also typically weigh less than men, so alcohol becomes concentrated in a smaller body mass. Also, as women age, they may develop more body fat, so alcohol can have a more potent effect on older women. Women metabolize alcohol less efficiently than men, so women get drunk more quickly than men on the same (or smaller) amount of alcohol," explains Dr. Nicholas Pace.

Indeed, researchers at the Mount Sinai School of Medicine and the Alcohol Research and Treatment Center at the Bronx Veterans Affairs Medical Center in New York discovered that women produce half as much of a stomach enzyme called *alcohol dehydrogenase*, which breaks down alcohol before it enters the bloodstream and can damage other organs, such as the brain and the liver.

"We also found that alcoholism, both in men and women, decreases this gastric protective mechanism. But alcoholic women end up with no protection to speak of, because they started out with lower levels of the protective enzyme to begin with," says Charles Lieber, M.D., director of the Alcohol Research and Treatment Center. Dr. Lieber says that this may explain why the long-term complications of alcoholism, such as cirrhosis of the liver, hit women earlier and harder. Because the liver detoxifies alcohol, chronic abuse can cause inflammation and scarring.

Alcoholism is a chronic disease that can be fatal. It can cause brain damage, impair memory and mental function, aggravate high blood pressure and increase the risk of stroke, heart attack or kidney failure. Women alcoholics develop hypertension and cardiovascular disease sooner than men, says Dr. Geller. A postmenopausal woman who drinks heavily is at much higher risk than a man of cirrhosis, as well as of alcohol-related enlargement of the heart. Long-term alcohol use is also associated with oral cancer, and cancer of the esophagus, liver and pancreas. Some studies suggest that alcohol increases a woman's risk of breast cancer. Female alcoholics are up to twice as likely to die as male alcoholics in the same age group.

Dr. Wilsnack's surveys have found that a majority of women drinkers believe that drinking reduces their sexual inhibitions, and nearly half reported that drinking makes sexual activity more pleasurable. Contrary to stereotypes, she found very few women who were less choosy about sexual partners when they drank, and less than a quarter actually became more sexually aggressive. But 60 percent of women reported that drinking partners became sexually aggressive toward *them*. "Women who drink too much are considered sexually loose, and are often the targets of sexual abuse and rape," says Dr. Wilsnack. One study found that up to 74 percent of alcohol- and drug-dependent women reported incidents of sexual abuse. Alcohol is a factor in more than one half of all incidents of domestic violence, with women most likely to be battered when both partners have been drinking. One survey of college women found that 53 percent of rape victims had used alcohol or other drugs beforehand; 64 percent reported alcohol or drug use by their assailant.

Alcoholism has other damaging consequences for women. Over time, it can produce sexual dysfunction and sexual disinterest. Alcoholic women also have a higher rate than other women of gynecologic problems, including irregular menstrual cycles, miscarriage, infertility and early menopause. (Studies show that such problems can occur in any woman who consumes four to eight drinks per day.)

Alcohol abuse is also the leading preventable cause of birth defects, including fetal alcohol syndrome, a major factor in retardation in children (see box below).

Are all women who drink heavily alcoholics? Opinion is divided. Some people drink heavily on certain occasions or on weekends, and can go days or even weeks without taking a drink. Experts report a growing number of women with "subclinical" drinking problems—with symptoms of alcohol abuse, including increased alcohol tolerance, but not meeting the criteria for alcoholism—who may need help for problem drinking.

"In our survey, twenty percent of the women drinkers said that at some time they were worried that they were developing a drinking problem. This is considerably more than the number who qualified as alcoholics. So it's an area that certainly merits further study," comments Dr. Wilsnack.

Pregnancy, Alcohol and Drug Abuse

Up to one of every five pregnant women—at least 300,000 women a year—drink alcohol, use drugs or smoke cigarettes, which can have lasting effects on the physical and mental development of their children.

A 1995 report from the Centers for Disease Control and Prevention (CDC) showed that the percentage of babies born with health problems because their mothers drank alcohol during pregnancy increased sixfold from 1979 to 1993. Chief among those problems is *fetal alcohol syndrome* (FAS), caused by heavy drinking during pregnancy. FAS is the most common cause of mental retardation, and can lead to behavioral difficulties, growth deficiencies and abnormal facial features. It's estimated that more than ten thousand babies are born with FAS each year; up to one quarter of children born on Indian reservations may be affected.

As many as fifty-five thousand babies are born every year with a milder condition, *fetal alcohol effect,* which can cause deficits in hearing, speech and language, and behavior problems. Nursing mothers who drink may cause some slowing of their baby's motor development. Recent studies have also found that daughters of women who drink during pregnancy are more likely to have fertility and reproductive problems.

Sadly, the CDC says that, despite increasing awareness that avoiding alcohol prevents FAS, about one fifth of women continue to drink even after learning they are pregnant.

According to the National Association for Perinatal Addiction Research and Education (NAPARE), use of cocaine during pregnancy can cause spontaneous abortion, as well as cognitive and emotional problems. Cocaine-exposed infants show increased irritability and less interaction with those around them. Abuse of crack cocaine can cause prenatal strokes, seizures, premature birth and severe behavioral problems.

The CASA report remarked there are more "cigarette babies" than "crack babies." Smoking during pregnancy causes up to 141,000 miscarriages, 61,000 low-birth-weight babies, 4,800 perinatal deaths and 2,200 deaths from Sudden Infant Death Syndrome (SIDS), and may cause respiratory illness in infants and delay a child's cognitive development. The numbers are so alarming, some experts talk of a "fetal tobacco syndrome."

A recent federal report estimated the number of addicted pregnant women to exceed 280,000, and fewer than 12 percent receive treatment. One reason is that only a fraction of addiction treatment centers offers services specifically for pregnant women, especially child care.

"It's very hard for pregnant women to go into a drug treatment program where there are men, where there are nonpregnant women, because they take a lot of criticism. They'd rather not go at all than face the negative feedback they get," comments NYU's Dr. Machelle Allen. "Many of these women have a partner who is selling drugs, or have a history of abuse, and most treatment programs don't address those issues."

But given a supportive environment and proper follow-up, Dr. Allen says, many women are able to overcome substance abuse during pregnancy, and are able to stay off drugs or alcohol afterward.

❧ *Gail's Story* ❧

"When I first arrived in L.A. and got my first job in television . . . people did 'coke,' at business lunches, at parties. I never really thought twice about trying it. . . . Drinking used to make me feel more at ease socially. But cocaine made me feel like an insider, it energized me, it made me feel like I could do anything. Then I found I couldn't do without it.

"I was freebasing . . . blowing a hundred twenty dollars a gram on 'coke.' . . . I made a lot of money and I was broke all the time. At that time, I was working as an associate producer on a network sitcom. But cocaine made me unpredictable. One day I'd work like the devil, the next I'd be two hours late. Unless you're the star, no one puts up with that kind of shit. So I got canned.

"I couldn't find another job; later I was told that the word was out that I had 'personality problems,' which is like the kiss of death. I couldn't even find freelance work. . . . The bank foreclosed on my condo. I sold my car to raise cash. And in L.A. without a car, you're dead.

"I moved in with my boyfriend. He knew I had a cocaine problem, but after I stole some money from his wallet, he told me either I get help or I get out. . . . I camped out on a friend's sofa bed for a few weeks, but we had this big blowup and I was out. I had no place to go. I spent the night on the Venice Pier; then I tried a women's shelter downtown.

"It was like the last stop before hell . . . the stench, the noise. I used to spend seventy-five dollars just on nail tips, and now I only had five dollars in my pocket. I was terrified and humiliated. The next day, I got on the phone to a producer friend of mine who'd had the same problem. He pulled some strings to get me into a good treatment program. . . . Now I shudder to think where I would have ended up if I hadn't made that call."

❧❧

PRESCRIPTION FOR ABUSE

According to the most recent National Household Survey on Drug Abuse, conducted by the Substance Abuse and Mental Health Services Administration (SAMHSA), more than half of women aged 19 to 40 have used "hard" drugs at some point. Marijuana is the most commonly used illicit drug (used by about three million women), followed by cocaine and opiates like heroin. More than a third of women say a male partner introduced them to drugs.

However, more women than men abuse prescription medications such as tranquilizers, sedatives, painkillers and stimulants. The main reason is that women receive *two thirds* of prescriptions for these drugs. Nearly twice as many women as men regularly use tranquilizers; antidepressants and sedatives are used by more than three times as many women as men. Women are more likely to use these drugs for nonmedical purposes, and become addicted.

NICOTINE ADDICTION

According to the National Institute on Drug Abuse (NIDA), nicotine is as addictive as heroin, and five to ten times more potent than cocaine in its effects on mood and behavior. Along with alcohol, cigarettes are legal and accessible.

After inhaling on a cigarette, it takes only seven to ten seconds for nicotine to be absorbed into the bloodstream and travel to the brain (about half the time it takes for an injection of heroin to be felt). Nicotine stimulates the cerebral cortex, the brain's center of reasoning. It affects neurotransmitters, which improves cognitive performance, stimulates alertness and triggers feelings of pleasure and satisfaction. Nicotine can also temporarily calm anxiety or anger, and lift depression.

Researchers at the Brookhaven National Laboratory in New York have found an enzyme they believe may play a role in nicotine addiction. They reported in 1996 in the journal *Nature* that the enzyme, a form of *monoamine oxidase* (*MAO*) which breaks down neurotransmitters in brain cells (in this case dopamine), appears to be less active in smokers. As previously discussed, alcohol, cocaine and other addictive drugs increase levels of dopamine, which brings on feelings of pleasure; smoking may also have the same effect. The researchers say the enzyme *monoamine oxidase B* (*MAO B*) may be inhibited

by an as yet unknown substance in tobacco smoke and act along with nicotine to prevent the breakdown of dopamine, enhancing its pleasurable effects.

Lower levels of dopamine have also been implicated in depression. Not
surprisingly, people who have had persistent periods of depression are among
those most prone to nicotine addiction. There is also a strong association
between smoking and alcohol abuse (nicotine counteracts alcohol's sedative
properties) and drug abuse in general.

While nicotine addiction does not cause functional impairment as alcohol and other drugs do, smoking has serious health consequences: lung
cancer and cardiovascular disease. Lung cancer has now surpassed breast
cancer as the leading cause of death among women. Smoking also leads to
an earlier menopause (increasing the risk of heart disease and osteoporosis),
elevates a woman's risk of cervical cancer and may even boost her risk of
dying of breast cancer by 25 percent. In fact, a 1996 study from the Mayo
Clinic found that alcoholic smokers were more likely to be killed by cigarettes than liquor, and recommended that treating nicotine addiction should
be a key part of substance abuse programs.

While smokers are increasingly isolated socially and by local ordinances
banning smoking in restaurants and other public places, about one fourth of
American women still smoke.

Nicotine addiction is more complex than a chemical dependency. Smoking is a behavior that becomes woven into the fabric of a smoker's life,
connected with eating, socializing and even sex. For women, cigarette use is
also tied to weight control, body image and media-driven images of thinness
and sophistication. (Many "women's" cigarettes use the word "thin" or
"slim" as part of the brand name.)

The U.S. Department of Health says that women are more likely than
men to rely on nicotine's mood-altering effects, lighting up when under
stress or in situations characterized by unpleasant emotions like anger (which
women are expected to suppress).

Tobacco may also pack a bigger punch for women. Researchers at the
University of South Florida at Tampa say nicotine and other cigarette chemicals may affect women more strongly, increasing their craving and making
it harder for them to quit.

According to the 1993 National Survey on Household Drug Abuse, Native American women smoke more than any other group, 49.6 percent versus
27 percent of black women and 23.8 percent of white women. Among Asian-
American women, 12.6 percent smoke, compared with 19.2 percent of Latina

women. People who have only a high school education or who dropped out of high school are five times more likely to smoke than those with more education. Teenage girls are five times more likely to smoke if one or both of their parents or an older sibling smokes. Smoking has declined among black teenage girls.

THE "OTHER" ADDICTIONS

The thrill of gambling, shopping sprees and even sex can be addictive for some women. Psychiatrists view these as disorders of impulse control: A person cannot resist an impulse or temptation to do something that is harmful to themselves or to others (running up high debts, squandering savings).

COMPULSIVE GAMBLING: This has become a much more common problem in recent years with the spread of legalized gambling. Twenty-seven states now have some form of casino gambling, compared with just two states a decade ago; many more have state lotteries and legalized bingo. In 1975, 5 percent of casinogoers were women; today 55 percent are women.

Experts estimate that 2 to 6 percent of people who gamble become addicted. Compulsive gamblers mainly seek the "action" (the thrill, arousal and euphoria) produced by gambling. They may start out small (the average wager for a casino visit is $25 to $100), but eventually they need greater risks or higher stakes to produce that high, continuing to gamble despite the debts it produces, and despite repeated attempts to cut back or quit.

Many people find release from depression or anxiety in gambling. Their lives can revolve around planning the next gambling adventure or scheming ways to get betting money. Compulsive gamblers may lie to their family or commit forgery, embezzlement or theft to finance their habit. Many sacrifice their marriages and their jobs to their addiction.

"One in three compulsive gamblers are women," says Henry Lesieur, Ph.D., a professor of criminal justice at Illinois State University, who has studied women gamblers. "Five years ago, less than five percent of people in treatment were women, because women often got less family support. Today, the figures are higher, especially with the impact of video poker machines."

Dr. Lesieur recently surveyed members of Gamblers Anonymous in Illinois, and found that 18 percent were women, mostly hooked on riverboat gambling or video poker. Other studies show that slot machines are the number one choice of women gamblers.

"There are two kinds of women gamblers. There's the 'adventure seeker,' looking for a thrill in what they perceive as a man's world. They're into making money and the excitement," says Dr. Lesieur. "Then there are the 'escape seekers,' women who may have alcoholic or abusive husbands, or who had sexually abusive or addicted parents. They are extremely lonely and troubled. The action-adventure of gambling helps them forget and feel like a different person."

⟨ Casey's Story ⟩

"I was hooked on the risk, the thrill, the rush I got at the dog track, at Vegas. I was working as a data processor, and there is nothing duller than that. I was fifty, my marriage was going down the tubes, my kids were gone. . . . At the races . . . at the slots, I felt alive. When you're winning, you're on top of the world . . .

"Then I began losing. At first, you're really into denial. 'I can turn this around,' you say. 'All I need is one big score.' So you throw good money after bad. Before I knew it I was literally drowning in debt. Every addict has a moment when they hit 'bottom.' I had borrowed to the limit on all my credit cards; I got loans from friends. I was always going to win big and pay it all back. But it never happened.

"Then my husband left and everything collapsed. I couldn't pay the rent; I had no money for food. I was living out of my car. I was so desperate, I was on the verge of suicide. My sister really rescued me and forced me to go to Gamblers Anonymous."

According to Dr. Lesieur, "escape seekers" like Casey become compulsive gamblers more quickly than men. They gamble in an irrational way, almost in a trance. And when the debts pile up, they become reckless, using rent money, borrowing from friends. That leads to frenzied betting in a frantic effort to recoup.

Dr. Lesieur's survey of Gamblers Anonymous in Illinois found that over a quarter had separated or divorced and more than a third had lost or quit a job because of their gambling. Forty-four percent of the recovering compulsive gamblers had stolen from work to pay their gambling debts, 18 percent had been arrested on gambling-related charges and 16 percent had committed suicide. And that's just in *one* state with legalized gambling!

COMPULSIVE SPENDING: This can be an emotional stimulant. People who are unable to control the urge to spend money, despite overwhelming debts, are considered "compulsive shoppers." Some experts estimate that 5 to 10 percent of people may fit this description, and over *half* may be women.

The emotional problems that drive people to compulsive spending are common to other addictions, says Carole Lieberman, M.D., M.P.H., an assistant clinical professor of psychiatry at the University of California, Los Angeles. One of the most prominent is low self-esteem. Attentive salesclerks give compulsive shoppers a much needed feeling of importance. There's also the element of fantasy. Many compulsive shoppers have fantasies of being rich, gravitating to expensive stores. A credit card doesn't list one's income. There's also a need for approval; women often buy things for other people.

A 1994 study reported in the *Journal of Clinical Psychiatry* described the typical compulsive shopper as a thirty-six-year-old woman who had been obsessive about shopping since her late teens. Poor impulse control may have been present since childhood. One survey of compulsive shoppers reported that, as children, they never learned to control spending; their parents were often indulgent, allowing them to buy whatever they wanted, or buying it for them. Sometimes the reverse is true, says Dr. Lieberman; compulsive shoppers feel they were denied material things as children.

Clothes, shoes, jewelry and makeup are the biggest splurge items. Not surprisingly, many compulsive shoppers are overly concerned about their appearance, and may binge on buying when they're feeling bad about themselves. As with other compulsions and addictions, shopping relieves tension, prompting a person to shop even more to feel better, says Dr. Lieberman. Compulsive shoppers report more anxiety and depression than other people; shopping becomes a way to soothe themselves or salve hurt feelings or fill up the emptiness inside them.

There are two types of compulsive shoppers: the people who indulge in binges and those who feel a compulsion to shop every day, experiencing "withdrawal" symptoms of tension or nervousness if they don't go to the store. In some cases, compulsive shoppers may buy things they don't need and can't use; unworn clothing may accumulate in the closet, with the tags still attached.

As with compulsive gambling, these women juggle credit card bills like betting IOUs, and get mired in debts, paying only the minimum on credit cards.

COMPULSIVE OVEREATING: The other cross addiction likely to turn up in the file of a female addict is food.

Experts say compulsive overeating is part of a constellation of addictions that can include alcohol, drugs, shoplifting and sexual activity. A survey by the Renfrew Center, a Philadelphia-based program for eating disorders and addictions, found that 44 percent of the women being treated there for anorexia or bulimia had a problem with alcohol and 41 percent with drugs.

Compulsive overeaters most often binge on fatty sweets, and some experts say cravings for those foods may be linked to the same biochemical mechanism that sets off addiction to drugs. Research at the University of Michigan at Ann Arbor found that sweet, fatty foods (like chocolate) draw a reaction from heroinlike chemicals in the brain called *opioid peptides*. A 1995 study showed that blocking the action of those opioids with the drug *naloxone* reduced consumption of sweets in binge eaters. (For more on eating disorders, see Chapter 7.)

COMPULSIVE SEXUALITY: While the American Psychiatric Association does not classify sex as an addiction, compulsive sexuality shares many of the same underpinnings, observed the late Helen Singer Kaplan, M.D., former director of the Human Sexuality Program at New York Hospital–Cornell Medical Center.*

"Compulsive sexuality usually starts with high anxiety, a feeling of extreme vulnerability. You feel better when you have an orgasm. It's like taking a Valium or having a drink," remarked Dr. Kaplan. Sex "addicts" may also use promiscuity as a way to mask a fear of intimacy, or intense sex role conflicts, she said.

GETTING STRAIGHT

Treating addiction is a multifaceted process. First, a person must be helped through withdrawal, which can be difficult if their body has become used to high doses of drugs or alcohol. Treatment then focuses on the underlying

*Dr. Kaplan was interviewed for this book shortly before her death in 1995.

problems that led to the addiction, teaching behaviors that promote absti-
nence, and providing support to help avoid relapse.

Some people are helped by short-term, outpatient substance-abuse treatment programs, while others may need hospitalization, medication (see
page 129) and long-term psychotherapy. Other forms of treatment involve
halfway houses or support groups, or specialized residential treatment facilities. Many alcoholics and drug abusers require *detoxification*, a period of time
to allow the substance to be cleared from their system.

Statistics show that less than a third of all people being treated for substance abuse are women. One reason may be that most traditional treatment
programs are based on male patterns of addiction, and women require special, often separate, programs of treatment. (At some residential and hospital-
based programs, men and women are now put into separate therapy groups
after a standard twenty-eight days of detoxification.)

A study of programs funded by the federal Center for Substance Abuse
Prevention (CSAP) found that addicted women tend to have lower self-
esteem and higher levels of depression, anxiety and isolation than do men,
and have greater shame about their addiction. The study, presented at a 1994
American Psychological Association conference, said that women have difficulty speaking freely about their problems in groups that include men, need
more individual counseling, and especially need child care. Substance abuse
treatment programs also need to involve a woman's family to a greater degree than those designed for men.

Studies further show that alcohol-abusing women may perceive their
problem differently than men. They may not believe drinking is their main
problem, perceiving alcohol use as a coping response to stress or problems.
Women may feel more shame and fear of the social stigma attached to
addiction and may be afraid of losing their children.

Women also fall into subgroups by age, race, ethnicity, sexual orientation, socioeconomic status and prior history of battering or sexual abuse,
says Gloria Hamilton, Ph.D., an associate professor of psychology at Middle
Tennessee State University. "We can't just treat chemical dependency
among women, we also have to address their life circumstances. Battered
women may need shelter from abusive spouses; others may need permanent
housing. Most women have in common the responsibility for raising children
and they will need child care. This must be a critical component of treatment, but is seldom offered," she told the APA meeting.

Some experts also question the sole effectiveness for women of "twelve-
step" programs patterned after Alcoholics Anonymous. These programs

stress spirituality, the first "step" being an admission that you are powerless over your addiction to alcohol or drugs, and the second acknowledging there is a higher power greater than yourself that can help you fight the addiction. Programs like the AA's require attendance at weekly meetings to reinforce sobriety, with members identifying themselves as alcoholics (never as a former addict), and discussing past and present struggles. However, a recent report in the *Journal of Psychoactive Drugs* notes that "addicted women have a particular need to gain confidence in their abilities rather than be confronted for their failures."

Jean Kirkpatrick, Ph.D., a sociologist and founder of Women for Sobriety (WFS), agrees. "While AA is very effective in helping people get sober, it does not address the central issue why many women start drinking, which is low self-esteem," says Dr. Kirkpatrick, a former AA member who founded WFS in 1976. "Many women feel powerless and dependent on others to begin with, and twelve-step programs just reinforce this. Our New Life program is based on thirteen positive statements, such as 'I am a competent woman and I have much to give life,'" she explains.

In its thirteen statements, WFS emphasizes accepting alcoholism as a disease ("I have an addiction that once had me"), discarding negative thoughts and guilt, building a positive self-image and finding new ways to solve problems. In AA, members always refer to themselves as alcoholics; WFS urges women to put the past behind them. The program has been adapted for other addictions.

There is little research as yet on the effectiveness of such programs. One 1989 study looked at the outcomes of women in the early phases of alcohol dependence in traditional programs compared with those in women-only programs. The study found that, after two years, those in the women-only programs had better outcomes concerning alcohol consumption and social adjustment.

A new and controversial type of treatment program tries to help problem drinkers stop drinking (or learn to moderate their intake) *before* they progress to alcohol dependence, through education and short-term psychological counseling. Preliminary results among women in one such program, at the Research Institute on Addictions in Buffalo, New York, are encouraging. Among 120 women who completed ten weeks of treatment in the "Women and Health Program," there was a reported 55 percent increase in abstinent days, and a 75 percent decrease in heavy drinking. The report said the gains were maintained at a six-month follow-up.

However, the National Council on Alcoholism and Drug Dependence strongly opposes "drinking moderation" programs, warning they may give alcoholics "permission" to keep on drinking when alcohol presents a clear and present danger.

"The idea that people who are having problems with alcohol can drink a little plays right into the natural denial which is a symptom of alcoholism," argues Paul Wood, Ph.D., president of the NCADD. "People may be seduced into thinking they aren't really alcoholics, and they can once again become 'social drinkers.' Alcoholics have usually tried to abstain or cut back many times, and were ultimately unable to control their drinking. No alcoholic should be encouraged to drink."

ANTIADDICTION MEDICATIONS

There are a variety of medications to help treat chemical dependencies, used in conjunction with counseling and therapy:

NALTREXONE (REVIA): An opiate antagonist widely used to help speed withdrawal and ease symptoms in heroin addicts, naltrexone was approved in 1995 for treating alcoholism. The drug interferes with the brain's pleasure-producing chemicals to block the "high" induced by drugs, as well as reducing cravings. Studies show that it helped people quit drinking faster and stay sober longer.

A 1996 study from Yale, which followed eighty alcohol-dependent men and women randomized to receive either daily naltrexone or a placebo plus therapy for twelve weeks, found the relapse rate at six months was twice as high among those who received the placebo. The study also suggested that longer-term naltrexone treatment may be needed for some people. A randomized study of naltrexone among alcoholic women is now under way at Yale.

DISULFIRAM (ANTABUSE): This medication blocks the liver enzyme *acetaldehyde dehydrogenase*, which metabolizes alcohol. Disulfiram produces a host of unpleasant symptoms, including nausea, vomiting, headaches and palpitations, if a person drinks alcohol while taking it. Disulfiram is prescribed for short-term use in both inpatient and residential treatment programs and requires monitoring by a physician.

CLONIDINE (CATAPRES): A "central alpha agonist," clonidine is used to treat high blood pressure, which stimulates brain centers to lessen nerve impulses that cause blood vessel constriction. It blocks many symptoms of opiate withdrawal, and is mainly used for detoxifying heroin addicts, before switching them to naltrexone.

ANTIDEPRESSANTS: Medications that affect the brain's dopamine system (and some that affect serotonin) appear to help cocaine abusers. Some abusers may have low levels of both neurotransmitters, and use cocaine to alleviate depression. Antidepressants used include tricyclics and some selective serotonin reuptake inhibitors (SSRIs). *Wellbutrin* is expected to be approved shortly for use in smoking cessation. (For details on these medications, see chart on page 43.)

A small study reported to the American Psychiatric Association in 1995 suggests that the SSRI *fluvoxamine* may be effective for the treatment of compulsive shopping.

The antidepressant *sertraline (Zoloft)* is being tested in clinical trials to see if it helps depression-prone smokers kick the habit. Preliminary studies at the New York State Psychiatric Institute show that the drug may have doubled the quit rate. Studies of the drug *bupropion (Wellbutrin)*, which seems to affect neurotransmitters in ways similar to nicotine, are being conducted at the Mayo Clinic and elsewhere.

A number of experimental drugs have also been shown to reduce cravings for drugs in animal tests and limited trials in humans. A cocaine blocker called *flupentixol* is being tested with good results at Harvard and Yale. *Carbamazepine (Tegretol)*, a drug widely used to control seizures, is also showing promise as a way to block cocaine cravings.

The only drug available to counteract nicotine dependence is nicotine itself, in transdermal patches, gum or nasal spray.

NICOTINE PATCHES (NICO DERM, NICO DERM CQ): These are worn on the upper arm, and gradually deliver a small dose of nicotine through the skin into the bloodstream, affecting nicotine receptors in the brain, satisfying the craving for cigarettes. A 21-milligram nicotine patch delivers the equivalent amount of nicotine over a day contained in approximately one pack of cigarettes. Patches are changed every day and are used for three or four months in gradually lowered doses. Side effects can include insomnia and skin irritation.

Now available in nonprescription strength, nicotine patches work best as part of smoking cessation programs, aimed at changing smoking-related behaviors. A recent analysis of seventeen studies involving five thousand men and women smokers found that patch users were twice as likely to stay off cigarettes for six months, compared with those on placebo.

NICOTINE NASAL SPRAY (NICOTROL NS): This delivers 1 milligram of pure nicotine with one squirt up each nostril, with the nicotine absorbed through the lining of the nose into the bloodstream, eventually reaching the brain (but in lesser amounts than from cigarettes). The prescription-only spray, which went on sale in 1996, is designed to be inhaled no more than five times a day. (Overdosing can be dangerous; 40 milligrams of nicotine taken at once can be fatal.) Studies of 730 patients found that 25 percent were able to quit smoking for at least a year with the nasal spray, compared with 13 percent with the patch.

NICOTINE GUM (NICORETTE, NICOTROL): This delivers a gradual dose of nicotine through the mucous membrane of the mouth. Gum chewers must periodically "park" their wad of nicotine gum between the jaw and the cheek for a proper dose to be absorbed. Side effects include jaw aches, sore throats and hiccups. The gum, now available over-the-counter, may be used up to six months. It appears to be slightly less successful than the patch.

It's important to know that many recovering women addicts switch from one addiction to another, going from drugs to food or even exercise, for example. So the key to staying straight, say the experts, is making use of self-help groups for continuing emotional and behavioral support.

CHAPTER 7

Eating and Body Image

Eating disorders are a form of mental illness in which a person's body image becomes so distorted (usually because of an excessive fear of being fat) that their eating habits become dangerously abnormal.

Some experts blame the problem, in part, on society's obsession with being thin. According to the Centers for Disease Control and Prevention, as many as 40 percent of American women are *trying* to lose weight at any given time. More disturbingly, a recent Gallup Poll reported that 62 percent of women, including many who were *not* overweight, said they *wanted* to lose weight. Close to 20 percent said their weight caused them to be depressed or deeply worried, and that may contribute to disordered eating.

It's estimated that as many as 10 percent of women between the ages of thirteen and thirty may suffer from eating disorders (with the number as high as 20 percent among college-age women). New research indicates that some of these women may be genetically or biologically vulnerable to eating disorders.

Eating disorders fall into three categories: *anorexia nervosa*, in which people eat little or nothing at all to achieve and maintain a very low body weight; *bulimia nervosa*, where people eat too much, then try to rid themselves of the food by purging, fasting or excessive exercise; and *binge eating disorder*, compulsive overeating without attempts at purging. More than 90 percent of those afflicted with eating disorders are women. Approximately 1 percent of adolescent girls develop anorexia; 2 to 3 percent of young women develop bulimia.

Eating disorders can be deadly: One in ten cases of eating disorders lead to death from starvation, cardiac arrest or even suicide. While increasing awareness of the dangers of eating disorders has led many women to seek help, many more refuse to admit that they have a problem with food.

Quiz: Do You Have a Problem with Food?

If you answer yes to four or more of the statements below, you may have an eating problem.

- I always feel fat, even when my weight is "normal."

- I constantly worry about gaining weight, even though other people tell me I'm too thin.

- I am always on a diet; if I could lose weight I think most of my problems would be solved.

- I've bought lots of diet books, tried different weight-loss fads or joined and dropped out of several weight-loss programs, and regain any weight I've lost.

- I try to eat as little as I can to avoid gaining weight.

- I try not to eat when I'm hungry, as self-discipline.

- Sometimes I eat too much, and then eat nothing for several days, or try to exercise it off.

- I binge on junk food when I'm tense or unhappy.

- I have candies and cookies stashed all over the house so no one will see me when I binge.

- I have gone on eating binges where I feel I can't stop.

(continued)

- I have occasionally made myself throw up after a big meal to get rid of the calories.

- I frequently use laxatives or diuretics to lose weight.

- I exercise every day (or more than once a day) to prevent myself from gaining weight.

ANOREXIA NERVOSA

Individuals with anorexia literally starve themselves over long periods to achieve a body weight that goes far beyond any definition of "slender": at least 15 percent *below* the normal weight for their age and height. Yet these women see themselves as "fat" even when they are emaciated because of a distorted body image. Their self-esteem is tied to their shape and weight. They constantly weigh themselves, repeatedly check in the mirror for "fat" and even obsessively measure themselves.

The disorder usually begins between puberty (when girls typically begin to acquire more body fat around the hips) and age eighteen, when many girls begin college and typically gain weight their freshman year. Both periods can be stressful, which may trigger the onset of anorexia. Discomfort with a changing body, fear about changing roles and emerging sexuality may drive some girls to literally attempt to starve themselves back to the safe, small, androgynous body of their childhood.

A woman with anorexia doesn't set out to starve herself. She may begin by eliminating high-calorie foods from her diet, but eventually ends up eating only a few foods. Eventually, she no longer has normal signals of hunger or satiety, but feels full after eating only tiny amounts of food. She may induce vomiting, or abuse laxatives, diuretics or even enemas. Some women with anorexia also engage in binge eating followed by purging; in this case the diagnosis is *anorexia nervosa, purging type*.

People with anorexia often display obsessive-compulsive behavior, notes David L. Ginsberg, M.D., a psychiatrist who heads NYU Medical Center's Eating Disorders Program. For example, anorectic women may exercise compulsively because of their obsessive fear of being fat. A woman with anorexia may also develop strange, repetitive eating rituals, says Dr. Ginsberg. "Anorectics actually think a lot about food. They may collect recipes and even prepare gourmet dishes for their family and friends, but will never eat a bite themselves. They may refuse to eat even when they suffer intense hunger pains."

Anorexia involves a great deal of self-denial. A person may acknowledge that they have become thin, but will usually deny being malnourished. Sometimes they require hospitalization so that they do not starve themselves to death. Most often, it is concerned family members who bring the individual for help.

The medical consequences of eating disorders can be severe and, in some cases, life threatening (especially for women with the binge-purge type of anorexia). Dehydration lowers blood volume and contributes to constipation. Reduced body fat leads to lowered body temperature and the inability to withstand cold. Mild anemia, swollen joints and light-headedness are also common. Because the body produces less estrogen, menstrual periods may stop or (in girls not yet menstruating) be delayed; most anorectics stop having periods.

Starvation also causes loss of essential minerals like potassium, called "electrolytes," which help regulate the heart's electrical system, causing severe heartbeat irregularities, which can be fatal. Women also begin to lose calcium from their bones, resulting in premature osteoporosis. When body fat has been depleted, women begin to lose lean body mass, including vital muscle tissue in the heart, lungs, kidneys, liver and other organs, which can cause organ damage and failure. Many women with anorexia also suffer from major depression, anxiety, obsessive-compulsive disorder, psychosis, borderline personality disorder, substance abuse, and many are at risk for suicide.

❧ *Caroline's Story* ❧

"I first learned bulimic behavior when I attended . . . a girl's prep school. . . . Everyone was into achievement, perfection. We'd all been programmed that way from the time we were very young. . . . I was also a competitive swimmer, so I was very conscious of my body. You get that way when you spend so much time in a bathing suit. You never get away from the mirrors or from the coaches. . . . I was blond with that 'California look' that was so popular. When I look at pictures of myself, I realize I had a pretty normal body. But I was not 'perfect' in the way . . . models in the magazines looked. I became convinced that I was fat and ugly.

"The moment that I first started feeling bad about my body happened when I was about eight. I was having lunch with my family at a favorite restaurant. . . . I loved going there because my parents stressed healthy eating, three balanced meals a day, no snacks, et cetera. But there I would get all kinds of treats we never had at home, like french fries and shakes. When the waitress brought our order, my dad said, 'The milkshake goes to the heavy one.' It took a minute to sink in that he meant me. I was so humiliated. Heavy! No one had ever called me heavy before. In many ways, I think those seven words changed the way I felt about food for the next fourteen years. From that day on, I felt guilty eating anything that wasn't low-calorie. But I can't really blame my parents. I was the one who stuck my fingers down my throat and made myself throw up. . . .

"I was fifteen when I learned the 'secret.' I was having lunch with two friends in the school cafeteria. . . . Both of them were eating huge amounts of food . . . several big helpings. I was fascinated, since they were both so slim. . . . They ate until their stomachs were visibly bulging. I followed them upstairs to the bathroom, where both of them proceeded to throw up, actually cheering each other on! They looked awful afterward, their faces were red and puffy, their eyes watering. But they were both ecstatic at what they'd done.

"They told me that they'd learned the 'secret' from one of their mothers, who was a former model, who was incredibly thin and gorgeous. . . . I'd always had a problem controlling my appetite, and I felt throwing up meant I could finally be thin. . . . You start throwing up to control your weight. And you think that you'll do it only occasionally. But then . . . the behavior controls you. Within six months to a year, I was completely addicted.

"When I say bingeing, I mean like going to several ice cream stores in the space of an hour and eating quarts of ice cream, throwing up, and then shoplifting laxatives for an extra purge. Almost everyone I've talked to with this disorder also shoplifts. I would also exercise compulsively. It may be hard to imagine the mental agitation, how I couldn't feel calm until I could eat until I was just bursting. But that's how driven you are.

"The irony of it is . . . vomiting . . . often makes you gain weight, because eventually you're eating such huge quantities of food you can't get rid of it. . . . After a while your face becomes puffy, the salivary glands become swollen, you get chipmunk cheeks. And whenever I looked in the mirror, I would see this ugly, distorted face. . . . I would yell at myself in the mirror: 'You're fat and ugly. And a failure. And you'll always be fat and ugly.' And that propelled me to continue.

"I got married right after graduating from Harvard. My husband had no idea of what I was doing. I had binged and purged to the point of vomiting blood. But I wanted this tiny, Scarlett O'Hara waist for my wedding dress. I spent the two days before my wedding either sleeping or sick . . . from an overdose of laxatives. Not long after we got married, I called a self-help group.

"There was no real turning point; actually . . . it was probably the thousandth time I vomited blood, and vomited maybe for the fifteenth time that day. But something just clicked. Maybe I had gotten miserable enough to do something, and I guess I had enough fighting spirit to say, 'I'm not going to let this kill me.' "

Caroline Adams Miller has authored several books, including *My Name Is Caroline* (Doubleday 1988), an account of her struggle and recovery from bulimia, and *Feeding the Soul: Daily Meditations for Recovering from Eating Disorders*, (Bantam, 1994). The above remarks are from a personal interview and are printed with her permission.

BULIMIA NERVOSA

Unlike anorectics, people with bulimia usually maintain a normal body weight. They consume more food than people normally eat at one sitting (for example, wolfing down a whole pizza followed by a gallon of ice cream), then get rid of the excess calories by throwing up or by abusing laxatives or diuretics.

"Many women binge on foods that are easy to get down very quickly, such as ice cream, and which are soft and easier to bring up," remarks Melissa Ferguson, Ph.D., a psychologist who runs a support group for people with eating disorders at NYU Medical Center. Some women may not purge after a binge, but may fast or exercise excessively, adds Dr. Ferguson. This is *nonpurging bulimia nervosa*, according to new criteria in the *DSM-IV*.

A woman may binge and purge once or twice a week, or up to several times a day. Binges are characterized by a loss of control while eating, so that the woman eats rapidly and is unable to stop until she is painfully full. Then she will induce vomiting by putting her fingers down her throat to stimulate the gag reflex. Vomiting gives relief from physical discomfort and lessens her fear of gaining weight. Dieting heavily in between episodes of bingeing and purging is common. Bulimics are usually unhappy with their bodies, their self-esteem tied to their body shape and weight, says Dr. Ferguson. Because many individuals with bulimia do not become very thin, they often successfully hide their problem for years.

Bulimia often begins as a reaction to the self-starvation of anorexia. A woman revolts against the deprivation and begins eating anything and everything. But the frantic desire to control her weight remains, so she purges her body of the food. As many as half of women with anorexia will also develop bulimia.

Bulimia typically begins later in adolescence and young adulthood, sometimes during or after an episode of dieting. Some women hear about purging from friends as an "easy" way to control weight, as Caroline Miller did. The binge-purge pattern may be intermittent, or may become chronic over the years. Deeply ashamed of their eating habits, many women do not seek help until they reach their thirties or forties. By that time, their eating behavior is deeply ingrained and difficult to change.

Stomach acid brought up by frequent vomiting can cause cavities and damage to tooth enamel, and serious imbalances in important body minerals (electrolytes). Laxative abuse can lead to laxative dependence, interfering with normal bowel function. In rare instances, binge eating causes the stomach to rupture. The esophagus can become inflamed and torn, and the parotid glands (salivary glands below and in front of the ears) become swollen, giving the face a puffy appearance. Bulimia may also lead to irregular menstrual periods.

Some individuals with bulimia struggle with addictions, including alcohol and drug abuse. Others hoard food, almost like alcoholics maintaining their secret stash. Many people with bulimia suffer from clinical depression, anxiety, obsessive-compulsive disorder and other psychiatric illnesses. These problems, combined with their impulsive tendencies, also place them at increased risk for suicidal behavior.

BINGE EATING DISORDER

Binge eating disorder resembles bulimia, with frequent episodes of uncontrolled overeating. However, people suffering from binge eating disorder do not try to purge the excess calories. They will stuff themselves to bursting (even when not hungry), feeling out of control while eating, then disgusted, guilty and depressed by their behavior, says Dr. Ginsberg. Many binge eaters are solitary individuals, eating alone out of acute embarrassment over how much they consume.

Not surprisingly, most people with this disorder are obese, and have a history of weight fluctuations; they typically have much more difficulty losing weight and keeping it off than people with other serious weight problems. In fact, recent studies suggest that as many as a third of people in hospital-based weight-reduction programs meet the criteria for binge eating disorder, and 10 to 15 percent of people in nonmedical diet programs (like Weight Watchers) may also suffer from the problem.

Binge eating disorder is found in about 2 percent of the general population, more often in women than men (however, one third to one fourth are men). Five million Americans may be caught up in binge eating and weight cycling, increasing their risk for the serious medical problems associated with obesity: high cholesterol, high blood pressure and diabetes, as well as heart disease, gallbladder disease and some types of cancer.

They are also prone to major depression and anxiety, and have more psychiatric illnesses. However, because so little is known about binge eating disorder, it is not included in the formal diagnostic criteria in the *DSM-IV*, but is described in the appendix as a disorder that needs further study.

∽ *Caroline's Story, Continued* ∾

"Binges almost always happen when you're under stress, when you're very unhappy or angry about something. It's a lot like drinking . . . you just want to escape. You get incredibly sedated; you lose touch with reality during a binge. It gets rid of the feelings of self-hatred and failure. At least temporarily. For bulimics vomiting or laxatives is this incredible purge, you just feel empty and calm. Cleansed in some way. Afterward, people are usually very tired . . . like a drunk sleeps it off.

"The progression with an eating disorder is among the fastest of any addiction. Most people binge on high-fat, high-sugar foods; there's a definite mood alteration that goes along with these foods. There's a physical addiction and a behavioral addiction. Some doctors I've talked to say they've seen bulimics who are psychologically in as bad a shape as alcoholics who have been drinking for twenty years. . . .

"You don't have to starve yourself or make yourself throw up to have an eating disorder. You can be at the aerobics studio for hours every day, and society will applaud you. I mean, the highest compliment people pay you is to say, 'you look great. Did you lose weight?' That's kind of sad."

OTHER EATING DISORDERS

Many experts now view anorexia and bulimia as extremes in a spectrum of disordered eating. A number of problem eating behaviors do not meet the formal criteria for anorexia or bulimia, but, experts warn, may *progress* to these disorders.

For example, there are women who severely restrict their food intake, but who maintain a normal body weight and continue to menstruate. They may display some bulimic behavior for short periods, or may purge after eating relatively small amounts of food (like two cookies). Some women do not eat at all during the day, then binge at night. Others chew and spit out their food, so they're able to "eat" as much as they want and remain thin.

Experts say that millions of women may be suffering from such eating disturbances. "While approximately 3 percent of women are clinically bulimic, another 10 percent are 'dieters at risk.' They may engage in bulimic behaviors, bingeing and purging, but not sufficiently often to be diagnosed as bulimic," says Adam Drewnowski, Ph.D., professor and director of the Program in Human Nutrition, School of Public Health, at the University of Michigan at Ann Arbor. "Our studies show that, as women express a greater desire to lose weight, and the bigger the difference in their actual weight and their desired weight, the more likely they are to employ more drastic dieting strategies. We've found that drastic dieting puts women at risk for eating disorders over time."

THE BIOLOGY OF EATING DISORDERS

Many experts believe that some women may have a biological vulnerability to eating disorders. Certain neurotransmitters and peptide hormones, which help regulate anxiety and mood, also affect appetite and eating behavior.

The neurotransmitter serotonin helps control feelings of satiety in an area of the brain called the *paraventricular nucleus* (located within the hypothalamus). Serotonin in this area may be depleted or less active in people with bulimia, disrupting normal signals that tell people when they've eaten enough, speculates Katherine A. Halmi, M.D., a professor of psychiatry and the director of the Eating Disorder Program at New York Hospital–Cornell Medical Center, Westchester Division. When medications that boost serotonin or activate serotonin receptors are used in such patients, they reduce food consumption. People with anorexia may produce *too much* serotonin, blocking normal signals of hunger. When serotonin antagonists were used in some anorectics, it helped them begin to eat and gain weight, Dr. Halmi notes.

Norepinephrine, which can *increase* appetite, becomes depleted in people who drastically limit food intake or who are emaciated (but is normalized when weight is regained). Like serotonin, levels of norepinephrine are lower in people with major depression. People with anorexia and certain forms of depression also tend to have higher than normal levels of stress hormones, which also inhibit appetite.

Recent research indicates that eating fatty sweets can trigger the release of heroinlike chemicals in the brain called *opioid peptides*, triggering binges in vulnerable people. Levels of another brain chemical, *vasopressin*, are elevated in patients with anorexia, bulimia and obsessive-compulsive disorder. Normally released in response to physical and emotional stress, vasopressin may contribute to the obsessive behavior seen in some patients with eating disorders, enhancing the cycle of rigorous dieting, compulsive overeating and self-induced vomiting.

What all this means, says Dr. Halmi, is that some women may have an unstable chemical balance in their brain, which increases their risk of developing eating disorders when they are confronted with certain stresses. Once the cycle of eating disorders has begun, says Dr. Halmi, these chemical changes become more pronounced and either perpetuate the need for more dieting and weight loss, or sustain binge eating.

THE PSYCHOLOGY OF EATING DISORDERS

Besides an overwhelming fear of being fat, women with eating disorders share feelings of low self-esteem and helplessness. They constantly compare themselves (and their bodies) with other women, leading to a devalued self-image and depression. "Women with anorexia tend to be perfectionists, more rigid in their personality, overly concerned about their appearance to society, striving professionally," says Dr. Halmi.

Some girls with anorexia tend to be "too good to be true": obedient, good students, keeping their feelings to themselves. Many of these girls are socially withdrawn and almost suicidal in their refusal to eat. Some researchers believe that people with anorexia restrict food to gain a sense of control, especially during adolescence when so many body changes take place; the average age at which girls begin dieting is twelve, right after they begin having periods. "My belief is that, on a certain level, these girls do not want to grow up. It's too frightening for them," remarks Dr. Halmi. Many girls also gain approval from peers for becoming thin.

There may be a history of sexual abuse in young women with eating disorders. "I can't tell you how many bulimics have told me that the vomiting was a reaction to having to perform fellatio as a child on an uncle or other adult male. Almost to expel the act itself," remarks Caroline Miller. "They also express a loss of boundaries around their body, and almost want to deny their femininity and sexuality . . . they want to stop the whole process."

The stress of leaving home for the first time, and a typical weight gain during the freshman year of college, can put girls at risk of bulimia. "Drastic dieting is not so much a response to being overweight as it is to stress," observes Dr. Drewnowski.

In fact, women who develop bulimia (and binge eating disorder) typically consume large amounts of junk food to relieve stress and anxiety. "Somewhere along the line in these people's lives, eating became associated with comfort. They say, 'Food is my friend,'" adds Dr. Melissa Ferguson.

But bingeing brings on guilt and depression, with purging providing only temporary relief. This may be why severe dieting and eating disorders are linked to alcohol and drug abuse. Like substance abuse, bulimia may have a compulsive quality to it.

Eating disorders appear to run in families; behavioral and environmental factors in families may also play a major role. One recent study found that mothers who are overly concerned about their daughters' weight and attractiveness may put them at increased risk; girls with eating disorders often have fathers and brothers who are overly critical of their weight.

Women pursuing activities or professions that require low weights for optimal performance—especially ballet, gymnastics and modeling—are more susceptible to eating disorders.

And while a 1995 report in the *American Journal of Psychology* suggests that eating disorders may have declined slightly among college-aged women since the 1980s, the authors said that "body dissatisfaction and the desire to lose weight were still the norm for more than 70 percent of young women."

One reason may be the continuing tyranny of fashion.

The Unattainable "Ideal" Female Body

Our slavery to slenderness got its start around the First World War, when men marched off to the trenches and women marched off to work, and constricting corsets gave way to practicality. Hemlines rose and hourglass figures became passé. The first best-selling diet book for women, *Diet and Health, With Key to the Calories*, was published in 1918—and an industry was born.

During the roaring 1920s women acquired what had previously been a privilege reserved to men—the right to vote. They also adopted traditionally male vices: smoking and drinking. They cut their long tresses and tried to achieve a decidedly boyish figure, helped by "Elfin Fat Reducing Gum Drops" and "Every Woman's Flesh Reducer" for the bath.

Hard times during the 1930s made being too thin a badge of poverty, so female curves made a comeback (albeit less curvaceous than they once were). "Rosie the Riveter" may have worn pants during World War II, but when the men came home the hourglass figure and new versions of the corset were in vogue again, as women were once again consigned to the "domestic sphere." The "mammary movie goddesses" of the era would be considered overweight by today's standards; Marilyn Monroe wore a size 12.

The tumultuous 1960s ushered in a new cult of slenderness, as women once more claimed their "freedom" from domesticity. The slender ideal has remained firmly entrenched ever since and the diet industry has became a multibillion-dollar business, promoting everything from calorie-controlled milk shakes to thigh-reducing creams.

The irony is that as the "ideal woman" became thinner, real-life women did not. Over 60 percent of American women wear a size 12 or larger, while a typical fashion model weighs 16 percent less and is 9 percent taller than the average woman.

A 1994 study of 238 women in the *Journal of Abnormal Psychology* confirmed what many experts have long suspected: Repeated exposure to images of such "fashionably thin" models and movie stars "is related to eating pathology and suggests that women may directly model disordered eating behavior presented in the media." Although most women are exposed to these images, the authors of the study found that only a small percentage develop anorexia or bulimia, indicating that factors like biology, personality and culture play a major role in disordered eating.

↫ Shanetta's Story ↬

"I'm proud to be a black woman. But I hate the idea that it's culturally okay for us to be large. . . . I hate those T-shirts showing black women with big butts. . . . I'm a dancer and I'm proud of my body. It's long and lean, like a beautiful African sculpture. I worked hard to get that body . . . but in a lot of unhealthy ways. . . . I am a recovering anorectic and bulimic.

"When I was growing up, I always had this obsessive fear of becoming fat like my momma and my aunties. They are big, big women. They like to cook and eat. To them, food says love. Saying no to their cooking . . . would be like rejecting them. So I'd take a little of everything and pick. Which, of course, would never satisfy them. . . . I didn't realize at the time how big my hang-up was, or how wrapped up it was in unconsciously rejecting my background. I didn't have the pride then that I have now. . . .

"I first heard about throwing up from other dancers I was taking class with. . . . One Christmas, I remember very vividly, I was just sixteen, there was this big dinner . . . ham, fried chicken, biscuits, candied yams, grits, smothered okra . . . all loaded with butter . . . and the pies, three kinds, sweet potato, pecan, and coconut. I'd been so good at dinner. And I was only going to eat one bite of pie. But when they put that piece of pecan pie with whipped cream in front of me, before I knew it, it was gone. And then I said, what the hell, I'll have the coconut, too. I was so disgusted. So I went into the bathroom and stuck my finger down my throat. And that made me feel better about myself. Like I hadn't lost control. . . .

"After that, everyone remarked how I'd finally 'gotten some appetite.' They had no idea that after I ate, I'd be in the bathroom, throwing up. What started to scare me was the bingeing . . . chips, cake, and ice cream, a gallon at a time. Sometimes, I would work out till I would drop trying to work off the extra food. Or I'd take lots of laxatives, which gave me cramps and made me sick. . . . Then my body rebelled. My face got bloated, my belly was bloated, I started to gain weight . . . and that made me twice as disgusted with myself. . . . So I'd go on these starvation diets. And then I'd binge again. It was taking a toll on me professionally. . . . I was with a major dance company . . . if I lost that, I'd lose everything. . . . I said, 'Girl, you've got to stop before it kills you.' . . .

"The treatment was hard, partly because there were no other black women in the therapy group, and partly because I was terrified that if I stopped throwing up I'd get fat. And fat to me meant so many negative things I unconsciously associated with being black. I hated myself for feeling that way. But I had to admit that I did. . . . I had to make peace finally with who I was, where I'd come from, and who I wanted to be. It's been a long road. . . . Don't think for a minute that black women don't do this. They do, honey, they do."

IN THE EYE OF THE BEHOLDER

In some cultures, being well fleshed is a sign of good health, making a person more resistant to disease. African Americans and other groups have often regarded big hips or an ample rear end as being more feminine and sexy. Studies show that African-American, Latina and Native American women are more satisfied at higher weights than middle- and upper-income white women; less than 40 percent of black women have ever tried a weight-loss diet, compared with 62 percent of white women.

Most tellingly, a three-year study of three hundred adolescents by researchers in the Department of Anthropology at the University of Arizona found that 70 percent of black girls were satisfied with their current weight, *even if they were significantly overweight*, while 90 percent of their white counterparts expressed dissatisfaction with their weight, *even when it was normal.* In fact, 64 percent of the black girls felt it was better to be a little overweight than underweight.

"African-American girls were notably less concerned with the beauty standard of the ideal girl depicted in the media," says Mimi Nichter, Ph.D., an anthropologist and an author of the study. "For these girls, beauty was flexible, not dependent on a particular size or body statistics. For them, 'looking good' or 'got it going on' entails making what you've got working for you, creating and presenting a sense of style, an attitude, no matter what your size or shape."

In contrast, the white girls interviewed for the study had one, specific standard of beauty they tried to measure up to: being tall, slender, with blond hair, blue eyes and long legs. "White girls who measured up to this idea were admired, but also envied, there was a great deal of competitiveness. However, the black girls described themselves as being supportive of each other, getting and giving positive feedback for 'looking good,' rather than for meeting one prescribed ideal," she comments.

That doesn't mean that women of color don't fall prey to eating disorders. More economic opportunities are available to women of color who conform to the social standards of white society, including the preference for slenderness. Eating disorders may also show themselves differently among women of color. For instance, studies show that Native American women have a much higher percentage of compulsive eating than bulimia or anorexia.

Recent studies show that eating disorders are on the rise among women of color, especially when ties to one's ethnocultural heritage loosen, says Sue A. Kuba, Ph.D., coordinator of Behavioral Medicine and Health Psychology at the California School of Professional Psychology. In a preliminary study of 150 college-aged white, African-American, Latina and Asian-American women, Dr. Kuba and Diane Harris, Ph.D., an associate professor at San Francisco State University, found a high correlation between symptoms of eating disorders and how acculturated the women were to American mainstream values and standards of beauty.

Interestingly, a 1996 update of the study data found that among Latina and Asian women, strong peer relationships seemed to be *protective* against eating disorders, no matter how acculturated the women were. "But Latinas whose families reacted strongly to their efforts to adopt nontraditional roles were more likely to develop eating disorders, suggesting that issues of control were a factor," adds Dr. Kuba.

Obesity is often related to socioeconomic status, with higher weights being a product of poverty, poor diet and stress, Dr. Kuba points out. Obese individuals are discriminated against on many levels, especially in employment. Studies show that fat women suffer enormous social and economic consequences, with more discrimination at lower weights than their male counterparts.

A 1993 study by the Harvard School of Public Health, which followed over ten thousand men and women between the ages of sixteen and twenty-four for a period of eight years, found that fat women were 20 percent less likely to marry, had lower household incomes and were 10 percent more likely to be living in poverty. A typical woman in the study was five feet three inches and weighed two hundred pounds. The effects on overweight men in the study were more modest.

Fear and loathing of fat and eating disorders are not unique to America. Anorexia and bulimia are common in other industrialized countries, including Canada, Europe and Japan, where being attractive is also linked to being thin.

✐ *Caroline's Story, Continued* ✐

"I think eating disorders have some parallels with . . . addiction. [When] the problem starts to impede your work, you're losing sleep over it, if you've given up hobbies and activities, if you binge eat to sedate yourself, if you're hoarding food, buying food in secret, hiding grocery bills. That kind of thing. Don't wait till you find yourself bent over the toilet trying to get rid of dinner . . . to get help.

"At a good treatment program there's a lot of education about food, unlearning fears about food, how to cook it, touch it. How to eat in restaurants. What kinds of situations set you off. Shopping for clothes and not freaking out at buying a particular size. The recovery process involves dealing with those fears and behaviors. . . . I eventually went into therapy and found antidepressants very helpful. I did suffer an episode of clinical depression during my recovery."

TREATING EATING DISORDERS

If an eating disorder is suspected, particularly if a woman has undergone a drastic weight loss, the first step is a complete physical examination to rule out other illnesses. In extreme cases of anorexia, emergency hospitalization may be needed, especially if weight loss has reached a danger level of 25 percent below normal weight. Hospitalization may also be needed to treat serious metabolic disturbances, clinical depression, psychosis and the risk of suicide. The longer the disorder remains untreated, the harder it is to treat, because the behaviors and distorted thinking become so entrenched.

The hardest obstacle to overcome in anorexia is getting the patient to eat. To women with anorexia, food is the enemy; they have developed a feeling of mastery over not eating. They often deny there's a problem. "Because of their illness . . . they have no energy, they are not sleeping well, and they are physically weak. You need to point out that once they gain some weight they will be physically stronger, they can be more active, and that is often the one thing they respond to," says Dr. Halmi. "A person who is suffering from the physical effects of starvation cannot begin to deal with the emotional problems underlying the disorder."

However, the focus of treatment should not be on food and eating, stresses Dr. Halmi, but on replacing the anorectic behaviors and the thinking behind them with healthy patterns. Patients need constant emotional support to understand their illness (and the self-hatred that often drives it). Some may need round-the-clock medical supervision to overcome the self-destructive behavior of anorexia. "One has to spend a lot of time with an anorectic patient, helping them to understand the reality of their medical situation, while acknowledging their fears about food and what has driven them to starve themselves," says Dr. Halmi. "Therapy involves a cognitive restructuring of their distorted perception of themselves and their self-esteem. Therapy teaches the patient to place less emphasis on thinness for measuring self-worth, and to modify her all-or-nothing thinking."

A woman's treatment team may include a psychotherapist and a family therapist to work with family members, physicians to treat the medical complications and prescribe medications if needed and nutritionists to help a woman learn how to eat normally again. This process can be complicated by metabolic changes that take place in anorexia, which may make it harder to maintain a stable weight. Preliminary evidence shows that antidepressant medications may be helpful when combined with other treatments.

Treatment can be a lengthy and difficult process, with frequent relapses. In a ten-year follow-up of seventy-six patients, Dr. Halmi reports that only one quarter could be regarded as being "cured"; five patients had died. About half of the patients were able to stay within a normal weight, but many were still preoccupied with their body image and displayed abnormal eating behaviors. One quarter remained quite ill.

Bulimia is generally less resistant to treatment than anorexia. For one thing, it is usually the woman herself who seeks treatment, often because of the emotional distress accompanying bulimic behavior and fear of the medical consequences of constant purging. Women are hospitalized less often with bulimia than with anorexia, and if they are not seriously ill, they can be placed in a group therapy program, says Dr. Halmi. For women who have a more serious illness, use of individual cognitive-behavioral therapy to change distorted thinking patterns about body image, self-esteem and disordered eating behaviors is often the most helpful form of therapy.

A change in diet may also help. A recent study by Dr. Halmi found that bulimic patients reported less feelings of satiety after a high-fat meal than after a low-fat, high-carbohydrate meal, and compared with nonbulimic controls. So, she suggests, bulimic patients should avoid high-fat foods and try a low-fat, higher-carbohydrate diet, which may reduce the urge to binge.

In 1994, the selective serotonin reuptake inhibitor *fluoxetine* (see page 43) became the first drug approved to treat bulimia; it is also useful in treating some patients with binge eating disorder. In addition to the action of increasing serotonin (which helps restore normal satiety signals), these antidepressants can help treat co-occurring depression, which may occur in as many as three fourths of cases of bulimia nervosa. Other antidepressant medications commonly used to treat bulimia include the tricyclics *desipramine* and *imipramine* (see page 44).

Drugs that block the action of the brain's natural opioids may also have promise for treating binge eating. The University of Michigan's Dr. Adam Drewnowski tested the drug *naxolone* in forty-one women, half of whom met the criteria for either bulimia or binge eating disorder, and found that it helped reduce consumption of sweet, fatty foods in binge eaters, compared with nonbinge eaters. A six-week clinical trial of a similar drug at Wayne State University reduced the number of binges in a small group of bulimic and anorectic binge eaters.

Recent studies indicate that combining medication with intensive group therapy or cognitive-behavioral therapy is especially helpful for bulimic patients, especially in preventing relapse once medications are discontinued. Relapses are most common within the first year after treatment.

The Eating Disorders Research Team at the Massachusetts General Hospital has followed 225 patients for the past six years. Data at one-year follow-up found 50 percent of the bulimic patients fully recovered (asymptomatic for eight weeks), while only 10 percent of the anorectic patients were considered fully recovered. Of the recovered bulimics, a third relapsed.

For women who engage in occasional bulimic behavior, or who find themselves occasionally bingeing, NYU Medical Center's Dr. Melissa Ferguson advises contacting a self-help group, such as Overeaters Anonymous. Such a support group may provide enough intervention that a full-blown eating disorder can be prevented. Says Dr. Ferguson: "As with alcohol and drug abuse, if food or an obsession with weight loss has become the focal points in your life, or are interfering with your life, it's time to get help."

CHAPTER 8

Sexuality

Experts in human sexuality stress that the *mind* is our major sex organ. You may have all the equipment in working order, but if your mind isn't willing, your body won't be, either. Which is why sexual dysfunction is included in the psychiatric diagnostic manual.

Based on what we see in the movies (or read in certain novels), you'd think everyone was "doing it" all the time and having earthshaking orgasms. Not true.

Researchers at the University of Chicago interviewed 3,432 men and women aged fifteen to fifty-nine about their sexual habits and found that people were not having sex as often as we thought. The data, published in 1994, revealed that one third of American adults make love two or more times a week, one third have sex once or a few times per month, and another third only a few times a year (if at all). Married people have sex more often than singles.

The survey also found that sexual problems were fairly common among women. One in three women reported a lack of interest in sex for at least two months over the past year; one in five had trouble reaching orgasm. Some 13 percent of women had pain with sex for several months. The most common sexual problem is lack of desire. Many of these women never discussed these problems with their partners, much less sought professional help.

Most of us were never really educated about sexuality; quite the opposite. Religious, cultural and social beliefs about sex and sexual roles all contribute to sexual ignorance and inhibition. Moreover, both men and women are often unable to communicate their sexual feelings and needs, says Virginia Sadock, who heads the Program in Human Sexuality and Sex Therapy at NYU Medical Center. "A certain amount of sexual activity, and certain amount of sexual satisfaction contributes to emotional well-being," she stresses. "Unfortunately, we seem to be reluctant to discuss sexual issues or difficulties, even though as a society we're fascinated by sex."

Medical problems, medications and substance abuse can all cause sexual dysfunction, says Dr. Sadock. But more often it is depression, anxiety, troubled relationships, dissatisfaction with body image and past sexual abuse or assault that contribute to women's sexual difficulties.

Sexual dysfunction is defined clinically as a disturbance in sexual desire, and in the psychological and physical mechanism of sexual response. In women, it can take the form of low sexual drive (libido), avoidance of sex, failure to achieve orgasm, involuntary muscle spasms so strong they prevent intercourse (*vaginismus*) or pain during sex (*dyspareunia*).

But before discussing the things that can go wrong with sex, let's discuss what should go right, starting with the basics.

UNDERSTANDING SEXUALITY

A woman's physical organs of sex are the *vagina* and *clitoris*. The *clitoris is the only human organ that has no function other than bringing pleasure.* There are more free nerve endings on the clitoris than any other part of the body.

The vagina and clitoris, and even the upper thighs, buttocks and lower back, are eroticized by nerves extending from the lower spine. But the clitoris is the sexual nerve center. The word *clitoris* comes from the Greek word for "key," suggesting that even ancient anatomists considered it the key to a woman's sexuality.

This small, sensitive shaft is hidden beneath the mound of protective tissue called the *mons*, covered with pubic hair. Branching out from the mons are two outer lips of the genitals, called the *labia majora*. Within the labia

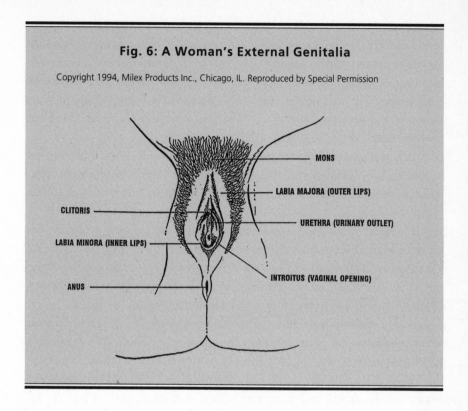

Fig. 6: A Woman's External Genitalia

MONS

LABIA MAJORA (OUTER LIPS)

CLITORIS

URETHRA (URINARY OUTLET)

LABIA MINORA (INNER LIPS)

INTROITUS (VAGINAL OPENING)

ANUS

are the inner lips (*labia minora*), which protect the vagina and the opening of the *urethra* (the urinary outlet). Inside the vagina is the *cervix*, the opening to the uterus. The clitoris is sheathed in a tiny hood just above where the inner lips meet.

Tactile stimulation of the clitoris (by penile thrusting, by manual stimulation or by oral stimulation by a partner) results in an erection somewhat similar to that of the penis. Stimulation of nerve endings causes increased blood flow to the spongy erectile tissue in the shaft of the clitoris; contraction of tiny muscles compresses a tiny vein, trapping blood in the erectile tissue, making the clitoris firm and exquisitely sensitive. Unlike an erect penis, which moves up and out, the clitoris moves back and up beneath its hood during arousal.

There are four phases to the sexual response cycle: desire, excitement (arousal), orgasm and resolution. When we're aroused, the brain sends signals to the clitoris and vagina through the nerves in the spinal column, causing blood congestion in the pelvis and genital tissues. This *vasocongestion* causes the labia to swell and darken in color, and triggers lubrication and dilation of the vaginal walls and engorgement and sensitization of the shaft of the clitoris. As the uterus becomes engorged, it balloons upward and the cervical opening widens slightly (the better to admit sperm). The breasts also become congested with blood and the nipples become erect and sensitive. During the excitement phase, the heart beats faster, blood pressure increases and breathing speeds up. The skin may become flushed, and you may perspire.

As sexual excitement increases, the muscles around the entrance to the vagina become swollen and the opening to the vagina narrows, the erect clitoris slides beneath its hood and muscle tension increases throughout the body.

If clitoral stimulation continues, orgasm occurs. During orgasm, repeated pleasurable contractions pulse through the lower third of the vagina. Contractions also ripple through the uterus, beginning at the top and working their way down to the cervix. Some women may have more intense orgasms due to the pressure of penis on the cervix and uterus, or by the conscious contraction of their pelvic floor muscles. To a certain degree, every muscle in the body contracts during climax. That's one reason you feel totally relaxed after making love. It's a whole-body workout.

In the resolution phase, the vasocongestion and muscle contractions dissipate, our breathing and heart rate return to normal, and we feel relaxed and peaceful.

For generations, traditional concepts of women's sexual responsiveness all but ignored the clitoris. Freud taught that a woman became sexually mature only when she progressed from her "infantile" focus on the clitoris (her inadequate "substitute" for a penis) to having vaginal orgasms. Many women believed they were inadequate (or even abnormal) if they didn't have vaginal orgasms, notes Dr. Sadock. This notion was dispelled in 1953 by Alfred Kinsey in his landmark study on sex, based on interviews with nearly six thousand women. *Sexual Behavior in the Human Female* revealed that the vast majority of women could not have orgasms without direct stimulation of their clitoris. More recent information from the Kinsey Institute for Research in Sex, Gender and Reproduction shows that less than half of women are able to climax through penis-in-the-vagina intercourse alone.

Men and women are also programmed a bit differently in the timing of sexual arousal and release, notes Dr. Sadock. A man can become aroused and come to climax in three or four minutes, simply by physical stimulation (though it's possible to prolong erections). A woman's time from arousal to orgasm can be almost four times longer, because her excitement phase is prolonged. Women generally need more stimulation than men to climax; longer kissing, caressing and other forms of sexual expression, including oral sex.

Once aroused, women can have multiple orgasms; men have to wait to "recharge" after climaxing (this *refractory* period gets longer as a man ages). Many women also have higher cycles of arousal linked to the hormonal changes of the menstrual cycle, some peaking at mid-cycle or ovulation, others premenstrually and still others just prior to menstruation.

The famous sexual research team of William Masters and Virginia Johnson first studied the mechanics of orgasm and identified the arousal cycles of men and women in *Human Sexual Response*, published in 1966. During their studies of more than eight hundred men and women, Masters and Johnson also uncovered some of the hitherto "hidden" aspects of a woman's sexual response, including vaginal lubrication during arousal.

The works of Kinsey and Masters and Johnson proved that any woman can achieve orgasm through clitoral stimulation. One of the best ways is through masturbation. An electric vibrator can produce very intense orgasms. Unfortunately, many of us were taught that masturbation is shameful or harmful.

Once a woman learns how to achieve orgasm, experts say, it's rare for her to *lose* that capacity unless she experiences a trauma like rape, or unless there's poor sexual communication or conflict in a relationship. Women can have just as intense orgasms with a female partner as they can with men.

The trouble is that popular fiction and movies often depict women having spectacular, multiple orgasms, *every* time they make love. When reality doesn't measure up, many women believe they are abnormal, or "frigid." It can be distressing if you expect a major earthquake and get only a small tremor. Many women are reluctant to tell their partners they need more stimulation of their clitoris to climax.

About 10 percent of women say they have *never* experienced an orgasm by any means. But orgasm may not be the sole measure of sexual satisfaction or happiness in a relationship. Indeed, for most women, what fuels sexuality is a drive for intimacy and emotional connection with a partner. For a woman, making love is about making connections on many levels, not just the physical.

A 1995 study of 541 male and female college students in the *Archives of Sexual Behavior* found that over 70 percent of the sexually active men, but only 36 percent of the women, said they'd had sex at least once with a person for whom they felt no emotional attachment. It is no surprise, then, that a recent survey of four hundred heterosexual men and women aged eighteen to fifty-nine found that women were more likely than men to prefer activities associated with "romance," such as talking, holding hands, wearing sexy clothing, hugging, kissing and engaging in petting that doesn't necessarily lead to intercourse, and wanting continued hugging and kissing after intercourse. On the other hand, the men were more focused on the physical, exploring new sexual positions, performing and receiving oral sex, having both partners climax at the same time and looking at erotic movies and books.

The same holds true for sexual fantasies. A recent review of some two hundred studies of sexual fantasies found that women's fantasies involved touching, caressing and feelings, whereas men's fantasies tended to be more sexually graphic and impersonal. Another study found that while women were *physically* aroused by X-rated movies, they became *mentally* aroused by those scripted from a "feminine" point of view, with less graphic sex and more emotional content.

Our cultural background, religious beliefs and upbringing may also inhibit sexual functioning. For example, in traditional families, Latina women are raised to be submissive to men, sexually pure, viewing sex as for making babies, not for pleasure. Women who are outwardly sexual, or enjoy sex, are viewed as promiscuous. This madonna/whore conflict is actually shared by women in many cultures, and can result in an inability to reach orgasm and other sexual problems, experts say.

While just about every woman is physically capable of orgasm (barring some disease or anatomical problem), some women may not be *psychologically* capable of being aroused or coming to climax. Many psychological factors, such as sexual or physical abuse, depression, stress and anxiety, can interfere with a woman's sexual desire and responsiveness, as can a lack of perceived intimacy.

"The entire life experience of a woman comes into play in her sexual response," says Dr. Sadock. "Was she conditioned to be ashamed of her sexuality, or of her body? Does she perceive her partner as loving and concerned with her pleasure? Does she feel emotionally connected to or distant from her partner?"

If a man doesn't have an erection, he can't have sex (impotence has many causes, including vascular disease, medications, smoking, depression and anxiety). A woman can have intercourse with moderate vaginal lubrication and "fake it," without her partner ever knowing something is wrong, unless there's pain, notes Dr. Sadock.

Lack of female hormones (and the male hormone testosterone, produced in small amounts by the ovaries) can change sexual responsiveness after menopause. The vaginal tissue thins and becomes drier. The vagina itself may shrink, making sex uncomfortable. If testosterone levels are also low, it can dampen a woman's libido. Lack of lubrication can also be caused by diabetes and other chronic medical conditions. Vaginal lubricants, estrogen cream or estrogen therapy and, if needed, small doses of testosterone can all help. (For more on sexuality in later life, see page 160.)

The urethra and bladder are less cushioned by atrophied vaginal tissue after menopause, so there can be irritation or frequency of urination after sexual contact (not to mention the problem of urine leakage, or *stress incontinence*). Kegel exercises, which strengthen the muscles at the base of the pelvis, can help overcome the embarrassment and disabling symptoms of stress incontinence. Kegels can also improve the "grip" of the vagina during intercourse.

But for pleasurable sex at any age, experts stress that the mind and body must work *together*. And that means maintaining healthy relationships as well as mental wellness.

∽ *Elaine's Story* ∾

"Finally after years of trying to have a baby, Camille arrived. My husband comes from a big Irish family and they were beside themselves. My parents were thrilled; Camille was their first grandchild. . . . So it was a very happy time for all of us.

"I was able to get an extended maternity leave . . . until Camille was six months old. . . . Because I was the one who was home, all the housework got dumped in my lap. Before the baby, Ryan used to help with the laundry and the cooking . . . but suddenly I was Mrs. Housewife. . . . On top of that, we seemed to have guests every weekend. Ryan invited every distant cousin to see the baby. . . . So there I was, cooking breakfast, lunch and dinner, taking care of Camille, doing all the laundry, shopping. . . .

"Before Camille came along, we used to have sex three times a week, maybe more. . . . My ob-gyn said I could start making love six weeks after giving birth, but honestly I wasn't up for it. I was just too damn tired . . . it hurt a lot . . . and after a few times, I ended up in tears. . . . Ryan was upset, I was upset. It was like our sex life was over. Totally. My ob-gyn said there was nothing wrong with me internally to make sex painful. She gave me the name of a sex therapist. At first Ryan refused to go. He said it was me that had a problem. . . . Finally, I persuaded him.

"In therapy, I learned that even though I wasn't able to restrict access to my home, I could restrict access to my body. If Ryan wouldn't share the housework, he couldn't share my body . . . and that's why sex hurt so much. I simply closed up.

"So I had to confront Ryan and tell him, not ask him, to do his share. He grumbled, but he did. Especially when he understood that these issues were keeping us from making love."

SEXUAL CONCERNS ACROSS THE LIFE SPAN

A 1994 survey by the Alan Guttmacher Institute found that more than half of women (and three quarters of men) have had sexual intercourse before their eighteenth birthday. The Guttmacher survey found that a majority of teens who had had intercourse before age fourteen said they had been forced to have sex. Experts say one of the biggest challenges is to help adolescent girls develop enough self-esteem and self-confidence to say no. These days, sex education must also include a discussion of sexually transmitted disease and safe sex.

Adolescence and early adulthood are also the times when "our sexual self-esteem can be eroded by dislike or shame about our bodies. We may love and desire someone who doesn't love us back, which makes us feel undesirable," says Dr. Sadock.

Healthy sexuality can also be damaged by sexual abuse during childhood or adolescence, by rape or by domestic violence (see Chapter 9). Young adulthood is often the time when some women come to terms with their homosexuality (see page 164).

But often sexual ignorance leads to sexual dysfunction in younger women. "The most common sexual dysfunctions I encounter among younger women are vaginismus and anorgasmia. Many young women don't know what to expect from sex. Some have had poor sex education. Some have guilt about their sexuality, or are unable to communicate with their partners," noted the late Dr. Helen Singer Kaplan, former director of the Human Sexuality Program at New York Hospital–Cornell Medical Center.*

Some women may have satisfying sex lives until they become pregnant. Most studies show a decline in sexual interest as pregnancy progresses. While some studies suggest that hormonal shifts may be at fault, cultural and psychological factors are more likely to blame. There are still physicians who believe that sexual intercourse during pregnancy, especially the first trimester, isn't a good idea, and there are still men who are afraid to touch their wives for fear of "hurting" the baby. While a few women who have suffered repeated miscarriages might be advised to refrain from sex, for the majority of women sex during pregnancy is safe and pleasurable. In fact, during the second trimester increased blood flow to the genital area (and breasts) can greatly increase their sensitivity . . . even to the point of a feeling of heightened readiness for orgasm! There's no clinical evidence that sexual activity right up until the time of delivery is harmful, or that it triggers the onset of labor.

Most women can resume making love three to six weeks after delivery. But the round-the-clock care of an infant all too frequently hampers desire. And experts stress that couples need to *make* time for sex after becoming parents. If they neglect their sex lives, or if sex becomes hurried and routine, interest wanes.

◈ *Miranda's Story* ◈

"I know that many couples find in vitro fertilization messes up their sex lives . . . you have to keep track of your cycles, when you're ovulating and . . . when you have to 'do it.' That's fine if it's only for six months . . . but if this is going on for years, it can really interfere with your sex life . . . and we had a good one.

"When we decided to try intrauterine insemination, my husband found it very hard to produce sperm on demand. It was terribly difficult for him to go into an empty room . . . and [ejaculate] into a test tube. He just couldn't do it . . . so we ended up essentially making love at home, and then I would take his sperm in a container and stick it under my armpit and take a cab up to the clinic. We had to be there within an hour. And they would

---

*Dr. Kaplan was interviewed for this book shortly before her death in 1995.

do the insemination. . . . In many ways, I liked it better than IVF, which I found very intrusive . . . because they had to retrieve the eggs and put the embryos into the uterus. . . .

"But overall, for me, the mechanics of IVF were a positive. . . . It divorced the issue of making a baby from making love. And it made our sex life normal again. It made it much easier for me, psychologically."

The emotional stress of infertility, as well as the intrusiveness of using assisted reproductive technology, can take a toll on sexuality. "There's a loss of privacy and control, people are looking at the most intimate part of your life. Sexual problems are very common. Sex ceases to be spontaneous and pleasurable; it becomes something that is done by the calendar," says Gail Erlick Robinson, M.D., professor of psychiatry and obstetrics and gynecology at the University of Toronto, and chair of the American Psychiatric Association's Committee on Women. "The husband may get a call at work, that this is the day, come home right now. And nothing is more guaranteed to make a man impotent than to be told he *has* to perform."

Some women who have had their ovaries removed find they lose interest in sex and have difficulty achieving orgasm; and lack of hormones causes vaginal dryness. Other women who have had their uterus removed report less intense orgasms. Experts say they may be among those who experienced orgasms not only from clitoral stimulation but also from the pressure on the cervix and the movements of the uterus. Chemotherapy can also result in premature menopause and reduced sexual desire.

The pressures of two people working and handling home and family responsibilities can lead to low sexual desire, a common problem among today's dual-career couples. "It's unrealistic to think that you can have sex after working twelve, fourteen hours a day. Sex happens when the body is rested. Couples who have this problem don't necessarily have a sexual disorder; they may just have unrealistic expectations. They think sex should just happen, and they become worried when it doesn't," Dr. Kaplan observed.

After menopause, a woman's problems with sex are related not only to estrogen insufficiency but to her partner's not taking the related physical changes into account. Vaginal tissue shrinks, thins and dries, leading to painful sex and, consequently, loss of desire. The physical problems can be avoided by hormone replacement and/or use of lubricants.

However, many women find themselves sexually revitalized at midlife, while men find their sexual responsiveness somewhat slowed. Testosterone production gradually declines in men, perhaps by 25 percent by age sixty, but it's not clear whether this affects libido. More important, changes in blood flow and muscle tone can make a man's erections take longer to achieve, they may not be as firm as he ages, and the "refractory" period between periods of arousal also lengthens. Cardiovascular disease, smoking and diabetes also cause circulatory problems with erections; depression as well can lead to sexual dysfunction.

"All of this can make a man anxious and concerned about his virility, which can be accentuated by the changes in his partner that accompany menopause, such as the diminished lubrication and slower arousability," remarks Dr. Malkah Notman, clinical professor of psychiatry at Cambridge Hospital and Harvard Medical School. "A man's emotional and sexual withdrawal can certainly affect the woman's feelings of sexual vitality and self-esteem."

Some men blame their spouse, and seek out other partners or have an affair with a younger woman. The idea that a younger woman can rejuvenate a man is fairly widespread in our culture, observes Dr. Notman, but the woman is likely to blame *herself*. "That can make a woman feel as if she has diminished capability sexually, and the rejection and marital split take a toll on her self-esteem."

๑ Pat's Story ๑

"When my husband was alive, I would say we had a very satisfactory sex life. We were both very young when we married. He was the only man I've ever been with, so I don't have anything to compare it to, but that part of our lives got better over the years. . . . It wasn't something we talked about much.

"It's hard for me to imagine being with another man at this stage in my life. . . . My husband has been gone ten years, and I am now seventy-one. So I feel that part of my life is over. I have other friends who have lost their husbands, but they are much younger and they might remarry. I don't think I would, but who knows?"

According to Robert N. Butler, M.D., a noted expert on aging and director of the International Longevity Center at Mount Sinai Medical Center in New York, the age-related decrease in vaginal lubrication during arousal does not seem to occur in women who are able to maintain regular sexual stimulation once or twice a week from youth onward. This may mean masturbation, which some older women may not be comfortable with.

"In later life, men often get trapped in performance anxiety. Women, on the other hand, are trapped in what might be called 'appearance anxiety,' " Dr. Butler told a 1994 conference sponsored by the American Federation for Aging Research (AFAR). "Our culture promotes the image of a sexy woman as a young woman, so as women age they may become trapped by the notion that older women are not sexual. But that is simply not true."

There is, however, a wide range of sexuality in people as they age, and personal health and the availability of a healthy partner are key factors. Around 80 percent of Americans aged sixty-five and older have at least one chronic disease that can potentially affect their sexual functioning. (In diabetes, for example, 50 percent of people will have sexual dysfunction due to the disease's effects on blood vessels and peripheral nerves.) Medications commonly taken to treat chronic diseases, such as high blood pressure drugs, digitalis and diuretics, can also interfere with sexual functioning (see page 165).

An older woman's sex life can also be disrupted by the illness of a partner, who may require special care, or the death of a partner. One survey found that after age sixty-five, only about a third of unmarried women are in an ongoing sexual relationship.

Divorced or widowed women (and men) also may have to confront their children's reactions to their dating again. "Some of it relates to shock that there was such as thing as parent sexuality," says Dr. Butler. "There's also loyalty to the deceased parent. There may be an unrealistic enshrinement of a former mate that interferes with sexual function."

But overall, older age does *not* have to shut the door on sexuality. Masters and Johnson have found that 30 percent of 70-year-olds continue to have sexual relations (not necessarily intercourse) once a week; 60 to 70 percent make love at least once a month. A recent study of healthy, upper-middle-class people aged 80–102 living in a residential retirement facility indicated that the most common activities were touching and caressing without sexual intercourse (a majority of the men and women still fantasized about sex).

There are special qualities of sex and intimacy that emotionally healthy people seem to discover in their later years, what Dr. Butler calls "the second language of sex. That is, a more respectful, mutual intimate concern with a partner and their needs, as opposed to only being concerned with our own selfish needs, as we sometimes were in our youth."

In fact, age-related changes can be a plus. For one thing, because men now need more time to achieve orgasm, that gender gap in timing of arousal and climax becomes much narrower. Experts say slowing the pace of love-making, experimenting and restoring a sense of play can help women and their partners enjoy an ever better sex life in later life. "We know that in general, the principle holds: 'use it or lose it,'" concludes Dr. Butler.

⤴ *Judy's Story* ⤵

"When I met girls in school for the first time, I knew that I was attracted to them. Nothing seemed wrong with it. I don't think I put it in a sexual context; who could at that age? I just knew that when I was around girls, I couldn't talk, I would blush. All the awkward stuff that teenage boys go through when they fall for girls, I was feeling in first and second grade. . . .

"I didn't realize what was 'wrong' until I was in high school, and everybody started dating the opposite sex. . . . I dated guys and I enjoyed it . . . but when the pretty, blond, cheerleader types came near me, I would start to melt. With boys, even sexually, I always felt totally cool, in total control. . . . I was very promiscuous for a while. . . . I enjoyed the feeling of power I had over the guys . . . but I was never comfortable with girls, especially the ones I was attracted to. . . .

"As for telling anyone else about myself, I didn't have the words to even tell myself. . . . Sexually, I felt like a normal teenager at the time. . . . That changed once I went out into the real world. Going to college . . . meeting other gay women . . . I would have 'come out' if people came out in those days. But remember, this was the early 1960s. I didn't even know there was a 'gay lifestyle' I could have. . . .

"My parents found out when they read some love letters of mine. . . . First there was screaming . . . they said things like 'Why did you do this to us?' . . . It was pretty terrible. After that, they never wanted to talk about it again. . . . That was sad. And it made me angry. Because once they denied what was one of the most important parts of my life, I felt that my parents, from that moment on, lost their daughter. . . .

"Sexually, I think gay women are much more knowledgeable about their bodies and sexual responses . . . because we're not out to please men, we're out to please ourselves. . . . I don't know a gay woman who has ever faked an orgasm. . . .

"I am very comfortable with being gay, and saying that I am a lesbian. . . . But it is really a very small part of who I am. My identity in terms of my profession is much more central to me, and always has been . . . I'm not political. I don't see my sexuality as a cause. . . . I do get pissed off at some homophobic women . . . who, as soon as they found out I was gay, were afraid to be my friend. . . . That's their own sexual insecurity. I've wanted to grab them by the shoulders and shake them and say, 'Just because I'm gay doesn't mean I want you. Get over the ego trip.' . . . I hate it when people automatically judge you, assume things and treat you differently. That's just fear and stupidity."

LESBIAN SEXUALITY

It's estimated that between 4 and 10 percent of individuals in the United States are, or will become, predominantly or exclusively homosexual. One sexual survey of nearly six thousand women found that 2 to 3 percent identified themselves as exclusively lesbian, and 13 percent said they have had lesbian sexual experiences. Lesbians come from all age groups, cultural backgrounds, religions and nationalities, and work in every occupation. But not every woman comes to terms with her sexual orientation as easily as Judy did.

"Behavior doesn't equal identity. Women who are in sexual relationships with women may or may not call themselves lesbian," emphasizes Marla Jean Gold, M.D., an assistant professor of medicine at the Medical College of Pennsylvania and a member of the advisory board of the Lesbian Health Fund. "Lesbian is more than just a sexual orientation; it has to do with psychological and emotional responses. While it's not a choice in *orientation*, it is a choice in *identity*."

No one really understands how sexual orientation develops. Many women and men simply seem to be born with an innate sexual preference for members of their own sex. Researchers have been trying to find the genetic components of homosexuality for some time; some have been looking for physical differences in the brain. Whatever the source, homosexuality (or bisexuality) can emerge during adolescence or later in life. The 1994 University of Chicago survey found that a majority of lesbian women began same-gender sexual activity after age eighteen.

Lesbian women experience the same physiological responses to sexual arousal and orgasm as heterosexual women, but concentrate more on caressing, on specific erogenous zones, and clitoral stimulation. Some may have more partners, but in monogamous relationships their sex lives are not that different from heterosexuals.

But it's not really important what goes on behind closed doors. What *is* important to understand is that gay women want in a relationship the same things heterosexual couples want: love, commitment, mutual respect, caring, and someone to share life experiences. Most gay women are in monogamous relationships. And many want society to acknowledge them in the same way as heterosexual couples (conferring the same rights and benefits, including sharing medical coverage).

Between one and five million lesbians have chosen to become parents, some by artificial insemination or, less frequently, by adoption. An estimated 6 to 14 million American children have one or more lesbian or gay parents. Recent studies comparing groups of children raised by homosexual and heterosexual parents find *no* differences in psychological or social adjustment and development of sexual or gender role identity, nor do they find that children raised by gay parents grow up to be homosexual themselves. One study found that children of gay and lesbian parents are *less* likely to be victims of sexual or physical abuse, says Dr. Gold. Unfortunately, some women who came to terms with their homosexuality later in life have had to fight bitter legal battles over child custody because of society's ignorance.

Indeed, the major problems faced by lesbians are prejudice and discrimination. Many women continue to stay "in the closet" for fear of jeopardizing jobs, alienating families or losing their children in a divorce.

Experts stress that homosexuality is *not* a mental disorder; nor is sexual orientation alone associated with emotional or social problems. (So-called conversion therapies, attempting to change sexual orientation, do *not* work.) A 1993 report in the *Journal of General Internal Medicine* notes that "psychological illness is no more common in lesbians than in heterosexual women, but lesbians have unique psychosocial issues and often limited support to help them cope." The researchers at the Good Samaritan Hospital and Medical Center in Portland, Oregon, observed in the report that "the quality of the relationship with a partner can be particularly important to a lesbian's psychological well-being. Discord in a lesbian couple can be even more stressful than it is for a married heterosexual couple because of lack of social support."

Some women, especially adolescents and older women, may have a rougher time emotionally than others coming to terms with their sexual orientation, fearing rejection by family, friends and coworkers. The National Lesbian Health Survey found that almost 20 percent of women had not told their families of their sexual orientation; almost a third kept their orientation a secret from coworkers. But a position paper from the American Psychological Association stresses that for many homosexuals the process of "coming out" is important to their mental health: "The more positive the gay male or lesbian identity, the better one's mental health and the higher one's self-esteem."

SEXUAL DYSFUNCTIONS IN WOMEN

Sexual dysfunction doesn't happen suddenly or all by itself. "Sexual difficulties can result from psychological conflict or interpersonal problems, and may reflect relationship difficulties, environmental stresses, chronic anxiety or depression, be caused by medical illness or medications . . . and even a lack of sexual knowledge," says Dr. Sadock.

Sexual dysfunction can affect desire for sex, sexual excitement and the physiological changes that occur when we're aroused, and the ability to have an orgasm. Sexual dysfunctions can be lifelong or acquired, and can be due (or not due) to specific situations or partners. They can be caused purely by psychological factors, or by a combination of things. They can affect adults at any age, of any sexual orientation.

There is no way to tell whether a woman has lost her desire due to low hormones or because of depression. So a person experiencing sexual difficulties should have a complete medical and physical evaluation. For a psychiatric diagnosis of sexual dysfunction, the problem must be persistent, recurrent and cause mental distress and interpersonal problems.

Types of sexual dysfunction listed in the DMS-IV include the following.

HYPOACTIVE SEXUAL DESIRE DISORDER: Is characterized by the absence (or deficiency) of sexual fantasies and desire for sex. It can affect all forms of sexual expression, or may be limited to one sexual activity. A person with low sexual desire usually will not initiate lovemaking, and may only take part reluctantly, when it is initiated by a partner.

SEXUAL AVERSION DISORDER: Is an aversion to sex and an active avoidance of any sexual contact with a partner. People with this disorder may feel disgust, anxiety or fear when faced with making love; some may even react with symptoms of panic attacks. People may go to great lengths to avoid sex, from staying late at work to refusing to bathe.

FEMALE SEXUAL AROUSAL DISORDER: Occurs when a woman is unable to become excited and cannot maintain the physical responses, such as vaginal lubrication. The disorder should not be entirely due to menopause (such as vaginal dryness and atrophy), medical conditions or the effects of medications. Occasional problems of arousal do not fit this category, nor does inadequate sexual stimulation by a partner.

FEMALE ORGASMIC DISORDER: Involves recurrent delays in achieving orgasm or the absence of orgasm following a normal sexual excitement phase, in which all the physical signs of arousal are present. It's estimated that 10 to 15 percent of women may never have experienced an orgasm. Most female orgasmic disorders are lifelong, rather than acquired (the problem may be more common in younger women).

VAGINISMUS: Is a recurrent, *involuntary* spasm of the muscles surrounding the vagina, resulting in a constriction of the outer part of the vagina, which prevents penetration (by a penis, by a finger or even by the insertion of a tampon or gynecologist's speculum). The muscle spasm can be mild or quite severe; it can occur in response to pain, or it can be psychological.

DYSPAREUNIA (SEXUAL PAIN DISORDER): Results in genital pain associated with intercourse, usually during penile thrusting. Symptoms can range from mild discomfort to sharp pain. Thirty percent of women suffering from pain during intercourse have physical problems, including lack of vaginal lubrication due to menopause, or vaginal or urinary tract infections, endometriosis and pelvic inflammatory disease. But dyspareunia is not exclusively related to those conditions.

Medications That Can Cause Sexual Problems

Medications used to treat high blood pressure, angina, cardiac arrhythmias, ulcers and irritable bowel syndrome may all cause sexual dysfunction. Antihistamines that dry out the mucous membranes of the nose also dry the membranes of the vagina, and inhibit sexual function, notes Dr. Sadock.

Among psychotropic drugs: *Selective serotonin reuptake inhibitors* (SSRIs) (see chart on page 43) can reduce sexual desire and functioning in women (and in men). *Monoamine oxidase inhibitors* (*MAOIs*) can cause vaginal dryness. *Tricyclic antidepressants* do not appear to cause sexual dysfunction in women. However, since depression is also associated with sexual dysfunction, reduced desire and other symptoms may be related to the disease and improve as a result of medication, says Dr. Sadock.

Antianxiety drugs can actually improve sexual function since many women may find themselves inhibited by anxiety. Barbiturates (which act as sedative-hypnotics) can enhance sexual responsiveness in people suffering from anxiety. Antipsychotic medications can inhibit vaginal lubrication.

WHEN YOU NEED HELP IN THE BEDROOM

Let's face it: None of us has a sex life that matches the movies. Studies show that almost half of all couples experience some waning of desire and sexual interest over the years.

We all have to adjust to the disappearance of the first euphoria of falling in love and the intense sexual desire of early intimacy, says Dr. Sadock. But we *don't* have to lose emotional intimacy. "In order to maintain a healthy sex life, partners must maintain a sense of intimacy by talking and sharing. If we close down emotionally, we can't make love."

Occasional sexual failure, lack of desire or even an unsatisfactory sexual experience is not uncommon. Today's busy lives often result in fatigue, which is not conducive to passion. However, when a problem continues for weeks or months, impacting on the relationship, professional help may be needed.

The process usually begins with a detailed history of a person's current sex life, as well as a medical evaluation to uncover any physical problems. If no medical problem is found, a referral may be given to a sex therapist.

Because many women see their gynecologist on a regular basis, they will often be the first person consulted about sexual difficulties. Most men do not visit a physician regularly, and when they do, they are often reluctant to discuss impotence. Men who do consult a urologist about sexual problems all too often will come in alone, so the information a man is given may never get to their partner, notes Andrew McCullough, M.D., an assistant professor of urology and director of the Male Sexual Health Program at NYU Medical Center. In addition, a recent study found that men with "nonorganic" impotence may often be reacting to a partner's sexual problem, such as pain during intercourse.

"Whenever possible, I like to see the couple as well as the individual. Whether the problem is purely physical or psychological, the couple invariably develop increasing fear and self-consciousness about their sexual performance. Sexual problems are frequently the pressure valve of other problem areas of the relationship," says Dr. McCullough.

For this same reason, couples usually undergo sex therapy together. "The relationship as a whole is treated, but the emphasis is on sexual functioning as a part of that relationship," adds Dr. Sadock.

Sex therapy does not involve making love (or engaging in any sexual activity) in front of the therapist. Couples are usually seen once a week and are given special exercises to do at home (depending on the nature of the problem), including masturbation. "The overall goal of sex therapy is to educate people about the physical and psychological aspects of sexual functioning, to diminish fears about performance. And to establish or reestablish communication verbally, as well as in sexual terms," emphasizes Dr. Sadock.

The initial focus of therapy is not on intercourse, but on getting partners to focus on each other sensually (called *sensate focusing*), by touching and caressing, openly talking about desires and sexual fantasies. Through a gradual process of learning how to communicate and to understand each other's needs, partners progress through sensual exercises to the point where they can have intercourse.

Older couples can also benefit from sex therapy, adds Mount Sinai's Dr. Butler. However, while self-stimulation can help preserve potency in men and sexual lubrication and functioning in women, many older people were brought up to believe masturbation is physically and mentally harmful. And while that barrier may need to be overcome, there's no reason for any older person to live out the rest of the life span with sexual dysfunction.

Some therapists' strategies for maintaining a healthy sex life at any age include the following.

- Talk to each other. Express your feelings and needs. While it's not always possible to put sensitive topics into words, try.

- Renew intimacy. Sex doesn't just happen in the bedroom. Intimacy is an ongoing process, involving sharing and expressing affection. Don't forget the Valentine cards, the little notes and gifts that say, "I love you."

- Learn to enjoy kissing and touching again. Remember how much fun necking was when you were courting? The less focused you are on intercourse, the more you can explore another's needs in bed.

- If you'd like some changes in the way your partner makes love, start out by making positive statements like "I love it when you do this, but I'd also enjoy . . ."

- If your partner expresses a need that's different from your own, don't dismiss it as selfish or abnormal. If something makes you uncomfortable, speak up. But be open to new things.

- If your partner has lost interest in sex, don't blame yourself or get angry about it. Voice your love and concern in a tender way, and try to find out what may be wrong.

- If sex hurts for any reason, say so.

Each one of us has uniquely individual emotional and sexual needs. In a fulfilling sexual relationship, both partners need to be aware of, and accommodate, those needs, stresses Dr. Sadock. Remember, there is no "right way" to have an orgasm, or "normal" way to make love. What feels right for both of you *is* right.

CHAPTER 9

Violence and Victimization

The scope of abuse of women is broad, encompassing childhood sexual abuse, domestic violence, date rape and sexual harassment. The roots of violence against women are many, from cultural and social emphasis on male dominance to alcohol and drug abuse. Acts of violence cut across every social, racial, economic and age group. The psychic aftershocks recur throughout a woman's life.

The link between violence against women and mental illness is just now beginning to be studied and understood. Experts now realize that women with a history of abuse are vulnerable to depression and anxiety, and often suffer from posttraumatic stress, as well as substance abuse and eating disorders.

The statistics are horrifying.

- Every fifteen seconds a woman is beaten in North America; every six minutes a woman is raped.

- More than one million women annually seek treatment for injuries inflicted by husbands, ex-husbands or boyfriends.

- Fifty-two percent of all women murdered each year are killed by spouses or intimate acquaintances.

- Homicide is the most common cause of death among African-American women.

- Twenty to 30 percent of women will be physically assaulted by a partner or ex-partner during their lifetime.

- Perhaps one fourth of American women (some 21.7 million women) may have been victims of rape or attempted rape. More than half of rape victims are girls under age eighteen.

- Almost three million cases of child abuse or neglect are reported each year; one in five girls have been victims of childhood sexual abuse.

- Between 4 and 10 percent of older Americans may be victims of "elder abuse," by a family member, usually one of their own children, or by health care attendants.

The sheer number of violent acts against women qualifies it as an epidemic, Dr. Susan Blumenthal, deputy U.S. assistant secretary for women's health told a 1994 federal conference on Women, Abuse and Mental Health. "For all too many years, abuse has taken a tremendous physical, emotional and economic toll on our nation's women and children. And for all too many years, the scope, even the existence of the problem, has been concealed or denied," Dr. Blumenthal says. "The emotional consequences of abuse sometimes arise years later. They cost countless women their jobs, their families, their mental and physical health. And tragically, all too often, their lives."

Until recently, victims of such violence were sometimes revictimized by the legal system, which did not view domestic violence or marital rape as crimes and allowed the sexual history of rape victims to be used against them in the courtroom, effectively putting the *victim* on trial. And some survivors tell of having their trauma bizarrely reenacted by forced medication or restraints while in the mental health system.

IN THE CONTEXT OF CULTURE

Violence against women is deeply rooted in many cultures. "Violence is an extreme variation of what is occurring between men and women in society. Despite the successes of the women's movement, the balance of power favors men," remarks Mary Zachary, M.D., director of the Women's Emergency Care Program at NYU-Bellevue Hospital Center. "The media, movies and television constantly show us violence as a means of conflict resolution.

"We still tend to view the family as a private sphere. Beating a woman in the home has been traditionally regarded as a private matter, not a public concern," she says. "Families which use alcohol or drugs as a way of handling problems also incorporate violence as a way of handling problems."

Culture can foster violence against women. "The traditional *machismo* ethic among some Latino groups, for example, dictates that men have to be in control of the home. . . . The extension of that is violence to express that dominance," she observes. "At the same time, it can also shield a woman from violence, if the man's role is seen as protective."

Economic conditions also contribute to abuse. "For example, the history of African Americans is that in the past women have been more able to find . . . jobs and black men have had more of a struggle. So the balance of power in black homes is somewhat different. A man may act out his impotence and rage, and a black woman may find herself a target," adds Dr. Zachary.

Some white women, especially those in high-profile jobs or higher-income groups, may feel less able to ask for help. Women from Asian cultures may feel that revealing abuse—even by a stranger—will shame their family. Immigrant women may have less information about their legal rights and access to medical care, and fear exposure and deportation. One study found that over half of lesbians may be victims of abuse either by a partner or as the result of antigay violence.

⨎ *Gina's Story* ⨍

"I was raised to be a subservient type of woman. . . . Inside there was a more aggressive person, but that was suppressed by my parents. . . . My father was the sole breadwinner, and my mother's job in life was to shop and serve my father. . . . I met my future husband when we were sixteen years old . . . He had a strong and dominant personality . . . like my father, whom I greatly admired and loved. He was also extremely charming. . . .

"Two incidents stand out in my mind . . . I was nominated for homecoming queen, but he made me decline because he was afraid other boys would look at me. . . . I also remember being in his home on several occasions when he was extremely physical with his younger brother. He would pound his brother's head into the tile in the bathroom. . . . I had never seen anything like that before.

"As our own relationship grew, he became mentally abusive toward me, although I didn't really understand it then. He made all the decisions, he made it understood that he knew more of life. . . . I thought, 'He's going to take care of me.'

"As soon as our child was born, the mental abuse became worse. He told me that I was stupid, worthless and fat. . . . I truly started to believe it. . . . It seemed like the more domesticated I became, the more he disliked me.

"After our second child was born, he started hitting me. . . . And I would keep saying, 'I'm sorry. I'm sorry.' . . . The beatings went from bruised ribs to split lips to black eyes. One of the last times he beat me, he woke up my eldest daughter, and said, 'Let me show you how I hit Mommy.' He then took my head and pounded it into the ceramic tile in the bathroom, just like he had done with his brother years before. . . .

"After some of the beatings, I would call shelters. But because I had no money of my own to pay for them, they could offer me absolutely no help. . . . Although my husband earned a good living, he said he could not give me any more than a dollar a day . . . to spend on food and essentials and clothes. My parents bought most of the children's clothes, and I would take food from them. . . . My husband would go out for dinner every night. His reason was that he was working and he had to relax.

"It wasn't until he went to hit my youngest daughter that something in me snapped. . . . I remember scooping her into my arms and telling him that I couldn't go on like this. Our marriage ended the next morning. . . . We moved in with my parents. . . . One night, I remember, I went out on the balcony (of my parents' home) and just kept staring down at the ocean and wondering what falling would feel like. . . . My mother came out, and she asked me what I was doing. I told her. She said something I will never forget. That I was not alone in this world, that I had two children to think of and that no one could replace their mother's love. . . . That saved my life. . . .

"I met and married a wonderful man, who supported my efforts to educate myself and to start my own business. I know I am lucky to be able to tell my story. Many of the women who have been in my situation are not alive to tell just how horrible their own lives were."

DOMESTIC VIOLENCE

Partner abuse can be physical, involving pushing, hitting, sexual assault and rape, burns, broken bones, knife or gunshot wounds and even murder. Or it can be psychological, with threats and isolation used as a weapon instead of fists.

Between 1.8 and 4 million women are victims of domestic violence each year. U.S. Justice Department statistics show that 95 percent of assaults against partners are committed by men against women, although in one study of lesbians, 37 percent of respondents said they had been or were currently involved in an abusive relationship (either as the victim or the perpetrator).

Instances of wife abuse have been on record in the United States since the 1830s. A husband's right to hit his wife was actually sanctioned by U.S. law until 1874—citing the English common law "rule of thumb," that a man could physically chastise his wife (and children) so long as the instrument he used was no thicker than his thumb. It took one hundred years for battering to be labeled a crime by the legal system, and to be regarded as a problem by the public.

Perhaps the most widely publicized case of domestic violence was that involving former football star O. J. Simpson, who in 1995 was acquitted of criminal charges in the murders of his former wife, Nicole Brown Simpson, and a male friend, Ron Goldman. While many were surprised that the mostly female, African-American and Hispanic jurors appeared to discount Simpson's history of battering, some experts in the field pointed out that domestic violence is often seen through the prism of race for many women of color, who may be willing to overlook violence on the part of their men, whom they feel have been victims of a racist society.

Still, as a result of the Simpson case, calls to battered-women's shelters increased by 25 percent, and police are taking domestic violence calls more seriously. But a lingering problem persists. Even when they do call police, many women often refuse to press charges, or to testify against their partner. A 1993 study found that reports were filed in less than a third of the annual 200,000 domestic violence calls to police; arrests were made in only 7 percent of those cases.

Those women who do report battering may risk escalating the violence, often at the risk of their lives. One study found that 85 percent of spousal assault and homicides occurred after at least one previous intervention by police.

Many terrified women stay in abusive relationships because they have nowhere to go, have little money and fear for their children. Women who do leave have found that court orders of protection (legally barring any contact) often afford little real protection from a violent partner; many women murdered by partners were under orders of protection.

Over half of all men who batter their wives also beat their children; perhaps a third of battered women beat their children. And experts say that men who have witnessed or experienced family violence as a child are more likely to abuse a partner as adults.

Understanding the Cycle of Abuse

There's no typical profile of a battered woman, but there are some shared characteristics among batterers: Many are between eighteen and thirty years of age, in blue-collar occupations or unemployed, use illicit drugs, have a different religious background from their partner, saw their own father hit their mother and may use violence against their children. Pregnancy is considered a high-risk period; some surveys find as many as 15 to 25 percent of pregnant women may be abused. Women with disabilities are also at greater risk.

A man who abuses his partner may be filled with anger, suspicion and tension. He may be insecure, with low self-esteem (especially if he is unemployed). One 1994 study from the University of California at Berkeley found that people who had been laid off within the past year were six times more likely to show violent behavior than those who were employed.

As Gina's story shows, a batterer may suffer from pathological jealousy and a need to control his partner, or, less commonly, abuse may occur in the context of antisocial personality disorder. Both partners may have a family history of domestic violence, physical or sexual abuse. "It also happens in a progression, so the first time it's a shove. So he says, 'Oh my God, how could I do this, I'm so sorry. I'll never do this again.' And she, like many women, wants to protect the relationship, and she forgives him. And then it increases," says Dr. Gail Erlick Robinson of the University of Toronto, chair of the American Psychiatric Association's Committee on Women.

Recent studies suggest there are two types of batterers. "Type One" is a man for whom intimate violence is a deliberate act, part of a larger pattern of violence toward family, friends or coworkers. During a fight their heart rate doesn't even rise. They react with calm, cold fury, and tend to be insulting and threatening toward their partner. "Type Two" are those men for whom violence is an infrequent, impulsive act, associated with a loss of control, increased heart rate and anger. These men are jealous, dependent on their wives and fear rejection, leading to intense arguments. Only a small percentage are violent outside the relationship; many are separated or divorced.

Experts say that therapy can help Type Twos learn how to control their anger. If batterers are jailed and such therapy is mandated, its chances of being effective are greater. Type One men may be difficult, if not impossible, to help.

"Marital therapy may be very dangerous for a couple in which active violence is taking place," Dr. Robinson remarked to the 1995 Annual Meeting of the American Psychiatric Association. "Because often what will happen is that a woman may venture to speak up in therapy about something he has done. And then he'll go home and beat the tar out of her for doing that."

"In addition to the social stigma, a battered woman has real physical fear. Men who abuse their partners will threaten them, saying, 'If you tell anybody, I'll get you. If you try to leave me, I will come after you and kill you,' " adds Dr. Virginia Sadock, director of the program in Human Sexuality and Sex Therapy at NYU Medical Center.

Dr. Sadock says there are many similarities between a battered woman and a hostage. "She's in an intimidating situation; there is generally the constant threat of physical abuse if she doesn't obey whatever rules there are (and the 'rules' can change from moment to moment). In addition, there's physical isolation so brainwashing can occur," she explains. "The battered wife is frequently prevented from working, to keep her from having her own economic resources and developing independence. She's discouraged from having friends, for fear she will reveal her secret, and gain support to leave her partner."

On top of physical abuse, there is usually emotional abuse. "The woman has been told she is stupid, that she can't do anything right . . . that she brings the abuse on, and until very recently that message has been reinforced totally by the culture, which tolerates violence and male aggression," says Dr. Sadock.

Moreover, until recently, police have refrained from getting involved in domestic disputes and the clergy may discourage divorce. "For years, women have gone to their ministers and they have said if you were a good Christian, or Jewish (or whatever) woman, you would go home and look after him. You're the only one who can save him. You can make it better if you only hang in there and be strong," comments Dr. Robinson. "Women in some racial and ethnic groups may also find it more difficult to come forward; they may fear authority figures more than their husbands. In some groups, it may be regarded as a particularly terrible betrayal of the husband. So we have a whole group of factors that keeps women tied to abusive relationships."

Many battered women deny the danger they are in, or believe they can control or end the violence. Many live for the calm that follows the storm. In a typical battering cycle, there is a period of increasing tension, then an explosion of violence, then a period where the batterer feels guilty, and acts loving and contrite. The good sex and attention a woman receives during this conciliatory phase, as well as promises that the abuse will never happen again, keep her believing that her partner can change, says Dr. Sadock. Some women leave (or force their partner to leave), only to return to the relationship.

This storm cycle eventually wears down the woman emotionally. Like a hostage, she becomes preoccupied with survival and avoiding more abuse. She may become dependent, depressed and apathetic, feeling intense anxiety, loss of control, shame and self-blame. Lack of financial resources, available shelters and a husband's threats to take the children also hamper a woman's ability to leave a violent marriage.

Women in poor communities may be surrounded by other violence and crime, compounding their sense of helplessness and hopelessness. High-achieving, high-income women may be too ashamed to reveal the reality behind the social facade of their lives. All of this hampers a woman's ability to make decisions or take action to change her situation, says Dr. Sadock.

Some women snap after years of abuse, retaliating with violence of their own. According to the Bureau of Justice Statistics, about one third of women in prison for homicide have been convicted of killing an intimate partner.

Elderly women may be more helpless to stop abuse, which can range from battering to stealing money or possessions. Perpetrators are most often the spouse, a child or a caregiver.

Acknowledging Intimate Abuse

It's estimated that battering accounts for up to 35 percent of all emergency room visits by women, for 25 percent of women seeking emergency psychiatric help and for one quarter of female suicides. In 1992 the American Medical Association declared domestic violence a "major public health problem," and issued guidelines for physicians to identify and treat victims of abuse. The March of Dimes urges doctors to screen all pregnant women for abuse. Hospitals cannot receive accreditation and qualify for Medicaid and Medicare reimbursement without meeting federal standards for identifying and caring for victims of abuse.

The mental health profession is now recognizing and treating the problems of victims of domestic violence, which include posttraumatic stress disorder, major depression, anxiety and substance abuse. Special treatment and counseling programs are available to women, as well as their partners.

Law enforcement and the legal system are also changing, albeit slowly. Prior to the 1970s, batterers were seldom arrested and, when an arrest was made, the charge was usually a misdemeanor. At least sixteen states and many cities now have laws or policies requiring felony arrests for serious battering. Some twenty-seven states mandate an arrest if there is probable cause that abuse has occurred (even if the wife denies it).

Every state now allows victims to transfer cases between family and criminal courts, where penalties are stiffer. Courts are trying to bring cases of domestic violence before judges more quickly. About two thirds of big-city prosecutors follow "no drop" policies to pursue cases against batterers, even if victims demur. Laws are being proposed and passed in many states for mandatory jail sentences and long-term counseling for abusers.

Changing laws does not mean changing attitudes, however. Some police, prosecutors and judges still do not view partner violence as a serious issue, and mandatory arrest laws are not universally enforced. Until recently, in many courtrooms, testimony about prior abuse was not admissible in cases where a battered woman was charged with assaulting or murdering her abusive partner. Some attorneys are now using the controversial "battered-woman syndrome" as a defense, claiming a woman's actions were necessary to protect herself (and her children) from further harm. In 1990, Ohio Governor Richard F. Celeste granted clemency to twenty-five women convicted of crimes while they were abused, citing acceptance of the battered-woman syndrome by the state's supreme court and legislature.

The first emergency shelter for battered women in this country opened in St. Paul, Minnesota, in 1974. There are now over two thousand shelters, but still not enough temporary beds for all the women who need them, and few shelters accommodate children. Therefore, the trend in many places is now on forcing the man to leave the home, putting him into therapy and/or prison. But while forty-nine states and the District of Columbia have laws allowing judges to evict violent family members from the household, many fail to do so because of concerns over an accused's right to due process.

The federal Violence Against Women Act, which took effect in 1995, provides $1.6 billion over six years for state and local grants to fund local domestic violence agencies, shelters and a national family violence hot line. The law also mandates states to respect each others' court orders, increases federal penalties for repeat sex offenders, permits federal prosecution when batterers cross state lines, funds restitution programs for victims of sexual assault and even allows women to bring suit.

Breaking the Silence/Getting Help

Experts say the first step for battered women to escape the cycle of violence is to admit to herself that she is being abused and to reach out to people who can help as well as protect her. Call a women's shelter or someone who can help formulate an escape plan. Recognize the signs of impending danger, to avoid a violent incident before it happens. Warning signs include: a partner acquiring or threatening to use a weapon (particularly a gun); extending violent threats or acts to children, other family members or even household pets; forcing a woman to have sex; a decrease in remorse or guilt. Formulate an escape plan to use when you feel you are in danger:

- Pack a suitcase in advance and leave it at a friend or neighbor's house. Include extra cash, credit cards and extra clothing for yourself and your children. Pack a favorite toy for each child.

- Keep important papers in an easy-to-locate but safe place so you can take them with you on short notice. These include: birth certificates, social security cards or numbers, driver's license or photo ID, pay stubs, health insurance cards, medication, checkbook and extra checks, and deed or lease to your house or apartment.

- Hide an extra set of house and car keys outside your house in case you have to leave quickly.

- Know exactly where you will go, and how to get there at any time of day. Explain to the friend or family member whom you trust that you may show up without warning.

- If you are hurt, go to the emergency room, call your doctor and notify the police. Get copies of medical records; they will be needed if you file charges.

Battered women seeking help can call a toll-free national domestic violence hotline: 1-800-799-SAFE (7233). There are also local and state hotlines, referral services and support groups, such as the National Coalition Against Domestic Violence. (For information, see Appendix I.)

⤳ *Jill's Story* ⤶

"I met the man who was to become my rapist at an adult education course in French. . . . He was an executive, well dressed and very charming. We both were planning a vacation abroad . . . and we liked to practice together. . . . Before the night he raped me, he had never even touched me or tried to kiss me. . . .

"One night after having dinner at a French restaurant with some other people in the class . . . we went back to his place. We had a glass of wine; we talked about our failed marriages. He expressed a lot of bitterness and anger about his two ex-wives. . . . What happened next seemed to come out of the blue. He had gone to get his car keys to drive me home. . . . The next thing I know, he came over, grabbed my shoulders and said with absolute, total calm, "I'm going to rape you. . . ." His face looked totally different; his features were wild, like an animal's. His eyes were cold, vicious and brutal.

"I tried . . . to fight back. But he pinned me down and started hitting me. . . . He ripped at my clothing . . . and then he rammed inside me. . . . When he finished, he tried to strangle me, saying he hated all women, we were bitches and whores, and he hated me in particular because I thought I was so smart. . . . I must have passed out a couple of times. I didn't try to get away; the door was locked, he had security gates on the windows. . . . Finally, the next morning about ten o'clock, he opened the front door and pushed me out.

"I didn't go to the police. . . . I was convinced that I should have seen it coming. . . . I sat in the tub for hours; I couldn't wash enough to feel clean. . . . I finally called my sister, and told her what happened. She made me report the rape to police. Because I'd waited a week . . . there was no physical evidence except my bruises. It was really my word against his. Of course, he said I willingly had sex with him. . . . The police said there wasn't enough evidence. So nothing ever came of it.

"I never went back to the class, or attended night school again. I was just too afraid. I take a lot of cabs . . . I don't walk alone . . . I still have nightmares. I don't really date anymore. I can't bear to have a man touch me, hold my hand . . . I never told anyone else before. I'm going to therapy now. . . . My whole life has been changed. It's like I'm this different person. Nothing will ever be the same. Nothing."

SEXUAL ASSAULT AND RAPE

It's hard to come by precise figures on rape because, like Jill, many women are ashamed (or afraid) to report their assault. In 1995, the U.S. Justice Department *doubled* its estimates of rapes or attempted rapes that occur each year, to 310,000, saying that previous crime questionnaires failed to ask direct questions about such assaults. As many as 500,000 American women may be victims of sexual assaults. But some experts say even those numbers may be *underestimates*. According to the Law Enforcement Assistance Administration, for every rape that is *reported* to police, 3 to 10 go unreported (especially marital rape and date rape).

The National Crime Victims Survey reports that rape incidence is highest among single, divorced or widowed women, under twenty-four years of age, who have less than a high school education and family incomes below $25,000 a year. A 1994 FBI survey found that girls younger than eighteen are victims of 61 percent of rape cases reported to police; girls under age twelve are victims 16 percent of the time (usually raped by family members). Victimization rates for African-American and white women are about equal; rates are somewhat lower among Latina women. Little data is available on lesbian women. More than one million women have been victims of forcible sex by their husbands.

The FBI defines rape as "carnal knowledge of a female forcibly and against her consent." But state laws vary in what *acts* constitute rape, whether husbands can be charged with rape, and what constitutes "nonconsent" (verbal or physical resistance) or "force" (physical assault, verbal threats, psychological coercion, use of drugs or alcohol to impair judgment). If the woman knew her assailant (as is often the case), it often lessens the perception that rape even took place.

Persistent cultural myths about rape can influence reactions by a woman's family, friends and law enforcement officials—and even by the victim herself. "Myths include notions that women were raped because they 'asked for it' by dressing provocatively or by going out alone late at night, that women secretly enjoy it," says Dr. Mary Zachary.

Traditionally, a woman who has been raped is often seen (or fears being seen) as "damaged goods," by her family and the men in her life. She may feel "soiled" and shamed (especially women of Middle Eastern or Asian heritage, since those cultures view rape as a stain upon the woman's and the family's honor). "Some Middle Eastern countries still have the practice of murdering women if they've been raped," says Dr. Zachary.

Other persistent myths are that most rapes are of white women by black men. In most cases, the attacker and victim are of the *same* race. However, recent studies show that African-American women are more hesitant than white women to report rape, feeling they will be disregarded by the criminal justice system.

There is also a myth that rapes are random acts by disturbed individuals who are carried away by a sudden, uncontrollable urge. In fact, most rapes are planned in advance, by men known to the victim, men who appear normal and who are often involved in other, nonviolent sexual relationships. According to the National Women's Study, only 22 percent of rape victims were assaulted by a stranger, and half of all rapes occurred in the victim's home. Nine percent of victims were raped by a husband, or ex-husband; 11 percent by their fathers or stepfathers; 16 percent by other relatives; 10 percent by boyfriends or ex-boyfriends; 29 percent by friends or neighbors.

Most women who are raped suffer extreme fear and suspicion of men. They also fear retaliation if they press charges. "In many places, the average length of time a rapist serves in prison is about six months, sending them back on the street to do it again, or to take revenge," notes Dr. Zachary.

The Consequences of Rape

Rape is a violation that is *both* physical and psychological, with a lasting impact on women's mental and bodily health, stresses Mary P. Koss, Ph.D., professor of family and community medicine, psychology and psychiatry at the University of Arizona, and a noted expert on violence against women. "Women with a history of rape and other crimes . . . report more symptoms of illness than non-victimized women," Dr. Koss told a 1994 conference by the American Psychological Association on Psychosocial and Behavioral Factors in Women's Health.

Some 30 percent of rape victims report at least one major depressive episode. Within two weeks of being raped, 90 percent of women meet symptom criteria for posttraumatic stress disorder. Nearly one third have PTSD symptoms a year later; for some, the symptoms persist for years. The National Victim Center reports that rape victims with PTSD were thirteen times more likely to abuse alcohol and twenty-six times more likely to abuse drugs, than women who have never been raped.

Other persistent psychological symptoms include lingering fear and mistrust, guilt, diminished enjoyment of everyday activities, anxiety and phobias, sleep disturbances, poor concentration, intrusive thoughts of the rape, fatigue, poor self-esteem, hypervigilance, anger, eating disorders and an increased risk of suicide, says Dr. Koss.

"Somatic postrape complaints include chronic pain syndromes, including chronic pelvic pain and headaches, and gastrointestinal problems such as irritable bowel syndrome. Rape victims are also at high risk for sexually transmitted diseases, unwanted pregnancies and reproductive problems," adds Dr. Koss.

Rape also causes sexual and social dysfunction. As a woman may "distance" herself mentally during an attack to blunt the psychic impact of what is taking place, she may continue to distance herself from men afterward. She may be unwilling to be touched or unable to function sexually. The men in her life may distance themselves, or even abandon a woman, after an assault.

Rape treatment should begin with immediate crisis counseling, in which women are encouraged to talk about the assault, relive the trauma, confront their fears and feelings, understand the myths about rape and how they affect thinking, and develop coping skills that will enable them to resume their normal activities, says Dr. Koss and coauthors in *No Safe Haven: Male Violence Against Women at Home, at Work, and in the Community* (American Psychological Association, 1994). Other therapies may include desensitization for women who develop situational phobias after an assault.

Unfortunately, too few women seek mental health treatment, despite the wide availability of rape hot lines and crisis services. The victims' rights movement has educated the public and the criminal justice system about rape and its consequences. Many states have enacted laws redefining rape, eliminating the need for proof of resistance and corroborating evidence, and "shield laws" prohibiting the use in trials of a victim's past sexual history. Laws making marital rape a crime are on the books in many states. Specialized sex crimes units exist within most police departments and prosecutor's offices.

ꙮ Ann and Anna's Story ꙮ

"My daughter Anna . . . was forcibly restrained and sexually violated by an adult male at the age of about three. In her own words: 'He tied me up, put my hands over my head, blindfolded me with my little T-shirt, pulled my T-shirt over my head with nothing on below, opened my legs and was examining and putting things in me and all that. Ugh. It hurt me. I would cry and he wouldn't stop. . . . I remember after he did that, I was walking toward the door out of the room, and I was feeling like I was bad. And why not my other sisters, and why just me? And I had this feeling in me that I was bad, you know, a bad seed. And I was the only one in the world.'

"The trauma Anna experienced then was compounded by the silence that surrounded her. She tried to tell us, but we couldn't hear her. . . . We saw her as a difficult to handle child. Her screams and cries were frequently punished by spanking and sending her to her room. In my ignorance, I did not see or hear her truth. . . . When she withdrew within herself, we attributed it to her artistic temperament or her independent personality. No one saw and understood what she conveyed in her childhood drawings or paintings, though I am told today that they are classic examples of a child traumatized by sexual abuse. . . .

"She broke at the age of thirteen. . . . Her isolation continued throughout her entire nineteen years in the mental health system. And her treatment . . . in spite of the genuine caring and good intentions of professionals, was a continual and almost bizarre reenactment of the circumstances, events and pain of her childhood abuse . . . invading, altering and disabling her mind, body and emotions. She once said to me, 'I don't have a safe place inside of me.' . . . I do not believe this is an issue of blaming. But it is absolutely essential to see and to say out loud what is real, if we are ever to stop this cycle of abuse."

Ann Jennings, Ph.D., directs the statewide Trauma Initiative for the Maine Department of Mental Health and Mental Retardation. Her career in public mental health began as a result of her daughter's psychiatric problems. Anna Jennings was institutionalized for over seventeen years, as a result of childhood sexual assault that was never recognized or treated. An accomplished artist, Anna took her own life in 1994. The above remarks were adapted from Ann Jennings's presentation to Dare to Vision: Shaping the National Agenda for Women, Abuse and Mental Health Services in July 1994 and are reprinted with permission.

CHILDHOOD ABUSE

It's estimated that more than one out of every four women have experienced childhood physical or sexual abuse. Every year almost three million children become victims of abuse by parents or other adults (sometimes even by other children), says Margaret McHugh, M.D., director of the Child Protection Team at NYU-Bellevue Hospital and a noted expert on child abuse. Tragically, some two thousand children a year lose their lives due to abuse.

As with domestic violence, it took more than a century for the problem of child abuse to be addressed by the medical and legal community. "Children were traditionally regarded as the virtual property of their parents, or as cheap labor to be used in factories and sweatshops. The actions of parents toward their children were never questioned," says Dr. McHugh.

It took the "Mary Ellen" case of 1874 for child abuse to attract public attention. Mary Ellen was a nine-year-old New York City girl, battered and malnourished by her adoptive parents. The Society for the Prevention of Cruelty to Animals brought the case to court, arguing that a child was a member of the animal kingdom and had the same right to be protected from cruel treatment. Shortly afterward, the Society for the Prevention of Cruelty to Children was organized.

In 1974, one hundred years after the Mary Ellen case, Congress passed the Child Abuse and Treatment Act, which provided funds to states and made it mandatory for health care professionals, teachers and others who suspect that a child is being abused (whether they see injuries or not) to report it to local authorities. All fifty states adopted such mandatory reporting laws, and developed child protection services. In the 1980s, child abuse cases were moved from family court to criminal court, where abusers were prosecuted.

Major efforts now need to be directed, says Dr. McHugh, toward prevention, identifying families at risk (such as those with drug or alcohol dependence) and using home visits to monitor those families. Parenting classes, for example teaching young, inexperienced women ways of handling frustration when colicky babies start crying (a frequent scenario for abuse) can be an important means of prevention. However, such classes are often pushed aside when women are sent home within twenty-four hours after giving birth, warns the American College of Obstetricians and Gynecologists, losing key opportunities for educating new mothers.

The Psychological Scars

Child abuse can leave lifelong emotional and physical scars. Psychiatric consequences can include depression, anxiety, posttraumatic stress disorder, dissociation, borderline personality disorder, somatization, substance abuse and eating disorders, as well as self-mutilation and suicide.

A recent review of forty-five studies examining nearly three thousand sex-abuse victims found that slightly half suffered from posttraumatic stress disorder in the first twelve to eighteen months after their reported abuse. Overall, more than one fifth of childhood abuse survivors suffer long-term psychiatric problems.

One of the most controversial is so-called multiple personality disorder.

Some experts believe this disorder stems from a person creating other selves as a protective mechanism to deal with trauma. Other experts believe that people repress memories of abuse, only to have them resurface in adult life (see box below).

Brain imaging studies at Yale and the University of California at San Diego, presented at the 1995 annual meeting of the American Psychiatric Association, suggest that repeated childhood abuse may damage the hippocampus, an area of the brain that helps to organize memory, possibly predisposing people to develop symptoms of PTSD (as well as dissociation). Moreover, recent research at the National Institute of Mental Health found that girls who had been sexually abused had increased levels of stress-related chemicals called *catecholamines* in their urine. Abnormally high levels of such substances in the brain may kill neurons in areas crucial for thinking and memory.

The Physical Scars

Abuse survivors can suffer many lingering physical complaints, including chronic muscular tension and pain, chronic back pain, asthma, chronic stress leading to hypertension and gastrointestinal problems, such as irritable bowel syndrome and Crohn's disease, says Christine A. Courtois, Ph.D., a psychologist and clinical director of The Center: Posttraumatic and Dissociative Disorder Program in Washington, D.C.

Women can experience chronic pelvic pain, physical damage to the vagina and urethra (which can lead to chronic cystitis and bladder problems), sexually transmitted diseases, pelvic inflammatory disease, as well as reproductive problems and sexual disturbances, Dr. Courtois told the conference on Psychosocial and Behavioral Factors in Women's Health.

The Controversy over Recovered Memory

The subject of recovered memories of childhood abuse has made headlines, and become frequent fodder for television talk shows and TV movies, not to mention lawsuits. The scenario usually involves an individual whose long-buried memories of sexual abuse surface during psychotherapy. Lawsuits are filed against the alleged abuser, frequently a relative or friend, and families are often torn asunder by the accusations. As many as three hundred lawsuits have reportedly been filed. Some people are able to obtain corroborating evidence from family members or others. But, given the complex nature of memory, there's no way to determine the truth of a memory if there's nothing concrete to back it up.

A 1994 conference at Harvard Medical School suggested that "miscoding" of memories (sometimes due to organic brain disease) may play a role in false memories. For example, it was reported that patients with damage to the frontal lobes and nearby areas often recall bits of past experiences, but confuse the context of the memory, so they fill in the gaps to make sense of it. There's also a constant process of reshuffling and decay of memories in the brain, and the *context* of a memory decays the quickest. Studies also show that each time you encourage people to conjure up a mental image, the more real it becomes. (Ideas can also be planted in the mind under hypnosis.)

A statement by the American Psychiatric Association also notes that some individuals who have experienced traumatic events nevertheless include some false or inconsistent elements when they recall the event. So there *is* a potential for people to have false memories of abuse. However, the APA stressed that the possibility of false accusations should *not* discredit reports by people who have been victimized.

The issue continues to be hotly debated. But experts agree that people should be wary of *any* therapist who has built a practice on recovering "lost" memories. "Ethical therapists try to elicit true memories during psychoanalysis or psychotherapy by asking neutral questions, not leading questions," stresses Arthur Zitrin, M.D., professor of psychiatry at NYU School of Medicine and chairman of the Dean's Committee on Medical Ethics. "And they will most definitely not suggest that past events may have taken place that the patient does not remember."

SEXUAL HARASSMENT

Mental health experts now view sexual harassment on the job as a form of abuse against women, with many of the same psychological consequences. Long a hidden problem tolerated by women who reluctantly traded silence for a paycheck and career advancement, the issue of sexual harassment burst into public consciousness in 1991, during Senate confirmation hearings on the U.S. Supreme Court nomination of then-Judge Clarence Thomas.

At the hearings, University of Oklahoma law professor Anita F. Hill accused Thomas of making sexual advances, pressuring her for dates and trying to engage her in sexually explicit conversations during the time she worked for him while he was chairman of the Equal Employment Opportunity Commission (EEOC) in the early 1980s. Thomas denied the charges, Hill's credibility was questioned by the all-male Senate Judiciary Committee, and Thomas joined the high court.

Barely one year later, a group of active and retired Navy pilots were accused of sexually assaulting at least eighty-three women at its annual "Tailhook" convention by, among other things, forcing the women to run a gauntlet of drunken aviators. The Tailhook scandal led to the resignation of the secretary of the navy and the reassignment of an admiral who ignored the initial complaint. Four naval officers were reprimanded or fined, but none was court-martialed. Former Navy lieutenant and helicopter pilot Paula A. Coughlin, who brought the assaults to light, was reported to have suffered from PTSD after the incident. She was awarded $5.2 million in damages by a federal jury in her lawsuit against the hotel where the Tailhook convention was held.

Sexual harassment was made illegal in this country under Title VII of the Civil Rights Act of 1964, which prohibits discrimination in the workplace based on race, sex, religion or national origin. But there was no legal definition of sexual harassment until 1980, when the Equal Employment Opportunity Commission issued guidelines on sex discrimination.

The EEOC defines sexual harassment as unwelcome sexual advances, requests for sexual favors and verbal or physical conduct of a sexual nature, which the victim is expected to tolerate or submit to in exchange for promotions or job security; and conduct that substantially interferes with work performance or creates an "intimidating, hostile or offensive work environment" (as prohibited in Title VII). The EEOC has since supplemented those guidelines, saying that harassment can also include conduct designed to denigrate or intimidate, such as taunts, threats or displays of pornographic material.

The U.S. Supreme Court affirmed in 1986 that sexual harassment violated Title VII, ruling that harassment that was so pervasive as to create a hostile work environment was a form of sex discrimination. Late in 1993, the high court ruled that workers suing employers under Title VII do *not* have to prove that they suffered severe psychological injury as a result of sexual harassment, as some lower federal courts had required.

As a result of increased public awareness, sexual harassment complaints to the Equal Employment Opportunity Commission nearly doubled between 1991 and 1993, from 6,883 to about 12,000. Case settlements also doubled, topping $25 million in 1993.

Still, the law is one thing, workplace reality is another. And that reality is that the workplace continues to be mostly male dominated, with women holding lower-status jobs; and experts say that sexual harassment has less to do with lust than with maintaining that balance of power.

"But She Knew I Was Just Kidding Around"

A recent report in the *American Journal of Psychiatry* estimates that half of all women will be subjected to some form of sexual harassment at some point during their working lives, from suggestive comments to coerced sex. But surveys show that only 1 to 7 percent of women who report harassment on the job actually file a formal complaint or seek legal recourse. Many women never even report offensive conduct for fear they will not be believed, or that their careers with suffer.

Such was the case with Anita Hill. During the Thomas confirmation hearings, several members of the Senate Judiciary Committee cited the fact that Hill did not report the harassment at the time it occurred, did not quit her job and, in fact, later moved with Thomas to another agency, as evidence that her claims of sexual harassment were false. At the time, surveys showed that many Americans agreed with that assessment. But as more attention was focused on the issue, the tide of public opinion turned in Hill's favor. And research now shows that Professor Hill's conduct was typical of many victims of sexual harassment.

Like Hill, many professional women and students depend on male mentors for educational and training experiences, references and aid in career advancement. A confrontation over sexual behavior may mean the loss of years of study and hard work. Limited opportunities to transfer out of a job, or find a new one, force some women to choose continued interaction with a harasser or suffer economic, educational or career losses.

Young, single women occupying "pioneer" positions in traditionally male professions (like the military), and women in workplaces where a majority of the employees are male, are at highest risk for harassment. A number of recent surveys show that sexual harassment is a common experience for female veterans, with many losing promotions or given poor assignments after refusing a superior officer's demands for sexual favors.

Some people still regard sexual harassment as merely a "miscommuni-

cation" between the sexes, or normal (and therefore excusable) sexual ban-
tering. Social and cultural norms decree that women are supposed to "enjoy"
flirting with men. If a woman rejects a harasser's advances, she may be seen
as challenging his masculinity, accused of being "unnatural" (i.e., a lesbian),
or labeled as "oversensitive."

A woman whose harasser is a member of the same ethnic or racial group
may feel that speaking out would draw negative attention to the group as a
whole. A gay woman harassed by another gay woman may also fear exposure
and negative reactions to her sexual orientation.

Recent studies show that women view sexual harassment as a serious
problem in the workplace, and believe that perpetrators should be held responsible for their conduct. But those same studies reveal that men are more
likely to believe that the problem is exaggerated, to disbelieve claims of
harassment and to hold the woman responsible for the situation.

Psychological reactions to sexual harassment can include depression,
anxiety, mood swings, posttraumatic stress, anger, damage to self-image, a
sense of violation, shame, feelings of loss and loss of control. A woman with
a history of rape or childhood sexual abuse can suffer more serious and
potentially damaging psychological reactions, especially posttraumatic stress
disorder. However, it's estimated that only 12 percent of victims of sexual
harassment seek professional psychological help. Common physical complaints caused by harassment include stress, poor concentration, sleep disturbances, lethargy, headaches and gastrointestinal symptoms.

The first step to ending sexual harassment is to keep an accurate record
of such incidents (and any retaliation by the harasser), identify potential
witnesses, contact others who have been harassed or find an advocate in the
workplace. A woman may choose to directly approach her harasser, file a
formal complaint within the work or educational institution or take legal
action.

Women also need to document their work achievements, while avoiding
absences, lateness or violations of work rules. If possible, explore possible
transfers to other work assignments and supervisors, as well as the feasibility
of changing jobs.

Treating the Trauma/Ending the Nightmare

To break the cycle of victimization, abused women must first break their
silence. Therapy requires that women talk about and confront their experiences. Therapy after sexual assault, rape or battering has as one of its main

goals the treatment (or prevention) of posttraumatic stress disorder, as well as treating depression, anxiety, phobias and other problems resulting from abuse. Therapy may also include crisis counseling, short-term psychotherapy, group or family therapy and cognitive-behavioral therapy. Battered women may also need social services.

For women who have been raped, cognitive-behavioral therapy may include the same type of "exposure" techniques used to treat phobias: A woman is helped to confront situations that remind her of the rape, as well as relive traumatic memories until they no longer produce intense fear reactions. Cognitive-behavioral techniques may help reframe distorted thinking caused by the assault, such as unjustifiably feeling unsafe, guilty, powerless and ashamed. Women may also be taught anxiety management (also called *stress inoculation therapy*), using thought-stopping, relaxation and deep breathing.

Edna B. Foa, Ph.D., professor of psychiatry and director of the Center for the Treatment and Study of Anxiety at the Medical College of Pennsylvania and Hahnemann University, developed a short-term exposure therapy for rape victims called *prolonged imaginal exposure* (*PE*). PE involves having the patient recount the memory of the trauma in detail, reliving the event over and over in her imagination, with the goal of reducing the anxiety and negative emotions associated with the assault. "A woman will always be upset about the memory of an assault, but it is not helpful to be so emotionally overwhelmed years later that you cannot go on with your life," says Dr. Foa.

Preliminary studies found that a majority of women diagnosed with PTSD (some as long as six years after being raped) who underwent five weeks of prolonged exposure therapy (or a combination of PE and stress inoculation) showed a 50 percent reduction in symptoms at three-month follow-up. Dr. Foa says that such therapies used immediately after an assault can help *prevent* chronic PTSD.

A controversial, experimental treatment for posttraumatic stress is called *eye movement desensitization and reprocessing* (*EMDR*). Patients are told to remember the assault, while they hold their head steady and fix their eyes on the therapist's finger held about twelve inches from their face. While the patient visualizes the distressing image, the therapist rapidly moves her finger twenty to thirty times across the patient's line of vision, and the patient tracks the movements with her eyes. After each set of eye movements, the patient reports any changes in the image and accompanying feelings, recording anxiety on a scale of 1 to 10. Depending on how the patient responds, therapy is repeated a dozen or more times. Each session takes about ninety minutes.

Studies presented to the American Psychiatric Association in 1995 reported that EMDR was as effective in reducing symptoms of posttraumatic stress in men and women as exposure therapy and other techniques. While EMDR is used in perhaps a dozen VA medical centers, experts caution that it has *not* been proven effective in randomized, clinical trials, and has not been accepted as a standard therapy.

For many women, experts say, joining efforts to aid other victims of childhood sexual abuse, battering or sexual harassment proves to be therapeutic as well.

CHAPTER 10

A Question of Hormones

What effect do female hormones have on brain chem-istry and on the incidence and symptoms of mental disorders among women? To ask—and attempt to answer—that question is extremely controversial. It raises the specter of negative gender stereotyping by virtue of women's biology that has taken place throughout history.

A BRIEF HISTORY OF THE "HYSTERICAL" WOMAN

For centuries, it was widely believed that women's reproductive organs ren-dered them psychologically unstable. In fact, the word *hysteria* is derived from the Greek word *hystero*, meaning "womb." Hysteria was first used per-haps two thousand years ago to describe mental afflictions allegedly caused by the dysfunctions or the physical "wanderings" of the uterus.

The Victorians believed that the instability of women's reproductive systems interfered with rational thinking, making them more vulnerable than men to mental illness. "With women, it is but a step from extreme nervous susceptibility to downright hysteria, and from that to overt insanity," wrote one physician in the *American Journal of Insanity* in 1866. No wonder that most patients in the mental institutions of the day were women!

"Psychiatric problems" in women (including hysteria, quarrelsomeness, erotic tendencies, suicide attempts and even masturbation) were often treated by hysterectomy, removing the uterus and ovaries. Many physicians believed that higher education might even cause damage to the uterus or drive women insane! Women were routinely given laudanum (tincture of opium) or addictive patent medicines containing opiates to treat "female complaints" (and, as a side benefit, render them more docile).

Well into the twentieth century, hysteria, hypochondria, depression, neurosis and other psychiatric disorders were thought of as "women's diseases" by therapists, says NYU's Dr. Virginia Sadock. (Freud believed hysteria was in part due to a woman's repressed sexual desires.) Laudanum gave way to lithium and then Valium for treating "neurotic," unhappy women. Women complaining of depression, anxiety or emotional distress were routinely prescribed tranquilizers, dubbed "Mother's little helpers."

Betty Friedan's landmark 1963 book, *The Feminine Mystique*, depicted the psychological effects of post-World War II society's insistence that women have no higher ambitions than being perfect wives and mothers. Friedan called it "the problem that has no name," but it might well have been termed hysteria one hundred years earlier: the psychic suffocation of a limited life, the despair at the loss of self, through ceaseless self-sacrifice to husband and children.

The women's movement set out to shatter the "feminine mystique," bury the myth of the hysterical woman and prove that women were equal to men. To some measure, it succeeded. Mental health professionals no longer view women as more vulnerable to mental illness by virtue of their hormones; "hysteria" is not listed as a diagnosis in the *DSM*.

But negative gender stereotyping persists, both in viewing women's behaviors and in treating women for mental disorders. Perhaps because of this, few people have wanted to explore the psychological differences between the sexes, much less the effect of "female hormones" on mental health. A case in point was the debate over including severe premenstrual mood problems, now termed *premenstrual dysphoric disorder* (PMDD), in the *DSM-IV* (see page 202). However, scientists are now actively investigating the role, if any, of female hormones in mental disorders.

THE BIOLOGICAL ROLE OF HORMONES

Female hormones are present in a woman's body even before birth, but begin to exert a strong biological influence when they are produced in higher amounts at puberty. Between the ages of eight and thirteen, the hypothalamus signals the pituitary gland to begin producing hormones called *gonadotropins*. These hormones, *follicle-stimulating hormone* (or *FSH*) and *luteinizing hormone* (or *LH*), signal the ovaries to begin producing estrogen, which triggers development of the breasts and other secondary sex characteristics, as well as monthly menstrual periods.

FSH and LH also regulate the menstrual cycle. FSH governs the *follicular phase*, stimulating increased estrogen production and the maturation of a follicle in the ovary that will produce an egg. Midway through the cycle, there is a surge in LH, causing the follicle to release the egg. The "shell" of that follicle becomes the *corpus luteum*, which produces progesterone (which peaks around seven days after ovulation). During the *luteal phase*, progesterone and estrogen stimulate the formation of a blanket of blood vessels in the lining of the uterus to prepare for implantation of a fertilized egg. If that does not occur, the corpus luteum degenerates and progesterone levels drop, the uterine lining breaks up and a woman sheds it as menstrual flow.

If pregnancy occurs, the corpus luteum continues to pump out progesterone, and the menstrual cycle is interrupted until after delivery. During pregnancy, the placenta takes over estrogen and progesterone production and produces other hormones as well, including *human chorionic gonadotropin* or *hCG* (pregnancy tests are designed to detect hCG in urine). There's a rapid rise in estrogen and progesterone before delivery, then a sharp drop, returning to pre-pregnancy levels around six weeks after the birth of the baby. The pituitary then assumes its normal role and ovulation resumes.

A normal ovulatory-menstrual cycle is twenty-six to thirty-two days long; it can be disrupted by illness, drastic dieting and even vigorous athletic training. Oral contraceptives contain continuous doses of synthetic estrogen and progesterone which interfere with production of FSH and LH and prevent ovulation.

As a woman approaches age fifty, estrogen production gradually starts to taper off. A woman's periods may become irregular and shorter and she may experience some of the symptoms of menopause. This is called *perimenopause*, or the *climacteric*. When the ovary produces only scant levels of estrogens, the hypothalamus desperately signals the pituitary to pump out extra FSH and LH in an attempt to stimulate the ovaries. (Menopause is confirmed by blood tests for the elevated FSH.) The resulting disturbance in the hypothalamus sets off a number of chemical reactions in the body. When blood vessels and the central nervous system are affected, it results in "vasomotor" menopausal symptoms, like hot flashes. Other tissues that have estrogen receptors, such as the bones, vagina and breasts, also undergo changes. Some women have more rapid declines in estrogen and, consequently, more symptoms.

All of this occurs as part of a delicate feedback loop called the *hypothalamic-pituitary-gonadal axis* (*HPG axis*). The HPG axis not only affects reproductive functions, it also interacts with other endocrine systems and brain chemicals (including stress hormones). An imbalance in one system can throw the others out of whack.

Possible Neurochemical Effects of Female Hormones

So far, clinical evidence that hormonal fluctuations may also influence systems that regulate neurotransmitters is scant.

As mentioned in Chapter 2, major depression has been linked to disruptions in the *hypothalamic-pituitary-adrenal axis*, or *HPA axis*, which regulates production of stress hormones like cortisol and norepinephrine by the adrenal glands. Some studies show norepinephrine activity increases shortly before ovulation and continues through the luteal phase; high norepinephrine levels are associated with anxiety. The HPA axis is affected by pregnancy (a possible clue to postpartum depression).

Some studies have also found that serotonin levels are lower during the luteal phase, especially in women who suffer from premenstrual depression. Low serotonin levels have also been linked to panic attacks and obsessive-compulsive disorder.

Excess serotonin has been linked to the "negative" symptoms of schizophrenia (social withdrawal and flat emotions). In some women with schizophrenia, symptoms may worsen when estrogen levels drop during or after pregnancy. Estrogen also dampens production of an enzyme called *tyrosine*, which reduces the amount of dopamine in the hypothalamus. Excess dopamine activity has been linked to the "positive" symptoms of schizophrenia (hallucinations and psychosis), so some experts believe that estrogen may lessen these symptoms in women.

It's also known that progesterone, which is increased during the premenstrual period, has depressive effects. Some population studies find that women who suffer premenstrual depression are more likely to have a major depressive episode during their lifetime, with prevalence rates ranging from 57 to 100 percent. Conversely, the prevalence of premenstrual depression has been estimated at 65 percent higher in women who had current or past diagnoses of mood disorders.

A number of studies find an increase in bingeing by bulimic women during the premenstrual period, but vary in the amount of depression and mood cycling reported. There is also some evidence of menstrual cycle-related fluctuations in symptoms of posttraumatic stress disorder and dissociative disorders in women who've had premenstrual syndrome (PMS).

Some experts believe that the drop in hormones after giving birth is partly to blame for postpartum depression (and possibly postpartum psychosis). Bipolar disorder worsens in some women after pregnancy. In studies of panic disorder, between 40 and 90 percent of women reported worsening of panic or anxiety premenstrually. During pregnancy, however, the course of panic disorder appears to be variable, with some women experiencing an improvement in symptoms, others getting worse. Forty percent of women with obsessive-compulsive disorder say they had their first symptoms while pregnant. Studies also show symptoms of agoraphobia and social phobia worsen during pregnancy.

However, the majority of the evidence linking shifts in female hormones to fluctuations in mood and behavior has come from studies that ask women to report symptoms, not from actually measuring neurotransmitters in the bloodstream.

One recent study used the "kindling" theory (in which repeated minor stresses make one more susceptible to depression), to suggest that repeated cycling of hormones each month, along with the behavior and mood changes that can accompany it, may make women more vulnerable to depressive illness.

So far, however, no direct cause and effect relationship between hormones or hormone fluctuations and any mental disorder (or its symptoms) has ever been clinically demonstrated. Much remains unknown about the effects of female hormones on the mind and body. A good example is *premenstrual syndrome (PMS)*.

⟨ᴓ Tina's Story ᴓ⟩

"I've always had premenstrual symptoms, but they never interfered with my life until a few years ago. . . . When I first got my period when I was around fourteen . . . I had bad cramps. . . . Later on, in my twenties, I also started to have bloating, weight gain and breast tenderness in the week or two before my period. ... I could gain as much as seven or eight pounds in 'water weight.' But my doctor gave me a diuretic. ... If I was a little more irritable before my period, I chalked it up to 'premenstrual tension.'

"But in my thirties, I started to have 'anxiety attacks' before my period ... feeling totally out of control, panicky, overwhelmed. I would be set off by the least little thing. ... At first, I thought it was because I had so many job pressures. ...

"I remember one instance very vividly. I had a business meeting in an area of the city I'd never been in before. I got lost, and I started to panic. ... I turned one corner and I couldn't find the street number. I turned another and couldn't find my way back to where I started. I stood there, right on that street corner, and screamed! I literally howled in frustration. People were looking at me! I made myself calm down. I went into a coffee shop, calmly asked directions ... and finally made it to the meeting. ... I never lost it like that in the office, thank God. ... But I began to worry about my career, and my sanity.

"My gynecologist was the one who suggested the anxiety might be premenstrually related, since I had a history of other symptoms. She said that I might have a very severe form of premenstrual syndrome, where some women get very depressed and others get really anxious. ... She told me to keep track of all of my physical and emotional symptoms for three cycles. I was really amazed to see the correlation between the bloating and weight gain, and these horrible episodes of feeling out of control and panicky. ... Just being aware of that made it easier to handle the anxiety the third month. ...

"My doctor gave me a prescription for antianxiety medication. She said to take it when I started to have anxiety symptoms in the days before my period. ... You can't imagine what a change this has made in my life. ... I no longer feel out of control, and other people don't see me that way, either."

☙

PREMENSTRUAL DYSPHORIA

The word "dysphoria" means a feeling of discomfort, unpleasantness or being unwell. For millions of women, the term aptly describes how they feel in
the week or two before their menstrual periods. The name commonly given
to this discomfort is *premenstrual syndrome*, or *PMS*.

No one knows exactly what causes PMS. Researchers theorize that some
women have a special sensitivity to normal hormonal (or physical) changes
in the luteal phase of their cycle. A 1998 study at NIMH suggests that these
symptoms stem from abnormal reactions in the brains of some women to
estrogen and progesterone; the first *real* indication that PMS may be
biological. The NIMH researchers suppressed ovarian function in twenty
women, half of whom had PMS, then gave them either estrogen,
progesterone, or a placebo. The hormones produced PMS-like symptoms
only in those women who had PMS.

Women with severe premenstrual mood changes, who have never had
panic disorder, are also likely to respond with extreme anxiety (or even a
panic attack) to chemical "challenge tests" used to induce panic attacks in
the lab. "Women who do not have PMS will have no reaction at all. This
indicates some biological vulnerability," notes Jean Endicott, Ph.D., chief of
the Department of Research Assessment and Training at the New York
State Psychiatric Institute.

But the dysphoria is quite real. Of the more than two hundred symptoms
associated with PMS, the most common are fluid retention, bloating, weight
gain, headaches, acne and breast tenderness, as well as cravings for sweets
or carbohydrates. Psychological symptoms include depression, anxiety, irritability, mood swings, tearfulness and changes in sexual drive.

Some women experience PMS with their first menstrual periods, but
the majority develop it during their thirties and forties, especially after a
major interruption of their ovulatory cycles, such as pregnancy or stopping
birth control pills. "It may well be that premenstrual syndrome occurs in the
thirties and forties as part of a process of hormonal and endocrine changes
leading up to menopause," suggests Sally K. Severino, M.D., professor and
executive vice chair of the Department of Psychiatry at the University of
New Mexico. Dr. Severino notes that women who experience severe
premenstrual symptoms are likely to suffer intense menopausal symptoms.

Many women who believe they have PMS do not actually have the severity of symptoms needed for a formal diagnosis. A National Institutes of
Health consensus conference in 1983 stated that symptom intensity must

increase by at least 30 percent during the premenstrual period for at least two consecutive months and interfere with functioning for a diagnosis of PMS. Around 75 percent of women have minor, occasional premenstrual symptoms, but only 20 to 30 percent have PMS by NIH's definition.

Perhaps 3 to 7 percent of women experience especially severe emotional symptoms every month, including depression. This problem is currently classified in the *DSM-IV* as a mood disorder called *premenstrual dysphoric disorder (PMDD)*.

Defining these severe premenstrual symptoms as a psychiatric disorder was rather controversial. Experts were divided over what to call it. It was initially termed *Late Luteal Phase Dysphoric Disorder (LLPDD)*, since some symptoms can occur in women who have had their uterus removed and therefore don't menstruate. Thus, some believed that the term *premenstrual* didn't apply. Others felt that including it in the diagnostic manual under *any* name would stigmatize women, implying that the menstrual cycle caused psychiatric problems. Some feared that the diagnosis could even be used inappropriately by the legal system, especially in child custody cases, as evidence of cyclical mental impairment or "diminished capacity." However, members of an advisory committee formed to study LLPDD argued that it would legitimize complaints many women have long sought help for.

After much debate, in 1987 LLPDD was listed in the appendix of the *DSM-III-R* under "Proposed Diagnostic Categories Needing Further Study." After a review of over five hundred published and unpublished studies, the name of the disorder was changed and the definition altered for the 1994 *DSM-IV*, emphasizing depressive mood and other psychological symptoms. Its inclusion (still only in the appendix as a proposed diagnosis) was meant to stimulate further research into the biological origins of PMDD. But it also served to finally acknowledge PMDD as an entity to be considered when evaluating women for premenstrual mood disturbances.

"The issue of stigmatization because of PMDD really reflects the continuing stigmatization of mental illness, not the stigmatization of women," argues Dr. Severino, who served on the PMDD advisory committee. "Women do seem to have a special vulnerability to developing certain disorders, as do men. So I don't believe that it's 'antiwomen' to recognize this disorder any more than it's 'antimen' to recognize the illnesses that are more common in men."

At the same time, Dr. Severino stresses that PMDD should not be confused with PMS. "Whereas PMS is mostly characterized by physical symptoms, with some associated mood problems, PMDD is primarily a disorder of mood, not just depression, but anxiety as well, with associated physical symptoms," she says.

The *DSM-IV* describes symptoms of PMDD as similar in severity (but not in duration) to major depression, and which must be present during most menstrual cycles throughout the year. Symptoms must be severe enough to interfere with school or work and social or marital relationships, and must be confirmed through daily diaries kept during at least two cycles.

Women who have had recurrent major depression, bipolar disorder (see Chapter 2), postpartum depression or postpartum psychosis (page 208), or who have a family history of affective disorders, may be at greater risk for PMDD. A number of medical conditions can exacerbate both PMS and PMDD, including migraine headaches, asthma and allergies.

Some experts characterize worsening of depression that occurs premenstrually as *premenstrual mood exacerbation (PME)*. This diagnosis is currently being investigated.

Symptoms of Premenstrual Dysphoric Disorder

Source: *Diagnostic and Statistical Manual of Mental Disorders, Fourth Edition (DSM-IV)*, 1994

For a diagnosis of PMDD, five (or more) symptoms must be present for most of the time during the luteal phase, subsiding within a few days of menstruation, during most menstrual cycles, with at least one of the following symptoms.

- Markedly depressed mood, feelings of hopelessness or self-deprecating thoughts.

- Marked anxiety, tension, feeling "keyed up" or "on edge."

- Marked affective lability (feeling suddenly sad, tearful, irritable or angry).

- Persistent and marked anger or irritability, or increased interpersonal conflicts.

Other symptoms can include:

- Decreased interest in usual activities (work, school, friends, hobbies).

- Difficulty in concentrating.

- Lethargy, easy fatigability or marked lack of energy.

(continued)

- Marked change in appetite, overeating or food cravings.

- Hypersomnia or insomnia.

- Feeling overwhelmed or out of control.

- Other physical symptoms can include breast tenderness or swelling, headaches, joint or muscle pain, a sensation of "bloating" and weight gain.

The *DSM-IV* is careful to point out that the mood changes many women experience premenstrually "should not be considered a mental disorder." But the image of PMS is often the opposite.

"The term *PMS* has traditionally been used in a pejorative sense in regard to women's behavior and competency. The general public perception is that women can be unreliably moody at 'that time of the month,'" says Judith H. Gold, M.D., a noted psychiatrist practicing in Halifax, Nova Scotia, who chaired the work group on LLPDD for the *DSM-IV* task force.

"Unfortunately, the lack of a consistent definition has made it difficult to study PMS. There has been a great deal of controversy over the actual existence of PMS, over the occurrence of disabling symptoms and their prevalence in populations other than white, North American women," she notes.

Women in cultures as diverse as Nigeria, Japan and Sweden all experience premenstrual symptoms. What differs is the type of symptoms, and whether women are distressed by them. For example, recent studies comparing American, Italian and Bahraini women in their twenties and thirties found that a third shared five symptoms: breast swelling, breast pain, irritability, mood swings and fatigue. However, the American women reported *more* irritability, mood swings and weight gain; the Italians said they had more breast swelling and pain; the Bahraini women complained more often of backaches. Interestingly, few women in Italy or Bahrain knew anything about PMS or premenstrual tension. In fact, the Italian women reported feelings of energy, well-being and orderliness before their periods! So while premenstrual symptoms may be common, some experts suggest that PMS as a "disorder" may be a concept confined to more affluent, American women.

Studies show that women who have more life stresses have more severe premenstrual symptoms; women socialized to have negative ideas about menstruation also report more symptoms. Premenstrual symptoms themselves may be a cause of stress. PMS seems to short-circuit the usual coping mechanisms, making some women more prone to social, marital or job problems. Women with better coping skills seem to suffer less from PMS.

Dr. Gold suggests that premenstrual dysphoric disorder (again, a more severe form of PMS) may, in fact, be related to "rapid-cycling depression," which also occurs in men (rapid cycling and PMDD are both associated with low serotonin levels). She believes that future studies of PMDD must include women of all racial, social and cultural groups, and men as a "control."

⤸ *Marcia's Story* ⤵

"When I had my first child in 1985, my postpartum illness came as a complete surprise to me. I was a teacher; I had been working with emotionally disturbed youngsters for years. I knew a lot about mental health issues. So I thought I would be the perfect mother. . . . But the minute my daughter was born, I felt absolutely nothing. I was crying on the delivery table . . . they were tears of emptiness: 'Is this all there is?'

"I never wanted to touch my daughter. . . . The only time I did anything with her was when she cried. Where most new mothers are cuddling their babies and holding them close and counting their fingers and toes, I felt none of that.

"I had a twenty-two-hour labor and was in the hospital for two days, but I never slept. I came home and never slept. . . . I would walk into a room and forget why I was there. At the end of two weeks, I became acutely suicidal. My husband found me in the kitchen with a butcher knife and writing a suicide note. . . . My obstetrician gave me Valium to help me sleep, but it made me worse. . . .

"I thought God was punishing me. I thought I was evil. . . . I also had a lot of magical thinking. I wanted my daughter to go away. I would think that when she was asleep, she wasn't really there. And when she would cry and wake up, I would be devastated that she was there and that this was real. And this was horrible because this was a very wanted and very planned for child. I was terrified. I told my husband to take the baby and leave me and go find a better life somewhere else. . . . Finally, my family got me to a psychiatrist and I was hospitalized.

"I was put on an antidepressant; it wired me like crazy. I discontinued it on my own, and discharged myself from the hospital against medical advice and then deteriorated rapidly. . . . I thought that God was punishing me . . . telling me that I was horrid and that I should give up my family. I was rehospitalized.

"I was finally put together with a female psychiatrist. . . . She was wonderful. She told me I was suffering from a postpartum illness and they are treatable. . . . I didn't know they had actually classified me as postpartum psychotic until two years later when I asked to review my records.

"I had never had anything you could consider depression before this happened. It took almost a year for me to completely recover. I had a wonderful therapist, but I want to emphasize that you have to treat the body and the soul. The medicine and the shock treatments . . . got me out of the severe biological depression and the horrible hopelessness. But I had a lot of emotional baggage to deal with . . . I felt horrible about missing my daughter's babyhood. I had . . . fears that I had somehow 'ruined' her. But that didn't happen . . . my daughter and I have bonded. She was getting what she needed from people who loved her.

"When I had my second child . . . I found a physician who gave me antidepressants right on the delivery table. I won't say I got away scot-free . . . I had mild postpartum anxiety and a brief depression. But in general I did great. I felt connected to my son from the minute I saw him; he slept the first night of his life on my chest."

Marcia B. Greco is the past director of education and outreach for Depression After Delivery, National. The above was taken from an interview and published with her permission.

PREGNANCY AND POSTPARTUM PROBLEMS

Pregnancy is usually seen as a time of well-being, but it can be a high risk period for some psychiatric disorders, including manic and major depression. Experts speculate that fluctuations in estrogen, progesterone, and pregnancy-related hormones like *oxytocin* (a pituitary hormone that initiates uterine contractions in labor and the release of milk during lactation), as well as other neuropeptides involved in reproductive changes may promote mood disorders and worsen anxiety.

"You have the highest estrogen levels that a woman will ever experience in her life, an increase of oxytocin at 36 weeks, then you have a very rapid drop of estrogen and progesterone within 24 hours. So there's something about this particular neurochemical situation that may have a kindling effect on the immune system and receptors in the brain," says Deborah A. Sichel, M.D., director of the Hestia Institute for Women and Families in Wellesley, .Massachusetts, and a member of the Perinatal Psychiatry Clinical Research Program at the Massachusetts General Hospital.

According to Dr. Sichel, risk factors for pregnancy or postpartum related disorders may include a history of depression, anxiety or premenstrual dysphoric disorder, and having mood or anxiety symptoms during pregnancy. Also at risk may be women who had depressive symptoms with oral contraceptives and/or severe mood problems with fertility drugs. "That suggests some women may have a vulnerability to hormonal change and may be susceptible to pregnancy or postpartum illness," says Dr. Sichel. Some women may have preexisting disorders, such as anxiety or obsessive-compulsive disorder (OCD), which may worsen during or after pregnancy, and they may also develop a coexisting depression.

DEPRESSION DURING PREGNANCY: May occur in 10 percent of women, as either major depression or *dysthymia*. However, symptoms like mood swings, appetite changes or insomnia may be attributed to the pregnancy itself and can be easily overlooked. Because of social expectations that pregnancy is a happy time, a woman may deny to herself and others that she's depressed.

Women most vulnerable to depression during pregnancy may be experiencing marital conflict, lack of partner support, stressful events during pregnancy, alcohol problems or problems resulting from lower socioeconomic status and education. Depression in pregnancy may have an acute onset in the first trimester with suicidal thoughts, or come on gradually. There is usually a worsening in the third trimester, with a woman not sleeping or eating, leading to inadequate weight gain, says Dr. Sichel. While therapy may help some women, treatment of severe cases can be a problem, since there have been no direct studies of the effect of antidepressants on the fetus (see page 283).

THE BABY BLUES: Is the most common pregnancy-related mood disturbance, affecting 50 to 80 percent of all new mothers for a short period after delivery. Between 10 and 15 percent of women experience *postpartum major depression* (PPMD), with symptoms lasting for weeks or months.

Traditionally, psychiatrists have viewed postpartum depression as a more severe form of the "baby blues." But some experts believe the "blues" may well be a *separate entity*. "The 'blues' may be a normal state of biological reactivity which facilitates bonding and maternal behavior," suggests Laura J. Miller, M.D., an assistant professor of psychiatry at the University of Illinois at Chicago. In preliminary research presented to the American Psychiatric Association in 1995, she noted that such normal biological "attachment systems" are seen in animals, where hormonal triggers such as the release of oxytocin create heightened responses to stimuli in the brain, activating maternal behavior. In humans, this may be comparable to a new mother being hyperalert to the noises and cries of her infant, even in another room.

"The predominant mood state of women with maternity blues is not sadness, but joy. However, through all that joy, they're tearful, they cry at the drop of the hat. It's a tremendously reactive state, but it's *not* the same as mild depression," says Dr. Miller. The "baby blues" typically occur three to five days after giving birth, and seem to be triggered by the birth of the baby itself, with its physical discomforts and the "letdown" that follows such an emotionally charged experience. The baby blues typically resolve quickly. In contrast, the sadness of postpartum depression deepens and lingers. It may be triggered by hormonal fluctuations and environmental stressors, like lack of support with changing diapers and 3:00 A.M. feedings.

Studies suggest that 25 percent of women who start out with a severe case of "baby blues" go on to develop true clinical depression, says Dr. Sichel. "I call this a 'complicated blues' phenomenon, where the blues seem to continue for a period of at least four weeks. These women should be monitored because they can evolve into major depression. This may, in fact, be a marker for recurrent depression after subsequent pregnancies. However, anything that occurs after four weeks is no longer the blues."

POSTPARTUM MAJOR DEPRESSION: Is classified in the *DSM-IV* as a distinct mood disorder that occurs within four weeks after delivery. However, it can also occur up to a *year* later, stresses Margaret Spinelli, M.D., director of the Maternal Mental Health Program at the New York State Psychiatric Institute. PPMD has some distinct features in addition to sadness and tearfulness: despondency, guilty feelings, lack of appetite and sleep disturbances, and feelings of inadequacy in coping with the baby.

"There may also be problems with concentration and memory, fatigue and irritability. Some women may worry excessively about the baby's health or feeding habits and see themselves as 'bad,' inadequate or unloving mothers," she says. "But many women are ashamed or guilty about feeling depressed at a time when they are expected to be happy, and may be reluctant to seek help, particularly if they experience thoughts about harming the baby."

Some cases of postpartum depression may also go undiagnosed because of lingering myths that women are somehow protected against depression or psychiatric illness during pregnancy. In fact, they're not. Just as many women become depressed *during* pregnancy as develop postpartum depression, notes Dr. Spinelli.

"Bipolar women are particularly at risk for having a severe episode during the postpartum period. There is a high incidence of postpartum hospitalizations among bipolar women, suggesting some hormonal effect. But this has never been proven. It could also be a thyroid or circadian disruption," says Dr. Ellen Leibenluft of the National Institute of Mental Health.

POSTPARTUM PSYCHOSIS: Occurs in one or two of every one thousand new mothers (especially those with a history of bipolar disorder). A woman with this disorder may seem perfectly fine for two to three days after delivery, but rapidly becomes depressed, confused and unpredictable, with wide emotional swings and sleep disturbances. A woman with postpartum "mania" may appear euphoric, overexcited, irritable and hyperactive, eating and sleeping very little. A woman may have difficulty caring for her infant. She may deny having given birth, become paranoid, hear voices or have hallucinations "commanding" her to harm the baby, or have delusions about the infant being dead or defective. Some women even try to kill their babies. Postpartum psychosis is a medical emergency, requiring immediate hospitalization, since the mother may be a danger to her child.

PREGNANCY/POSTPARTUM ANXIETY DISORDERS: May arise or worsen during pregnancy or immediately afterward, including panic attacks, obsessive-compulsive disorder and agoraphobia.

A 1992 report in the *American Journal of Psychiatry* found that almost 40 percent of women with obsessive-compulsive disorder first experienced symptoms during pregnancy; an earlier study put the number at almost 70 percent. A small Canadian study in 1993 found that a majority of women with social phobias reported more severe symptoms during pregnancy; a third of women with agoraphobia reported an increase in symptoms.

Dr. Deborah Sichel and colleagues at Harvard Medical School and the Massachusetts General Hospital followed 34 women with panic disorder during pregnancy and the postpartum period and found that while some had lessened symptoms during pregnancy, most continued to have panic attacks and needed medication.

The causes of postpartum anxiety are yet unclear. But new research has linked oxytocin to obsessive-compulsive disorder. "Recent studies have shown oxytocin to be increased in the cerebrospinal fluid of OCD patients," says Dr. Sichel. "Part of the role that oxytocin may have in OCD, or in the obsessionality that you often see postpartum, may be an effect of some kind by oxytocin on the monoamine system, which breaks down neurotransmitters in the synapse, and which may allow certain neurotransmitters to become overactive to produce anxiety."

THE MYTH OF "MENOPAUSAL DEPRESSION"

For many years it was believed that women suffered "involutional melancholia" at menopause, caused by shrinkage and atrophy of the uterus. But scientists never turned up evidence of such a malady. Still, the notion persisted that menopause caused depression, due to drops in hormone levels and to women's alleged grieving for their lost childbearing capacity (or because of the "empty nest"). That turned out to be bunk as well.

In fact, new data from studies around the world indicate an increase in depression and psychological distress in the *perimenopausal* period, not the menopause, in women seeking medical treatment for menopausal symptoms. This was shown in a small clinical study by Donna E. Stewart, M.D., the Lillian Love Chair of Women's Health at the Toronto Hospital. The 1994 study, involving 259 women (113 of whom were perimenopausal and 146 of whom had gone through menopause), found that women nearing menopause had much greater psychological distress, especially depression, as well as anxiety and somatization, than menopausal women, who had no more symptoms than the general population.

"It's likely that in common with other life changes, such as adolescence and childbearing, the transition period may be much more difficult than the final stage, in this case menopause," Dr. Stewart reports. "It may also be the changing levels of hormones, which may be fluctuating during perimenopause, may provoke psychological symptoms. Whereas low, but stable, levels of hormones as during menopause do not. And that psychological symptoms abate as physical symptoms settle down." Dr. Stewart and colleagues also found that women at greatest risk for perimenopausal distress were more likely to have had depressive symptoms with birth control pills; to have experienced premenstrual dysphoria, the "baby blues" or postpartum depression; or to have been treated for a previous depression unrelated to reproductive events.

Dysphoria during this period may be due to early, very subtle menopausal symptoms, says Lila E. Nachtigall, M.D., a professor of obstetrics and gynecology who heads the Women's Wellness division of NYU Medical Center Women's Health Service. She points out that hot flashes are actually clusters of symptoms (or "hot flash equivalents," as she terms them), which can include discomfort, nausea, dizziness, headaches and palpitations, as well as feeling hot, skin flushing and sweating. Women don't experience every symptom, and may not recognize what's happening, especially if they still have periods. "Other symptoms can include fatigue, irritability, changes in libido, poor concentration and memory, mood swings and anxiety," adds Dr. Nachtigall. "Some women are chronically tired because their sleep is disrupted by hot flashes; being tired makes you irritable. Hot flashes can disrupt your concentration; sweating makes you feel unpleasant. All of this may remind you that you're growing older, which can be distressing for some women."

Curiously, women in societies where age confers increased social, religious or even political status (or social freedom) report fewer menopausal symptoms (see page 238).

Physical symptoms of menopause can be treated with replacement hormones, which may also alleviate some of the psychological symptoms related to feeling "unwell."

Depression can occur during menopause, but experts stress that it needs to be treated as a specific entity, not as a menopausal symptom. Women who suffered clinical depression earlier in life may be more at risk for a recurrence.

Today, many women find that midlife and menopause are a time of renewed energy, optimism and sexuality, as well as of new interests and careers (see Chapter 11).

Fig. 7: Your Symptom Rating Chart

Reproduced by permission of Jean Endicott, Ph.D., chief of the Department of Research Assessment and Training, New York State Psychiatric Institute

Make extra copies of this chart so you can track your symptoms for at least three menstrual cycles. Fill in the date on the line under the day of the week when you start your daily ratings; start a new page each Monday. On the line under the date, note whether you are spotting (S) or menstruating (M). If you consistently rate your premenstrual symptoms in the moderate to severe range over several cycles (or if symptoms of depression or anxiety occur to a lesser degree throughout the month), and your ratings in the last three categories indicate symptoms are interfering with your life, it may be advisable to seek professional help.

If you have mild to moderate premenstrual symptoms, this chart may help you to better manage those symptoms.

Note the degree to which you experienced each of the problems listed below. Make your ratings each evening. Circle the number which corresponds to the severity as noted here:

1–Not at all 2–Minimal 3–Mild 4–Moderate 5–Severe 6–Extreme

Rate under correct day of week:	Mon	Tue	Wed	Thu	Fri	Sat	Sun
Note date under day of week	___	___	___	___	___	___	___
Note if *spotting* or *menses* with S or M:	___	___	___	___	___	___	___
1a. Felt depressed, sad, "down" or "blue"	1	1	1	1	1	1	1
	2	2	2	2	2	2	2
	3	3	3	3	3	3	3
	4	4	4	4	4	4	4
	5	5	5	5	5	5	5
	6	6	6	6	6	6	6
1b. Felt hopeless	1	1	1	1	1	1	1
	2	2	2	2	2	2	2
	3	3	3	3	3	3	3
	4	4	4	4	4	4	4
	5	5	5	5	5	5	5
	6	6	6	6	6	6	6

Rate under correct day of week:	Mon	Tue	Wed	Thu	Fri	Sat	Sun
Note date under day of week	——	——	——	——	——	——	——
Note if *spotting* or *menses* with S or M:	——	——	——	——	——	——	——
1c. Felt worthless or guilty	1	1	1	1	1	1	1
	2	2	2	2	2	2	2
	3	3	3	3	3	3	3
	4	4	4	4	4	4	4
	5	5	5	5	5	5	5
	6	6	6	6	6	6	6
2. Felt anxious, tense, "keyed up" or "on edge"	1	1	1	1	1	1	1
	2	2	2	2	2	2	2
	3	3	3	3	3	3	3
	4	4	4	4	4	4	4
	5	5	5	5	5	5	5
	6	6	6	6	6	6	6
3a. Had mood swings (e.g., suddenly felt sad or tearful)	1	1	1	1	1	1	1
	2	2	2	2	2	2	2
	3	3	3	3	3	3	3
	4	4	4	4	4	4	4
	5	5	5	5	5	5	5
	6	6	6	6	6	6	6
3b. Was more sensitive to rejection or my feelings were easily hurt	1	1	1	1	1	1	1
	2	2	2	2	2	2	2
	3	3	3	3	3	3	3
	4	4	4	4	4	4	4
	5	5	5	5	5	5	5
	6	6	6	6	6	6	6

(continued)

Rate under correct day of week:	Mon	Tue	Wed	Thu	Fri	Sat	Sun
Note date under day of week	___	___	___	___	___	___	___
Note if *spotting* or *menses* with S or M:	___	___	___	___	___	___	___

4a. Felt angry, irritable

	Mon	Tue	Wed	Thu	Fri	Sat	Sun
	1	1	1	1	1	1	1
	2	2	2	2	2	2	2
	3	3	3	3	3	3	3
	4	4	4	4	4	4	4
	5	5	5	5	5	5	5
	6	6	6	6	6	6	6

4b. Had conflicts or problems with people

	Mon	Tue	Wed	Thu	Fri	Sat	Sun
	1	1	1	1	1	1	1
	2	2	2	2	2	2	2
	3	3	3	3	3	3	3
	4	4	4	4	4	4	4
	5	5	5	5	5	5	5
	6	6	6	6	6	6	6

5. Had less interest in usual activities (e.g., work, school, friends, hobbies)

	Mon	Tue	Wed	Thu	Fri	Sat	Sun
	1	1	1	1	1	1	1
	2	2	2	2	2	2	2
	3	3	3	3	3	3	3
	4	4	4	4	4	4	4
	5	5	5	5	5	5	5
	6	6	6	6	6	6	6

6. Had difficulty concentrating

	Mon	Tue	Wed	Thu	Fri	Sat	Sun
	1	1	1	1	1	1	1
	2	2	2	2	2	2	2
	3	3	3	3	3	3	3
	4	4	4	4	4	4	4
	5	5	5	5	5	5	5
	6	6	6	6	6	6	6

Rate under correct day of week:	Mon	Tue	Wed	Thu	Fri	Sat	Sun
Note date under day of week	—	—	—	—	—	—	—
Note if *spotting* or *menses* with S or M:	—	—	—	—	—	—	—

7. Felt lethargic, tired, fatigued or had a lack of energy

	Mon	Tue	Wed	Thu	Fri	Sat	Sun
	1	1	1	1	1	1	1
	2	2	2	2	2	2	2
	3	3	3	3	3	3	3
	4	4	4	4	4	4	4
	5	5	5	5	5	5	5
	6	6	6	6	6	6	6

8a. Had increased appetite or overate

	1	1	1	1	1	1	1
	2	2	2	2	2	2	2
	3	3	3	3	3	3	3
	4	4	4	4	4	4	4
	5	5	5	5	5	5	5
	6	6	6	6	6	6	6

8b. Had cravings for specific foods

	1	1	1	1	1	1	1
	2	2	2	2	2	2	2
	3	3	3	3	3	3	3
	4	4	4	4	4	4	4
	5	5	5	5	5	5	5
	6	6	6	6	6	6	6

9a. Slept more, took naps, found it hard to get up when intended

	1	1	1	1	1	1	1
	2	2	2	2	2	2	2
	3	3	3	3	3	3	3
	4	4	4	4	4	4	4
	5	5	5	5	5	5	5
	6	6	6	6	6	6	6

(continued)

Rate under correct day of week:	Mon	Tue	Wed	Thu	Fri	Sat	Sun
Note date under day of week	___	___	___	___	___	___	___
Note if *spotting* or *menses* with S or M:	___	___	___	___	___	___	___

9b. Had trouble getting to sleep or staying asleep	Mon	Tue	Wed	Thu	Fri	Sat	Sun
	1	1	1	1	1	1	1
	2	2	2	2	2	2	2
	3	3	3	3	3	3	3
	4	4	4	4	4	4	4
	5	5	5	5	5	5	5
	6	6	6	6	6	6	6

10a. Felt overwhelmed or that I could not cope

1	1	1	1	1	1	1
2	2	2	2	2	2	2
3	3	3	3	3	3	3
4	4	4	4	4	4	4
5	5	5	5	5	5	5
6	6	6	6	6	6	6

10b. Felt out of control

1	1	1	1	1	1	1
2	2	2	2	2	2	2
3	3	3	3	3	3	3
4	4	4	4	4	4	4
5	5	5	5	5	5	5
6	6	6	6	6	6	6

11a. Had breast tenderness

1	1	1	1	1	1	1
2	2	2	2	2	2	2
3	3	3	3	3	3	3
4	4	4	4	4	4	4
5	5	5	5	5	5	5
6	6	6	6	6	6	6

Rate under correct day of week: Note date under day of week Note if *spotting* or *menses* with S or M:	Mon	Tue	Wed	Thu	Fri	Sat	Sun
	___	___	___	___	___	___	___
	___	___	___	___	___	___	___
11b. Had breast swelling, felt "bloated" or had weight gain	1	1	1	1	1	1	1
	2	2	2	2	2	2	2
	3	3	3	3	3	3	3
	4	4	4	4	4	4	4
	5	5	5	5	5	5	5
	6	6	6	6	6	6	6
11c. Had headache	1	1	1	1	1	1	1
	2	2	2	2	2	2	2
	3	3	3	3	3	3	3
	4	4	4	4	4	4	4
	5	5	5	5	5	5	5
	6	6	6	6	6	6	6
11d. Had joint or muscle pain	1	1	1	1	1	1	1
	2	2	2	2	2	2	2
	3	3	3	3	3	3	3
	4	4	4	4	4	4	4
	5	5	5	5	5	5	5
	6	6	6	6	6	6	6
At work, at school, at home or in daily routine, at least one of the problems noted above caused reduction of productivity or inefficiency	1	1	1	1	1	1	1
	2	2	2	2	2	2	2
	3	3	3	3	3	3	3
	4	4	4	4	4	4	4
	5	5	5	5	5	5	5
	6	6	6	6	6	6	6

(continued)

Rate under correct day of week:	Mon	Tue	Wed	Thu	Fri	Sat	Sun
Note date under day of week	___	___	___	___	___	___	___
Note if *spotting* or *menses* with			/				
S or M:	___	___	___	___	___	___	___
At least one of the problems	1	1	1	1	1	1	1
noted above interfered with	2	2	2	2	2	2	2
hobbies or social activities	3	3	3	3	3	3	3
(e.g., avoid or do less)	4	4	4	4	4	4	4
	5	5	5	5	5	5	5
	6	6	6	6	6	6	6
At least one of the problems	1	1	1	1	1	1	1
noted above interfered with	2	2	2	2	2	2	2
relationships with others	3	3	3	3	3	3	3
	4	4	4	4	4	4	4
	5	5	5	5	5	5	5
	6	6	6	6	6	6	6

HELP FOR PREMENSTRUAL PROBLEMS

Before premenstrual problems like PMS or PMDD can be diagnosed and treated, a woman must track her symptoms over several cycles. That establishes which symptoms are present and whether they only occur (or get worse) premenstrually.

"Some women report that within a day or two of starting their period, they have no symptoms. For others, it's almost the end of the menses before all the symptoms go away," says Dr. Jean Endicott of the New York State Psychiatric Institute, who developed the most widely used symptom rating chart. "If you get daily ratings, you see a consistency from cycle to cycle in individual women, and it helps to identify the timing of the problem and the early-warning signs. Most women get some physical symptoms before they get the mood changes."

Daily ratings also help determine when to start medication or adjust medication doses, as well as when to take other measures to minimize symptoms. "We also use the daily ratings to help women identify what are the *best* days of the month. For most women it's around the end of menses, around day six through day ten or eleven. So that she can take advantage of the good days, not just focus on the difficult days," says Dr. Endicott. In fact, 10 to 15 percent of women report *positive* changes premenstrually.

Treatment of PMS depends on the nature and severity of the symptoms. Medication may be reserved for severe cases, while women with moderate symptoms may be advised to make dietary changes and exercise. PMS management strategies include the following.

CAFFEINE AND ALCOHOL: Women suffering from PMS-related fatigue often up their coffee consumption, says Dr. Endicott, but coffee and other caffeinated beverages can increase anxiety and irritability (and may contribute to breast tenderness). Women are also cautioned to avoid alcohol, since they may be more sensitive to the effects of alcohol (and have higher blood levels) during the premenstrual period.

EXERCISE: While there's no clinical proof that exercise has any effect on PMS symptoms, most physicians recommend it.

Exercise has been shown to reduce depression and anxiety, and to boost energy and self-esteem. There's also some evidence that it raises serotonin levels and increases *endorphins*, the body's natural pain-reliever and mood-elevator. Some studies suggest that endorphin levels drop during the week before and the first few days of the menstrual period. Dr. Severino also says that exercise may help reduce some of the bloating.

DIURETICS: Diuretics such as *chlorthalidone* (*Hygroton*), *furosemide* (*Lasix*) and *hydrochlorothiazide* (*Hydro-D*) are prescribed to help the kidneys get rid of excess salt and water, reducing the fluid retention and weight gain. An over-the-counter product combining *ammonium chloride* and a small amount of caffeine (*AquaBan*) has somewhat less diuretic action, but studies show that it can relieve premenstrual bloating and act as a mild stimulant for some women. Other over-the-counter preparations, such as *Premensyn*, also contain mild diuretics.

BIRTH CONTROL PILLS: These can minimize premenstrual symptoms in many cases, but some women find that they cause depression.

FOOD—A "NATURAL" PMS TREATMENT?: Low levels of serotonin may not only produce premenstrual depression, but may also trigger the cravings for starches and sweets some women experience before their periods.

Research by Richard J. Wurtman, M.D., a professor of neuroscience and specialist in brain chemistry, and Judith Wurtman, Ph.D., a cell biologist and nutritionist, at the Massachusetts Institute of Technology, has found that women with PMS increased their intake of foods such as potatoes, rice, cookies, candy and pretzels by about 500 calories before their periods, apparently in an unconscious attempt to "medicate" PMS symptoms; controlled studies showed that such foods did indeed elevate mood and boost serotonin levels. A 1995 study by the Wurtmans tested an experimental carbohydrate-rich beverage designed to raise levels of serotonin, and found that women with PMS given the drink during the late luteal phase had fewer symptoms of depression, improved cognitive function and decreased carbohydrate cravings, compared with women given a placebo. While PMS symptoms can also be significantly reduced with drugs that boost serotonin levels (see below), giving in to cravings for chocolate or cookies (in moderation, of course) may well provide a nondrug approach to PMS for some women!

SLEEP: A good night's sleep can do wonders for PMS. Disruptions of the sleep-wake cycle, or circadian rhythm, may play a role in both PMS and PMDD. Some preliminary animal studies suggest that sex hormones may help regulate circadian rhythms (the body's twenty-four hour biological clock).

"Studies have shown that women with PMS have some sleep changes, and seem to sleep less efficiently in the premenstrual period. However, increases in tension and arousal during the premenstrual period, rather than hormonal shifts, may account for these problems," says PMS researcher Dr. Sally Severino. She believes that learning "sleep hygiene," regular sleep habits, which helps avoid insomnia and other sleep problems, may be an effective nondrug therapy for PMS (see page 307).

LIGHT THERAPY: Exposure to bright light (using special visors or light boxes) is being tested for treating PMS and PMDD. Barbara L. Parry, M.D., associate director of Consultation-Liaison Psychiatry at the University of California, San Diego, Medical Center, believes that hormone-related disturbances in circadian rhythms may also contribute to premenstrual depression. She has found that levels of *melatonin*, a hormone secreted at night by the pineal gland, which regulates sleep, are significantly lower in women with premenstrual depression; melatonin is derived from serotonin. In preliminary studies, Dr. Parry has found that light therapy (coupled with changing one's sleep patterns) reduces premenstrual depression.

ANTIDEPRESSANT/ANTIANXIETY DRUGS: These have recently been tested in large-scale, randomized trials for treating PMDD.

Selective serotonin reuptake inhibitors (SSRIs) have been found to be effective, presumably because of their serotonin-boosting effects. A major randomized clinical trial from Canada, reported in 1995 in the *New England Journal of Medicine*, compared the effects of *fluoxetine* (*Prozac*) and placebo in 313 women aged twenty to forty-five. The study found that both low and high doses of fluoxetine taken over six menstrual cycles helped to relieve tension, irritability and dysphoria in half of the women who took it, compared with less than a quarter of those who took the placebo. (The study was sponsored by Eli Lilly, which makes Prozac.) Smaller studies also found fluoxetine effective for PMDD.

However, women in all the studies complained of side effects (especially at higher doses) such as insomnia, headache, shakiness, dizziness, loss of sex drive and difficulty reaching orgasm. In fact, forty-seven women in the Canadian trial dropped out because of unpleasant side effects.

A recent twelve-site trial of the SSRI *sertraline* (*Zoloft*) among 162 women found that 70 percent of the women showed a significant response to treatment over three menstrual cycles, compared with less than 40 percent on placebo. Only a handful of the women dropped out due to side effects.

Several randomized, placebo-controlled trials have shown that the antianxiety drug *alprazolam* (*Xanax*) given during the luteal phase of the menstrual cycle helps relieve some PMS-related symptoms, as well as PMDD-related anxiety, irritability, severe tension and feelings of being out of control. Most recently, a 1995 study of 170 women at the University of Pennsylvania found that alprazolam reduced PMS symptoms by at least half in more than a third of the women who took it.

Ellen W. Freeman, Ph.D., director of the PMS Program at the University of Pennsylvania Hospital, says the findings support earlier research that progesterone, still given for PMS, is no more effective than placebo for women with severe PMS or PMDD.

Buspirone (*BuSpar*) is another anxiolytic drug shown to be somewhat effective in PMS, compared with placebo. Other studies have shown that the tricyclic antidepressant nortriptyline can relieve depressive symptoms associated with PMS. However, lithium has been found to be ineffective.

A preliminary study by the Medical College of Virginia found that women suffering *premenstrual mood exacerbation* (*PME*) can also be successfully treated with antidepressants.

TREATING POSTPARTUM DEPRESSION

Most cases of postpartum depression are treated similarly to major depression, with medication and/or some form of psychotherapy. Recent studies indicate that women with antepartum or postpartum depression can be treated with a modified form of interpersonal therapy (IPT), stressing role transitions and changes in priorities related to being a new mother.

At the New York State Psychiatric Institute's Maternal Mental Health Program, pregnant women are offered a special program of IPT for sixteen weeks, with maintenance sessions offered throughout the pregnancy. Close monitoring is also needed because some antidepressant medications can cause birth defects or developmental problems. Experts say that some antidepressants, including tricyclics, are secreted only in minute amounts in breast milk and can be safely given to nursing mothers (see page 283). However, even small amounts of medication may effect the developing central nervous system, cautions Dr. Spinelli.

Recent research also indicates that antidepressants started immediately *after* delivery may help reduce the recurrence of postpartum major depression. A pilot study by Katherine L. Wisner, M.D., now director of Women's Services, Mood Disorders Program, and an associate professor of psychiatry and reproductive medicine at Case Western Reserve University, found that women can sharply cut their risk by taking antidepressants within twenty-four hours of giving birth and continuing for three months afterward. The 1994 study, done at the Western Psychiatric Institute and Clinic in Pittsburgh, involved twenty-three pregnant women, all of whom had had at least one prior episode of postpartum major depression; fifteen of the women opted for prophylactic medication. Only one of the women on medication suffered a recurrence of PPMD after birth, compared with five of the eight women who did not take medication. (Two of the women became depressed *during* pregnancy and took medication.) The National Institute of Mental Health has begun a larger, placebo-controlled clinical trial to find out whether an antidepressant (amitriptyline) given immediately postpartum will prevent recurrent PPMD.

Previous research has also shown that lithium given after giving birth can help prevent postpartum psychosis. Lithium is not given during pregnancy (it can cause birth defects) or during breast-feeding. Treatment for postpartum psychosis may include other medications, electroconvulsive therapy and psychotherapy, as well as interventions to help family members. Once a woman has had an episode of postpartum psychosis, there's a 30 to 50 percent chance of a recurrence with each subsequent delivery, so prophylactic medication may be given.

There are recent indications that estrogen therapy may be helpful in treating PPMD. Researchers in Britain found that estrogen patches used after delivery helped lift postpartum depression. The study, reported in *The Lancet* in 1996, involved 61 women, 34 of whom wore estrogen patches and 27 who wore placebo patches for three months after delivery. Eighty percent of women using estrogen were no longer clinically depressed after 3 months, compared with 69 percent of the control group. Dr. Deborah Sichel has also studied the use of high dose estrogen in women with clear postpartum illness. "We had a really good success rate, with a relapse rate of only 10 to 20 percent. So there may be something in stemming the tide of the estrogen drop after delivery that may be protective in some way," she reports.

For treating OCD, Dr. Sichel and colleagues have found that SSRIs are very effective, but must be given in doses two to three times higher than used for treating depression. Treating anxiety and depression during pregnancy can be problematic, since medications may affect the fetus. For more on antidepressants and other medications during pregnancy and postpartum, see page 283.

EASING MIDLIFE DYSPHORIA

Certain drugs can help women with menopausal symptoms causing dysphoria. Chief among them is estrogen. But high-dose progestins and medications like *bellergal*, a combination of belladonna, ergotamine and phenobarbital, often used to treat stomach problems and certain kinds of headaches, can ease hot flashes and other vasomotor symptoms.

If a woman experiences depression at this phase in her life, she will be prescribed antidepressants. Some studies suggest that estrogen may improve mood in some women, perhaps by boosting serotonin, but estrogen is not a treatment for depression.

Some recent studies also suggest—but do not yet prove—that estrogen replacement therapy (ERT) may help improve memory. Studies at McGill University and at the Stanford University School of Medicine suggest that ERT may enhance short-term memory and the ability to learn new tasks in postmenopausal women, compared with women not taking estrogen. The researchers say the actual effects of estrogen, while not great, might be enough to enable a woman who takes estrogen after menopause to remember names, phone numbers and directions a little better.

Other recent studies hint that estrogen may offer some protection against memory loss and even Alzheimer's disease. In a study of more than twenty-five hundred women by the University of Southern California, Los Angeles, Alzheimer's disease was found to be 30 percent less common in women who had been taking estrogen replacement, compared with women who did not. Other studies have found that women on ERT scored higher on cognitive tests. Estrogen may foster increased blood flow to the brain due to improved cardiovascular health, increase energy uptake in the brain, and positively affect brain chemicals and brain cells themselves. Clinical trials of estrogen for both prevention and treatment of Alzheimer's are now under way.

Replacement hormones not only have the benefit of preventing coronary artery disease and reducing the discomfort of menopausal symptoms but also prevent vaginal dryness, genital atrophy and bone loss. At the same time, other drugs can also stave off osteoporosis and reduce the risk of heart disease. However, replacement hormones are *not* for every woman. They may slightly increase the risk of breast cancer; taking estrogen alone causes excessive cell growth in the lining of the uterus that can become cancerous, so progestins are added to prevent that. Some women have few or no menopausal symptoms and are not at high risk for heart disease or osteoporosis. Each woman should discuss the benefits and risks of hormone replacement with her physician.

CHAPTER 11

A Woman's Life Cycle

During each phase of a woman's life, there are many factors that can affect mental well-being. Some reproductive milestones carry their own special stresses: puberty, pregnancy and menopause. Those events are also affected by the way we perceive them, and further impacted by the society we live in. For example, at puberty, girls experience major changes in their body and body image at the same time that their social roles are changing, and they can suffer a marked decline in self-esteem. As many as one third may suffer from depression, and up to 3 percent develop anorexia or bulimia.

Rates of depression peak between the ages of eighteen and thirty-four, when important issues include finding satisfying work, making reproductive decisions and balancing work and family life. This stressful balancing act can lead to depression and anxiety.

New data indicate that depression rises again in women during the mid-life transition, ages forty-five to fifty-four. How a woman views the end of her reproductive years and aging can determine, in part, how well she copes. However, menopause itself is no longer seen as a cause for depression (or as a quasi-illness and the end of a woman's sexuality). In fact, many women see this period as a time of renewed energy and new directions.

The fastest-growing segment of the population is people over age sixty-five. While the rates of depression decline in later life, all of us must cope with aging, and more women than men will spend their older years alone after the death of a spouse.

New psychosocial stresses, such as the impact of infertility and the use of assisted reproductive technology, have only come into play in recent years. "Many of the people I see in my practice have what might be called 'adjustment reactions.' Their depression may be substantial, but it has been precipitated by a specific life event," says Veva H. Zimmerman, M.D., associate professor of clinical psychiatry and associate dean of the NYU School of Medicine. "These are people who have gone through a divorce, lost a job or are having trouble handling important transitions, such as infertility or as midlife," says Dr. Zimmerman. "While I may prescribe medication, what's usually needed is some form of psychotherapy to help them work through life issues which are causing emotional pain, and find ways to deal with them."

Experts suggest that while men and women respond in similar ways to life stresses, women may encounter more stressful situations in the months before a bout of major depression, and therefore experience more "situational" depressions.

This chapter will look at new views and new research into how life cycle events affect women's mental well-being.

ADOLESCENCE: THE AGE OF SELF-DOUBT

For many girls, the energy, optimism and self-confidence of childhood dissolve into agonizing self-doubt during adolescence. "Girls enter adolescence with an edge over boys. They have done better in elementary school, have better social skills and are generally bursting with confidence about the future. But these good feelings vanish, as girls are hit with the hormonal and physical changes of puberty amid very mixed sociocultural messages," says clinical psychologist Carol J. Eagle, Ph.D., head of Child/Adolescent Psychology at Montefiore Medical Center in New York, and coauthor of *All That She Can Be: Helping Your Daughter Maintain Her Self-Esteem* (Fireside, 1994).

While boys are taught to measure their success in strength, athletic and academic accomplishments, for girls success is often conferred by attractiveness and popularity. While boys gain muscle, girls gain fat around the hips and thighs, and their new bodies rarely conform to the dominant female ideal of being tall and slim, leading to constant dieting and eating disorders. Because of the emphasis on looks, girls often stop taking pride in more tangible strengths and accomplishments. Girls' devaluation of their capabilities is often reinforced by the increased attention boys typically receive in class, says Dr. Eagle. The resulting "silencing" fosters low self-esteem and underlies many cases of depression. Preliminary data from studies at Stanford University on coping styles show that girls begin to adopt a passive "ruminative response" to stress before puberty, leading to more adolescent depression.

Physical changes can also be abrupt and disturbing. Menstruation comes on suddenly; it can be painful and embarrassing. Breasts often develop before a girl is able to understand and cope with her own sexuality. Sexuality is often taught in terms of saying no, rather than making good choices. "Girls who don't feel good about their bodies and their sexuality don't feel good about themselves, and this can carry over well into adulthood," says Dr. Eagle.

Depression in teenagers can be hard to spot because teenagers often "act out," or cover their feelings with anger, rebelliousness, drinking or using drugs, breaking rules and even running away. Unfortunately, such behavior may often be seen as part of the "normal" turmoil of the teen years. But radical mood or behavior changes can be warning signs of depression, says Dr. Eagle. Depression may also show itself as boredom or apathy, with girls losing interest in friends or activities. And, experts note, because this decade of life is so full of energy, a child may be depressed but only show it intermittently.

Red Flags: Teen Depression

Source: National Institute of Mental Health, Depression/Awareness, Recognition, Treatment, (D/ART) Program

Warning signs of teenage depression include:

- Expressing feelings of sadness, emptiness, pessimism, guilt, worthlessness.

- Sudden behavior change such as restlessness, irritability, inability to concentrate, wanting to be alone all the time, withdrawing from friends, drinking heavily or taking drugs.

(continued)

- Losing interest or pleasure in hobbies, sports or ordinary activities like talking on the phone.

- Cutting classes; dropping out of after-school activities.

- Increased problems with school and family; a sudden drop in grades.

- Sleeping too much or having trouble falling asleep.

- Appetite problems: losing or gaining weight.

- Unexplained headaches, stomachaches, aches and pains in joints and muscles.

- Talking about death or suicide, giving away possessions, writing suicide notes.

Untreated depression increases the danger of suicide. The rate of suicide among fifteen- to twenty-four-year-olds has increased 200 percent nationwide in the past decade; it is the second leading cause of death among teenagers. Some surveys show that *half* of all teenagers have thought about killing themselves; 5 to 10 percent attempt suicide.

Many teens try suicide impulsively, viewing life as an all-or-nothing proposition, seeing every setback as permanent. Teenagers may also attempt suicide to get attention, or they may be influenced by a friend's suicide, or by drug or alcohol abuse.

Parents can play a vital role in helping their daughters avoid the downward slide into low self-esteem and depression. "Encourage preadolescent and teenage girls to achieve, to be assertive, to learn active coping and problem-solving skills, as well as develop her intellect and pursue her own goals, because these are the things which confer success in the adult world," advises Dr. Eagle. "By being advocates for our daughters, we can send confident, self-assured and, most importantly, happy young adult women out into the world."

Faye's Story, Continued

"I'm willing to bet anxiety and panic attacks are common among women my age. . . . We all came up believing that we could have it all. . . . But at some point, you realize this is not physically possible . . . and there's sort of a freedom that comes with that realization. . . . I'm at peace with the choices I've made. . . . You have to keep reinventing yourself and finding new goals instead of sticking to what you think you 'should' be doing. . . .

"Recovering from panic attacks was the most difficult thing I've ever had to deal with. But it . . . forced me to examine what I was about and what I was doing. . . . I think I'm better now at the things that are important to me, being a mom, being a wife. . . . Since I made the decision to work three days a week, I'm less conflicted . . . and I am much more able to cope with pressure."

A WOMAN'S WORKING LIFE

Women in their twenties, thirties, and forties face numerous choices and challenges as they juggle work and family responsibilities, often including the care of an aging or ailing relative. The much ballyhooed "superwoman" of the 1980s has given way to a more realistic appraisal of women's many life roles. Recent research indicates that "role overload" is less a matter of the *number* of roles a woman has than of the time, pressures and work they entail.

More than half of women with children under three years of age now work outside the home, compared with one in four women back in 1970. The number increases to 75 percent among women with school-age children and teenagers.

A 1993 survey by the Families and Work Institute (FWI) of 3,381 workers aged eighteen to sixty-four (half were in their thirties or forties)—the first survey of its kind since 1977—showed that among women with children under age six, more than half felt it would be difficult for their families to manage without their paycheck. And even though women now contribute half (or more) of a family's income, the FWI survey found that women's traditional role as the primary "caretaker" of the family has not changed.

An overwhelming number of women work a "second shift" at home—a factor high on the list of special stresses that working women face. The only area where men took on *more* responsibility was the traditional male bastion of household repairs. Men took on fewer household chores if their wives were homemakers. Younger men did about the same amount of housework as their older counterparts.

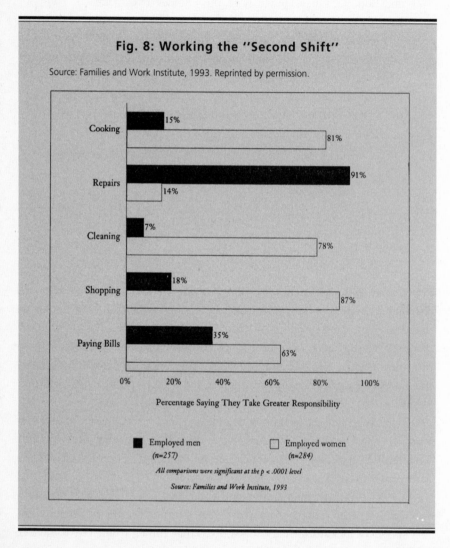

Fig. 8: Working the "Second Shift"

Source: Families and Work Institute, 1993. Reprinted by permission.

Percentage Saying They Take Greater Responsibility

■ Employed men
(n=257)

□ Employed women
(n=284)

All comparisons were significant at the p < .0001 level

Source: Families and Work Institute, 1993

Overall, the FWI study found that women spent almost forty-two hours a week on job-related activities (including overtime and commuting), and *another* twenty-one hours a week devoted to chores and children, five hours more than men. Men spent seven more hours a week than women on activities related to their jobs. A 1997 update found some things changing for the better, with men taking on somewhat more household chores and child care duties, and sharing equally in elder care. Still, 43 percent of the women said they wished men would do more around the house. Working mothers and fathers both complained that they don't have enough time to spend with their children, and wished that they could work fewer hours.

Working long hours at home *and* at the office was a major cause of role stress in studies presented at a 1994 conference on Psychosocial and Behavioral Factors in Women's Health sponsored by the American Psychological Association. Among the other causes of work-family stress:

- Having a high-prestige job (which often demands long hours).

- Working primarily because of financial needs.

- Having a spouse who is less available to help with family emergencies during working hours (and child care after hours).

- Dissatisfaction with child care arrangements. Sixty-two percent of parents in the FWI survey reported that finding reliable child care was a major problem.

But often it's the *quality* of a woman's home life that's the key in role overload, says Nancy L. Marshall, Ed.D., a senior research scientist at the Center for Research on Women at Wellesley College in Massachusetts. "When there are problems at home, either in the marriage or with the children, women are more likely to be depressed and in poor health," says Dr. Marshall.

A study of 250 working mothers (whose average age was thirty-seven) by the University of Montreal also found that satisfaction with child care helped reduce the stress felt by working women. Higher-income, better-educated workers have more access to quality child care, flexible hours, leave programs and dependent adult care assistance, as well as health insurance and pension plans, making their lives a bit easier (if not always less stressful), than people with fewer resources.

But women with hectic work schedules and work demands, low levels of control and fewer opportunities to make decisions and use their skills suffer more stress, anxiety, depression and other health problems. "The more control a woman feels at work, the more her sense of control over the environment increases. And this sense of control is linked to a sense of competence and self-esteem, and a lessened risk of depression," Lynn Weber, Ph.D., founder and director of the Center for Research on Women at the University of Memphis, reported to the APA conference.

Women also face different occupational stresses than men: They earn less than men with the same job titles and responsibilities, are usually restricted to low-paying service occupations (the "pink-collar ghetto") and are often faced with a work environment that does not acknowledge or support family needs, whose safety standards are based on the needs of men and that continues to tolerate sexual harassment.

While many women are locked into jobs for financial or insurance reasons, changing jobs (or reducing hours) may be a matter of preserving mental and physical health.

Interestingly, Dr. Marshall notes, while having children is associated with greater work-family strains, *not* having children was directly associated with greater depression, at least for some women. (Many studies do not find increased depression among women who choose to be childless.) "For women whose experiences at work and at home are, on balance, positive, the joys of having children, and the gains from combining work and family, make it possible to tolerate the strains from the demands of multiple roles."

ꙮ *Miranda's Story* ꙮ

"It took me quite a while to come to terms with my infertility, and mourn that loss. . . . The miscarriages were particularly hard. . . . You're thrilled to be pregnant . . . and then it's failure again, it's the loss of your hopes, the loss of your dreams. . . . You wonder, 'will this ever happen?'

"I always felt that if I worked hard enough, and tried different things, somehow I could overcome anything. And . . . here I was, struggling with my inability to conceive, feeling I had no control over anything. . . . And no one is saying to us, 'Enough is enough. Stop.' . . . It is simply how much can you afford, and when have you had enough. . . . You're also into the technology. We think technology solves everything. . . . If twenty percent of the people are getting pregnant, they tell you at the clinic, maybe my turn is up next. And it's very seductive. I would go through two months of being fine, and then maybe the third or fourth month, I would be so down in the dumps.

"We had finally decided to adopt just about the time I got pregnant. . . . We were in a support group with other couples who were infertile and were going to adopt. And a lot of people were struggling with the lack of genetic connection. . . . Because my parents had died . . . that was a hard thing for me to accept, that . . . I would never have a piece of my parents, somehow. But once I got through the mourning, and understood what I really wanted, and came out the other side . . . I realized that I can perpetuate my parents in other ways. I can pass along the family stories, the values. . . . So we went through with the adoption and we now have two beautiful children, ten months apart. And I cannot imagine my life without them."

A MATTER OF FERTILITY

Most women take their ability to have children for granted. But an estimated one in every twelve women have trouble conceiving a child after a year of trying. Infertility is on the rise partly because women are delaying childbearing, and also because of the effects of sexually transmitted diseases. Other factors include medical problems, such as endometriosis. Recent research also indicates that stress may also affect fertility.

In about half of the cases, a woman may have ovulatory problems, blocked or scarred fallopian tubes, endometriosis, inability to sustain a pregnancy or infertility associated with older age. A third of the time, there may be problems with the man (too few sperm, low sperm motility or production of antibodies to sperm). In 5 to 15 percent of couples, *no* cause can be found.

More than 2.3 million couples seek help for infertility every year. Over half can be helped to have children. But the emotional impact of not being able to conceive can severely stress a marriage; the guilt, sense of inadequacy and strain of having their sexual relationship under medical scrutiny can lead to depression, anxiety and sexual dysfunction. The emotional toll is usually greater on women; one study found that almost half of women considered infertility the most upsetting experience of their lives, compared with only 15 percent of men.

"A woman may have her life planned out, how much time she will spend on her career before she starts a family, and all of a sudden that changes. There is also mourning for the loss of the anticipated family," remarks Dr. Gail Erlick Robinson, professor of psychiatry, obstetrics and gynecology at the University of Toronto, who has coauthored a number of studies on the effects of infertility and miscarriage.

Treatments can be intrusive, with a major burden falling on the woman: monitoring of her temperature to predict ovulation, daily doses or shots of fertility drugs, early-morning visits to the clinic each day, retrieval of eggs, insertion of sperm, implantation of an embryo. If the problem is with the husband, he may feel inadequate (many men equate impregnating a woman with proving their manhood) and guilty that his problem is forcing his wife to undergo treatment.

Miranda's emotional roller coaster of anticipation and disappointment is quite common. Fertility drugs can also cause side effects such as nausea, headaches, abdominal bloating and, as has been recently documented, a possible increased risk of ovarian cancer. Fertility specialists are often unwilling to tell couples when to stop. And the financial burden can be considerable.

Even when a woman becomes pregnant, says Dr. Robinson, she worries about miscarriage, the effects of prenatal testing and the possibility of birth defects, or multiple births.

"Women are often shocked and amazed to find out that having worked so hard to get pregnant, they have ambivalent feelings when they *do* conceive. . . . And they often can't express those feelings to anyone, because everyone is so horrified that they should feel that way," Dr. Robinson commented to a 1994 meeting of the American Psychiatric Association. If assisted reproduction fails, there may be adverse effects on marital relationship and sexual functioning, and a high incidence of depression.

Counseling (or psychotherapy) before and during infertility treatments may help alleviate many stresses and help couples make informed decisions about treatments. Infertility support groups can connect couples with others encountering the same problems.

MISCARRIAGE:
THE SAD SIDE OF FERTILITY

Between 14 to 18 percent of pregnancies end in miscarriage, usually during the first trimester. The immediate aftermath of miscarriage has been associated with depression, feelings of emptiness, guilt and anger. Miscarriages later in pregnancy may provoke more severe grief reactions. However, says

Dr. Robinson, "miscarriage tends to be treated as a medical event, rather than something that has an emotional impact on women's lives."

One of the few studies that has followed women for a long period after miscarriage was done by Dr. Robinson, Dr. Donna Stewart and colleagues at the Toronto Hospital. The 1994 study followed thirty-nine women at three months, six months and a year after their miscarriage. The study found that depression was elevated twelve weeks after the miscarriage, symptoms decreased at six months and then increased again at one year (possibly due to an "anniversary reaction"). "This pattern may cause physicians to falsely assume that women have recovered from their grief after six months, when that may not be the case," says Dr. Robinson.

Over 40 percent of the group felt the miscarriage was their fault. Those who felt guilty, or who felt that others blamed them for the miscarriage, were significantly more depressed. "The impact of miscarriage was irrespective of age or other living children," Dr. Robinson adds. "So we should not assume that if a woman is young, can still have other children or has other children, she will get over her grief faster."

Hospital-based perinatal bereavement teams and support groups can often be a substantial help after a miscarriage. "Some women are able to get through their grief within a few months, while others grieve for years," says Susan Toms, R.N.C., M.S., cofacilitator of the Perinatal Bereavement Support Group at the Montefiore Medical Center, Weiler Division in New York. "It is a baby from the minute they find out they're pregnant, and they are grieving for the loss of that baby and the future that baby represents," says Ms. Toms. Perinatal loss usually causes a great deal of self-blame, which is most often unfounded.

Up to 80 percent of early miscarriages are due to chromosomal abnormalities, stresses Charles J. Lockwood, M.D., chairman of Obstetrics and Gynecology at NYU Medical Center. *Luteal phase defects* (low levels of progesterone needed to sustain a pregnancy) may contribute to many of the remaining losses, he adds. Later miscarriages are mostly due to uterine abnormalities, premature membrane rupture and labor or "incompetent cervix," where the cervix is unable to stay closed during pregnancy. (A woman may also have an *ectopic*, or tubal, pregnancy, which must be removed before it ruptures.)

Unless advised not to, working up until a due date will *not* cause miscarriage, says Dr. Lockwood. Nor will physical activity, most physical injuries or sex during pregnancy. "Most pregnancies are well protected. Miscarriage is *never* the mother's fault," he emphasizes.

Losing a pregnancy during the third trimester, losing a child to stillbirth or in the neonatal period can be much more traumatizing than early miscarriage. One study found that almost a third of women who lost a baby through stillbirth were so depressed they considered suicide.

Families are usually supportive for a while, but after a certain point, they expect couples to get on with life. In many cases people are simply not ready, says Ms. Toms. They need to find other people who will reassure them that their grief is normal. "Men and women tend to grieve differently. A man may try to busy himself in work, and may not want to talk about it much, whereas a woman may tend to focus on the pregnancy loss for a longer time and express her grief more openly. This can cause a real rift."

Most important, women need to know that they are not alone, and that they *will* be able to move beyond their pain in their own time.

In general, studies do not find lasting negative psychological effects in women who have undergone abortions, although they may suffer short-term emotional problems: conflict over their decision, mourning or guilt. However, a preliminary study of women at the University of Maryland Obstetrical Genetics Clinic who underwent abortions because of fetal anomalies found that they initially denied being depressed about the abortion, but later admitted feeling depressed. Most abortion providers stress that patients need counseling before and afterward.

What Is an Adjustment Disorder?

Source: *Diagnostic and Statistical Manual of Mental Disorders, Fourth Edition (DSM-IV)*, 1994, American Psychiatric Association

Behavioral or emotional symptoms that arise from a specific stressful life event or situation are aptly called *adjustment disorders*. Symptoms, including depressed mood, anxiety or both, must develop within three months after the onset of the stressors. The reaction can be either pronounced or in excess of what would be expected given the nature of the life event or stressor, and must cause significant impairment in social or academic functioning. Problems may be acute, lasting a short time, or chronic, lingering for months.

An adjustment disorder can be diagnosed in the presence of another disorder (such as major depression) if that disorder does *not* account for the pattern of symptoms that have occurred in response to a stressful event. However, the diagnosis does *not* apply when the symptoms represent bereavement.

Stressors can be a single event, such as the loss of a job or a divorce, or multiple problems, such as business difficulties and resulting marital or sexual problems. Some stressors may accompany life cycle events, such as leaving home, getting married or retirement.

❧ *Francie's Story* ❧

"I had absolutely no problem with menopause. . . . I was busy working . . . my marriage was in good shape . . . I had very few symptoms. . . . I never even considered taking estrogen.

"My problem began after my firm started 'downsizing,' and I was one of the ones downsized out. . . . They called it a 'voluntary buyout,' but my leaving was as voluntary as getting the flu. . . . And what a shock it was to start looking for a new job at age fifty-four! I got the runaround from most of the search firms I contacted. . . . I'm an upbeat person, but that kind of rejection makes you feel angry, your whole self-esteem gets shot to hell. . . . Finally, an acquaintance who happened to work for a headhunter told me that most search firms were not handling people over forty-five . . . companies were hiring younger, cheaper and less experienced people.

"I eventually became a freelance consultant in my field, more out of necessity than any burning desire to have my own business. I just wanted to keep working. . . .

"It *never* occurred to me that age would become a factor [in my work life]. . . . Now somehow I've reached this arbitrary cutoff where other people decided that I am no longer as valuable. . . . And I'm damn angry! I'm the best I've ever been. . . . I want to know who the hell decided that fifty-plus is a minus!"

NEW MIDLIFE PASSAGES

It was once thought that menopause was the main event in midlife for women. But that's far from true. "The complaints women often have in midlife are not menopausal, but may be caused by life cycle crises that are independent of their biological functioning. But because of the way our society operates, we merge the two for women," says Carol C. Nadelson, M.D., a professor of psychiatry at Harvard University and editor in chief of the American Psychiatric Press.

"Menopause is no longer regarded as a hormonal deficiency 'disease,' but as a normal biological stage in a woman's life. The way a woman experiences this stage is largely related to culture, and to a woman's own personal feelings about aging."

Population studies by researchers around the world suggest that it is during the *perimenopause*, the transition period, rather than after menopause, that women experience increased depression. Why that may occur is currently under study.

A 1996 update from an ongoing study of over five hundred women in the Seattle area (including African-American and Asian-American women) involved in a long-term investigation of aging found that the actual transition to menopause or experiencing menopausal symptoms had only *modest* effects on women's psychological well-being. However, Nancy Fugate Woods, Ph.D., R.N., a professor of nursing, and colleagues at the Center for Women's Health Research at the University of Washington, Seattle, found that stressful life circumstances, negative socialization for midlife and poor health status had *much* stronger effects on stress and depression.

"Positive socialization for midlife was directly associated with less severe vasomotor symptoms. Many contemporary lay publications about menopause project a positive image of midlife and have reframed hot flashes as 'power surges.' It may well be that women exposed to these images find their symptoms less distressing," Dr. Woods and her coauthors write.

On the other hand, negative socialization for midlife—for example, viewing changes in appearance as a threat to self-image—was very much related to emotional distress and to increased experience of symptoms such as hot flashes, reports Dr. Woods. Poor health status also had an effect on depression, as women perhaps felt sad about a diagnosis of chronic disease.

Women whose menopause was caused by removal of the ovaries or cancer therapy have a sudden, early menopause and more severe symptoms.

Symptoms of menopause also can be culturally influenced. In many nonindustrialized societies, older women are given greater authority, respect and social freedom. Such women experience few or no menopausal symptoms, even though they are undergoing the same biological process, Dr. Nadelson points out. By contrast, in most Western industrialized countries, where youth is valued over age, women experience more severe symptoms. Menopause becomes a symbol of loss, so women may feel less valuable . . . and suffer as a result.

In Asian cultures, age confers wisdom. Studies in Japan reveal that only 20 percent of women have ever experienced hot flashes, compared with 60 to 70 percent of American women. There isn't even a word for hot flashes in the Japanese language! Similarly, in studies among Navajo women, only 17 percent have hot flashes. In Native American culture, longevity also confers prestige; older women's wisdom and opinions are highly valued.

"With the availability of estrogen [therapy], many women pass through menopause with very little physical discomfort and loss of libido," observes Carol Feit Lane, Ph.D., a psychologist and women's midlife counselor at NYU Medical Center Women's Health Service. "However, menopause is a powerful biological marker which does signal the end to a woman's youthful, reproductive capacity. That marker is dramatic. And whether it functions on a conscious or unconscious level, it can have a powerful emotional effect," she says.

"The women who seem to have the most difficulty with menopause seem to be those who are most invested in their childbearing role. . . . This is particularly true if other roles and opportunities are not available," says Dr. Malkah Notman, clinical professor of psychiatry at the Cambridge Hospital and Harvard Medical School. If a woman is unmarried or childless, an approaching menopause brings a clear end to possibilities, says Dr. Notman, while for perimenopausal women, there may be an added push to have children. "However, for those who can find new roles, midlife and menopause can be a period of blossoming."

It was once believed that the "empty nest" caused depression in menopausal women. But that myth may be turned on its head these days. Women are having children later in life, many children go to school longer and young adults remain at home because of economics. Some adult children move back with their parents after a divorce or economic loss, so the nest may be *bulging*, rather than empty, and stress may be a result.

Many midlife women are also caught in the so-called sandwich generation, caring for children and aging parents at the same time. That can also cause added stress.

Another major concern for many midlife women is physical appearance, since society places such a high value on youthful beauty. Dozens of beauty products earn billions, marketed with promises "to minimize the visual effects of aging." The American Society of Plastic and Reconstructive Surgeons estimates that each year over 230,000 women undergo facelifts, eyelid surgery, liposuction and tummy tucks, as well as collagen injections to plump out sagging skin, among other cosmetic procedures.

"My own personal theory is that the more physically attractive a woman has been, or the more attention she has gotten for her looks when she was younger, the harder it is for her to adjust to changes that take place in the body during aging," says Dr. Lane. "But I think many women's perceptions that they are less attractive are often distorted. They often perceive physical changes as being much worse, or meaning much more, than they actually may mean to other people in their lives."

Career and employment changes are among the common issues seen in midlife women nowadays. "Some women may be feeling burned out in their jobs, or feel that they're not making enough progress, or they're afraid they may be phased out of a job because they are getting older," says Dr. Lane.

As Francie noted, many companies jettison their most experienced workers as part of economic "downsizing," because younger, less skilled workers simply cost less. It's more common for men to become underemployed, or unemployed, as they age; many women find themselves working more often in their later years (albeit in lower-paying service jobs) out of economic necessity. It's estimated that by the year 2005, over half of women aged fifty-five to sixty-four will still be in the labor force.

The good news is that women seem to have more flexibility than men to deal with midlife changes. One reason may be that they have been keeping close track of the passage of time and its cyclic events in their body through different stages of life, says NYU psychiatrist Virginia Sadock. "It begins when a woman has her first period. She keeps track of her monthly cycles. She may plan things around her period. She is aware of when she is most likely to conceive a child. When she becomes pregnant, she counts the months until the child is born. Then she marks the time when her periods stop. For men, time may be a work deadline, or a dreaded birthday. But women have a different sense of time."

This is one reason why men are often more likely than women to have a "midlife crisis," Dr. Sadock says. In some respects, men may be less aware than women of the year-to-year changes in themselves, until they hit forty, fifty or sixty, and suddenly perceive their lives as changed. An illness or a death in the family may make them acutely aware of their own mortality.

"Women may be looking ahead, see their potential expanding after years of child-rearing and juggling responsibilities. Men may be looking backward, seeing their roles as diminished, and wonder, 'Is this all there is? What have I accomplished in life?' "

While both sexes are sensitive to life's losses, the types of losses that hit harder at self-esteem and hope may be different. "Men are more profoundly affected by things that happen in their working life, while women are more profoundly affected by things that happen at home and in their social networks," says Dr. Sadock.

A woman often comes through midlife and menopause with a second wind, she observes. Some call it "postmenopausal zest." "A woman has the energy, ability and freedom to do things she didn't have before. She no longer has the monthly cycle to go through, and she doesn't have the children to raise. This may be the time of a woman's life when she begins to fulfill ambitions or interests kept on hold. If she's financially able, she may travel or continue her education. For many women, midlife can be a time of new beginnings."

THE CHALLENGES OF LATER LIFE

In *New Passages: Mapping Your Life Across Time* (Random House, 1995), Gail Sheehy comments that medical advances and longer life expectancies have opened up new territories for people in their fifties, sixties and beyond. She calls these years a "Second Adulthood," describing it as a "potential rebirth that offers exhilarating possibilities" rather than the "depressing downslide we have always assumed it to be." It is, she says, a time of mastery and knowing what's important in life.

Indeed, older age can be a time of change and challenges. Some changes are welcome. Retirement may be possible for some of us, but it is no longer a universal goal. Some women find new fulfillment in volunteer work, going back to school or even second careers. Grandparenting can bring special joy.

Other life events present major challenges. The physical changes of aging can be tough for some women to adjust to. There may be chronic illness in oneself or a family member, or the death of a partner or other loved ones.

Women are more likely to be divorced or lose their partners in later life. Women also have longer life expectancies than men, and many live out those extra years alone. In 1992, a third of all women aged sixty-five to seventy-five lived alone and about half lived with their spouses, compared with over 77 percent of men still living with spouses, and only 13 percent who lived alone.

However, the idea that the older years are mainly characterized by loss and depression is no longer totally true for most people, emphasizes Michael L. Freedman, M.D., the Diane and Arthur Belfer Professor of Geriatric Medicine and director of the Division of Geriatrics at NYU Medical Center. Many older people remain in robust health; only 10 percent of people over sixty-five have chronic health problems that restrict physical activity.

Women seem to do a better job than men of taking care of their health, notes Dr. Freedman. Women also seem to maintain more emotional resiliency in their later years. "Most women I have seen rebound from losses, and have many social networks to keep them going, friends, relatives. Women are much better at forming and maintaining these networks than men, and that's one thing that makes a big difference to their mental and physical health in later life," he says.

Recent studies emphasize that other secrets to staying "young" include keeping active physically (which can help stave off bone loss and heart disease), as well as staying active intellectually, says Dr. Freedman. "Many women I see who are in their eighties are still taking classes, going to museums, going to the theater, playing cards, traveling. These are all things that maintain vibrancy in older age."

For some women, replacement hormones can make a difference. "Estrogen replacement not only can relieve menopausal symptoms and some of the physical problems, such as urinary incontinence. But estrogen does seem to improve mood, and there are suggestions it may help improve or even preserve mental functioning."

DEPRESSION IN LATE LIFE

While the prevalence of major depression decreases with age, it is still more common in women. Experts say this phenomenon is mainly seen in the "cohort" of people born in the 1920s and, to some degree, in those born before World War II; rates may eventually rise as baby boomers reach older age.

Depression among older people is most often "situational," such as reaction to the death of a spouse or child. Women are more likely to be taking care of an ailing spouse or relative, and those pressures can take a toll. Late life depression may be a recurrence of earlier episodes, including postpartum or premenstrual depression. Americans over age 65 now account for one-fifth of the nation's thirty thousand yearly suicides.

Overall, perhaps 1 to 2 percent of elderly people suffer from major depression, and up to 12 percent have less severe, but still significant, degrees of depression. But, according to the American Association of Geriatric Psychiatry, less than half of those people are being diagnosed correctly. And half of those who *are* properly diagnosed are not getting help, says Ira R. Katz, M.D., Ph.D., professor of geriatric psychiatry at the University of Pennsylvania Medical Center.

"The signs of depression can be subtle in the elderly and they can be missed. But more often, they are considered by patients, families and doctors as 'normal.' If someone is eighty years old and disabled, why shouldn't they be depressed, people tend to say. But that's just not true. Depression in late life is an illness, just as in younger people," stresses Dr. Katz.

It's not uncommon for older women not to complain of *any* mood changes at all. Instead, they may see doctors for a variety of vague physical complaints, for which no cause can be found, although the symptoms are quite real. An older woman may complain of low energy, or that she no longer enjoys things she used to.

Classic symptoms of late life depression include withdrawal, loss of interest in normal activities, tearfulness, fixation with pain or disease, weight loss, sleep problems, preoccupation with death, a wish for life to end or even talk of suicide.

Many older persons with moderately severe depression complain of poor concentration. They are easily distracted and may misplace objects. Symptoms of depression, including memory problems, may also imitate disease, including Alzheimer's disease. However, less than 10 percent of depressed patients over sixty-five years of age have cognitive impairment that could be confused with dementia or Alzheimer's disease.

Many normal elderly people wake up earlier than they would like because sleep patterns become disrupted later in life. But depressed older people may complain that they cannot sleep through the night, awakening repeatedly and having trouble getting back to sleep.

Depression in later life often coexists with chronic illness or disability, or is brought on by disability or medical illnesses such as cancer or heart disease. So depression needs to be treated as a separate entity. "What's not as obvious is that depression can *lead* to disability. One study of older women hospitalized for hip fracture noted that those who were depressed in the hospital after their surgery were *less* likely to be up and walking a year after the surgery than those who were not depressed," says Dr. Katz. "Depression can also amplify medical symptoms in older patients, especially pain, and may make drug side effects less tolerable."

Depressed older people stay in the hospital longer and go to doctors more often. Studies also show they are more likely to die in the year after a heart attack, and die more quickly of other diseases.

An older person with depressive symptoms needs a complete medical evaluation, including all current medications, both prescription and over-the-counter, since many have depressive side effects. A complete blood count, a vitamin B_{12} assay, and thyroid-function studies can also help identify medical illnesses that may cause symptoms of depression.

Antidepressants must be used carefully, since many older patients are taking other drugs to control chronic conditions, such as high blood pressure, and elderly people often metabolize drugs more slowly (see Chapter 13).

Almost 8 percent of adults over age sixty-five may have a psychiatric disorder (including major depression) that requires treatment. But only about 40 percent receive treatment. Those who do are more likely to receive care from a primary care physician, and a majority receive psychotropic medications alone.

Some older patients may hesitate to seek help because of lingering stigmas about mental illness and psychotherapy. But in general, older people respond to treatment just as well as their younger counterparts. There is an increased risk of depression recurring after age sixty, perhaps as high as 25 percent—many older people benefit from some form of maintenance therapy.

At the same time, Dr. Robert Cancro, who chairs the Department of Psychiatry at NYU, cautions against associating *all* the emotional upsets of older life with depression. "There's a difference between being sad and being sick. Many people find aging upsetting, no one enjoys having arthritis, no one enjoys the loss of vigor, or of friends and spouses, or coming to terms with your own mortality. But that kind of sadness doesn't *always* mean you have a depressive illness."

⌖ Pat's Story, Continued ⌖

"For a long time after my husband died, I would start to cry every time I would drive by the place where he worked. . . . But I couldn't always avoid it. I couldn't go into the men's department of a department store—my throat would close up and I would feel a choking sensation. People who haven't been through it just can't empathize with that kind of thing. The best thing that happened to me was going to a grief recovery group.

"There were ten or twelve people who had all recently lost a loved one. . . . One woman told of how she kept seeing a car that she thought was her husband's. She would follow it for blocks hoping to get a glimpse of him. . . . It was the greatest relief to be able to spill out all these crazy feelings and see everybody nod and then tell their own similar stories. . . .

"At the last session, they brought back two 'graduates' from the year before. A man who had lost his wife told us something valuable: that we should not try to second-guess whatever actions and decisions we had made during the person's illness. That whatever we did was what we thought best at the time, and we had to accept that. Because we couldn't change it. That was a big thing, because almost everyone had some regrets about what they did or didn't do. . . .

"The grief recovery group also gave me someplace that I had to go. It made me get dressed and get out . . . among people, even at night. That helped to show me that I could do things by myself. . . . Little by little, I started doing more.

"My husband was the only man I'd ever loved. . . . We had been married for forty-one years when he died. It's been nine years, and I still think about him every day and miss him. You don't ever get over losing someone, you just learn to live with it and go forward. That's all you can do."

DEALING WITH LOSSES

There is no way to avoid loss in life. For women, the loss of a spouse (or a child) ranks as life's most stressful event. However, some studies indicate that women are less likely than men to suffer major depression or "complicated" grief after the death of a spouse (see page 247).

As the general population ages, some experts estimate that 75 percent of married women will experience widowhood and, because of women's longer life expectancies, may remain alone for an average of eighteen years afterward. Nearly half of women over age sixty-five are widows; more than 81 percent over age eighty-five are widows.

Unfortunately, because our culture is fearful of death, many people do not receive the emotional and social support they need to help them through grief and mourning.

Various religions and cultures have rituals surrounding death, which provide some comfort. Many Christians believe in heaven. People of the Hindu faith believe they will be reincarnated; other groups believe the dead will eventually be resurrected.

Even so, any death produces grief. And mourning is usually a solitary process. There are several stages to the grieving process. First, there may be shock and denial ("This can't be happening!"), followed by anger ("Why did this have to happen?"), depression and guilt ("If I had only done more . . .") and finally acceptance and adaptation ("I've got to get on with my life").

Most people equate mourning with depression, but they're not the same thing, says Dr. Freedman. The intense signs of mourning typically lift within a certain period of time, as do feelings of sadness and loss. Major depression caused by bereavement is usually diagnosed when depressive symptoms persist for at least two months. New studies indicate that anxiety can occur as a separate disorder in bereavement, and may predict later depression.

A typical grief reaction begins with numbness and inability to accept the loss. Then reality finally hits—often with physical force. There may be feelings of gnawing emptiness in the pit of the stomach, a feeling of suffocation, shortness of breath, difficulty swallowing or having a "lump in the throat," along with deep sighing, emotional distress and tearfulness. Some people feel a sense of unreality, and may even believe they see the deceased person (or act as if they were still there).

Normal activities are disrupted; the person wanders around aimlessly, often unable to work or make social contact, filled with anxiety and longing. There may be deep feelings of depression and despair. It's common to lose one's appetite, and to suffer insomnia or digestive problems. "Sometimes an older woman may come with physical complaints, when their real problem is unresolved grief. They may just need someone to talk to, and that person often turns out to be their physician," says Dr. Freedman.

In an "uncomplicated" bereavement, the acute phase generally lasts two to three months, and then slowly starts to lessen (although each individual is different, depending on their upbringing, ethnicity and culture). " 'Healthy grief' does not interfere with going on with your life. You are able to develop new strategies and remake your life without that person. It isn't that you're not sad, or don't think about the person, but you go on," says Dr. Freedman. "People who experience situational depression after the death of a loved one may well have an underlying biological vulnerability."

New research suggests that among the strongest predictors of depression after bereavement in women are anxiety, disturbed sleep and low levels of self-esteem and social support. Early intervention with medication can often help patients work through their grief without suffering depressive symptoms. However, it will *not* reduce the intensity of grief. For most people, time usually takes care of that.

Sometimes, however, time does *not* heal sorrow. Abnormal grief reactions can intensify over time, or even be delayed for months or years. A person may feel excessive guilt about the illness or death of a partner, and have a morbid preoccupation with death. Researchers recently identified a new form of bereavement-related distress, apart from depression or anxiety—a syndrome they call *complicated grief.* Complicated grief is a distinct disorder, often lasting longer than the situational (or reactive) depressions of bereavement, which have also been shown to have serious, long-term health consequences.

According to Holly G. Prigerson, Ph.D., an assistant professor of psychiatry at the University of Pittsburgh School of Medicine and the Western Psychiatric Institute, complicated grief may actually be a variant of post-traumatic stress disorder. "It has a lot of the same intrusive thoughts, the avoidance behaviors, in this case avoiding reminders of the deceased, the hypervigilance, the nightmares and hallucinations, poor concentration. And we have seen symptoms in people eighteen months to thirty-five years after they have lost a spouse."

Other symptoms of complicated grief include preoccupation with thoughts of the deceased, disbelief, feeling stunned by the death and an inability to accept it, obsessive yearning or searching for the deceased, even having "identification symptoms," such as pain in the same part of the body experienced by the person who died.

Researchers at the University of Pittsburgh followed eighty-two men and women for eighteen months after the death of a spouse. Those people who had been suffering from complicated grief had more signs of depression, anxiety, low self-esteem, insomnia and overall poor functioning and health. Men with complicated grief in the first few months after the death of their partner were more likely to abuse alcohol, be hospitalized or have a heart attack, stroke or a severe accident. In contrast, women with high levels of complicated grief in the first few months after a loss were more likely to have sleep problems, heart attack or stroke.

There were other interesting gender differences. "The men start off having fewer symptoms of complicated grief. But after three years, men begin having more symptoms, while the women have fewer, as they start adjusting to the death of their spouse," Dr. Prigerson says. "Many men become enraged and bitter over the death but are unable to express those feelings. Women tend to express their emotions. That's possibly why they adapt better."

Other reasons why women adapt better than men have to do with the social networks women traditionally maintain, which protect against depression, and with mastering tasks usually performed by their spouse. "Women seem to have less trouble assuming the tasks men may have been traditionally responsible for, such as finances, than men do learning how to cook, clean and do laundry. Such 'mastery experiences,' which promote a sense of competency and self-sufficiency, are very important in the recovery process, and may also help avoid depression. Maintaining regular routines also appears to be protective," remarks Dr. Ellen Frank, a coauthor of the bereavement research.

Complicated grief may need totally different treatments than bereavement-related depression. Tricyclic antidepressants help depression but don't work effectively with complicated grief, says Dr. Prigerson. She speculates that psychotherapy based on treatments for PTSD may help complicated grief. For uncomplicated bereavement, widows and women who have lost a parent or a child may be able to work through their grief in self-help groups, as Pat did, or in interpersonal therapy (see page 265).

Other strategies for dealing with losses:

- Realize that certain things are truly out of your control.

- Don't wallow in regret. You did the best that you could in the situation. There is no use ruminating over "what if."

- Don't enshrine the past. Don't idealize an absent partner, so that no one else can ever measure up.

- Stay active and avoid isolation. Continue to do things you enjoy with friends, or find an interesting new activity where you can meet new people.

- Help others less fortunate than yourself. Volunteer work gets you out of the house and away from rumination and self-pity.

- Rekindle your faith. Belief in a higher power (whatever that may be for you) has sustained many people through loss.

- Retain your sense of humor. While there's nothing funny about losing someone you love, there is still much in life that can please us and make us laugh. The ability to laugh can carry you over many of life's roughest spots.

Remember, too, that loss is often a growth experience. Many people emerge from their grief as stronger individuals with a renewed appreciation for life and for those around them.

CHAPTER 12

Getting the Help You Need

If your own attempts to solve problems are getting nowhere, and if life doesn't seem to be getting better no matter what you do, it may be time to seek professional help.

However, a 1996 survey by the American Psychological Association found that many people don't know when or how to look for that help. A majority of the one thousand survey respondents (two thirds of whom were women) expressed concern about the cost of treatment and its effectiveness, as well as how long it would take and what effect it might have on their job or career.

Experts stress that psychotherapy, "talk therapy," can be *very* effective in helping you understand and resolve the problems that led to depression or anxiety, deal with stressful life events and change how you think about yourself and others. Behavioral techniques used in therapy help build better problem-solving and coping skills, a key to emotional resiliency.

Medication can assist psychotherapy by alleviating symptoms that interfere with daily functioning, and may indirectly act on emotions, says Dr. Robert Cancro, chairman of the Department of Psychiatry at NYU Medical Center. "Our experiences can shape brain biochemistry, and brain biochemistry may affect future experiences. If that chemistry is off, it may skew the way we perceive and deal with the world. So the traditional view that therapy deals only with the root psychological causes of mental disorders is no longer accurate."

Also outdated is the image of all psychotherapy as Freudian analysis, where a patient explores the unconscious mind several times a week for years and years. While psychotherapy is based on insights gleaned from Freud's work, most therapy these days is short-term, and is usually less concerned with the unconscious than with consciously changing thinking and behavior. Therapy may also be conducted by a variety of mental health professionals, not just psychiatrists.

How do you know when you need help? The American Psychological Association suggests that you consider therapy if:

- You feel an overwhelming and prolonged sense of helplessness and sadness, and problems do not seem to get better despite your efforts and help from family and friends.

- You are finding it difficult to carry out everyday activities. For example, you can't seem to concentrate at work and your job performance is suffering.

- You worry excessively, always expect the worst and are constantly on edge.

- Your actions are harmful to yourself or others. For example, if you are drinking too much.

FINDING A THERAPIST

In your search for a therapist, it's important to remember that *psychotherapist* is *not a legal* term, and can be used by just about anyone. Any mental health professional you choose should be licensed, which means they have met minimum training requirements and passed state or national examinations, and must take part in continuing education programs.

There are three major types of *licensed* or *certified* mental health professionals: psychiatrists, psychologists and social workers. "These professionals are all interested in how people think and feel and helping them function emotionally and socially. The difference really is in their education and training," explains Dr. Bruce Rubenstein, who directs behavioral health programs at NYU Medical Center.

PSYCHIATRISTS: Are M.D.s, licensed physicians, who spend four years in additional specialized training after medical school. That includes a year-long internship and a three-year residency in psychiatry, with hands-on training in neurology, in treating mental disorders, in different forms of psychotherapy and in the use of medications, says Dr. Rubenstein. To become "board-certified," a psychiatrist must pass standardized written and oral examinations after completing a residency. Specialists in geriatrics or child psychiatry undergo additional academic and clinical training. Because they are physicians, only psychiatrists can prescribe medications.

PSYCHOLOGISTS: Have completed graduate, doctoral or postdoctoral studies in human psychology (theories of the mind and how the mind works); many have a Ph.D., a Psy.D. or an Ed.D. degree. They typically must complete one to two years of clinical training in treating patients, and a year of supervised postdoctoral experience; some may also have research experience. Many psychologists are trained in a variety of therapies, as well as in working with children and families. All states require a license for psychologists to practice independently.

CLINICAL SOCIAL WORKERS: They may be certified social workers (CSWs) or licensed clinical social workers (LCSWs). They have earned a master's degree (and sometimes a doctorate), completing a two-year graduate program in social work, as well as clinical training (some may have analytic training). Most states certify or license social workers, requiring two years of supervised postgraduate clinical work and a qualifying examination before they can practice as therapists.

Other mental health professionals may include the following.

PSYCHIATRIC NURSES: Are registered nurses (R.N.s), who have passed a special state examination and have extra training and experience in psychiatry. "Advanced-practice" nurses have a master's degree and can provide psychotherapy. In some places, no license or certification may be required to practice therapy.

MARRIAGE AND FAMILY THERAPISTS: They usually have a graduate degree (most often in psychology) and at least two years of clinical training in helping people with relationship problems. They are licensed in some, but not all, states.

SEX THERAPISTS: May be physicians or psychotherapists who specialize in sexual problems. The American Association of Sex Educators, Counselors and Therapists (AASECT) is a nonprofit association that certifies sex therapists, and will provide a list of therapists in your area for a small fee (see Appendix I).

PASTORAL COUNSELORS: Are members of the clergy who offer psychological counseling within a religious context. No licensing is required, but some pastoral counselors may have training in psychology, in addition to their clerical training, and they may be certified by the American Association of Pastoral Counselors.

A person doesn't need to be an M.D. to become an analyst, but they must be specially trained and undergo analysis themselves. Many psychologists or social workers take additional training at places such as psychoanalytic institutes, to become thoroughly versed in analysis or in psychodynamic therapies.

The appropriate therapist depends in part on what the problem is, and different therapists may often work together. For example, a psychologist seeing a patient for major depression may refer that patient to a psychiatrist for medication. Or, a patient being treated by a psychiatrist for bipolar disorder might be referred to a psychologist or social worker for family therapy.

You might begin your search for help with your own physician, a friend or a relative. Another good starting point can be a nearby medical center or teaching hospital that has a department of psychiatry, says Dr. Cancro. These centers often have mental health clinics staffed by residents in psychiatry. Universities may also have departments of psychology or social work. Senior citizens' centers, gay health organizations and the like can often provide referrals, as can your state's psychiatric or psychological associations and local departments of mental health. National organizations, such as the National Alliance for the Mentally Ill (NAMI), and local chapters of support and advocacy groups, may be able to refer you to therapists who specialize in specific disorders (see Appendix I).

People seeking psychotherapy might be wise to have a medical evaluation first, advises Dr. Cancro. "Some people may have thyroid deficiencies or other medical problems that can present as behavioral or mental problems."

Initial visits with a therapist are aimed at making a diagnosis, deciding on the best course of treatment and finding someone with whom you are comfortable. There will usually be a fee for this initial consultation, whether or not you choose to stay with the particular person.

The American Psychological Association recommends asking the following questions at that initial meeting.

- Are you licensed? How many years have you been practicing?

- I have been feeling (anxious, depressed, etc.) and I'm having problems (with my job, my marriage, sleeping, overeating, etc.). What experience do you have helping people with these types of problems?

- What are your special areas of expertise—for example, working with children or families?

- What kinds of treatments do you use, and have they been proven effective in dealing with my kind of problem?

- What are your fees? Do you have a sliding-scale fee policy? (Fees are usually based on a forty-five to fifty-minute session, and can be upward of $150 in big cities.)

- How much therapy do you recommend?

- What types of insurance do you accept? Will you accept direct billing from my insurance company? Are you affiliated with any managed care organizations? (See box.) Do you accept Medicare/Medicaid?

"You really do have to 'shop' carefully for a therapist, and meet with someone before making a commitment. Discuss their credentials, what treatment will consist of and, of course, what it will cost," advises veteran NYU psychiatrist Dr. Helen DeRosis. "But the most important criterion is personal 'fit.' Each therapist has his or her own personal approach, which may be more important than the form of therapy." A good "fit" is a therapist who you feel will understand and respect your particular issues, and with whom you are comfortable sharing your innermost thoughts, someone who seems genuinely interested in helping you, and whom you can trust, says Dr. DeRosis. For some women, that personal fit might be better with a woman therapist.

"Many women feel that it is more difficult for a man to empathize with some issues that are gender-specific," comments Dr. Carol Nadelson, a professor of psychiatry at Harvard University and Cambridge Hospital in Boston. "For example, women report that they do not tell male therapists details of menstrual-related symptoms, or even discuss concerns about hysterectomy or past histories of abortion, miscarriage or sexual abuse."

This is also true with racial or cultural matters; a black patient may not tell a white therapist something she sees as potentially reinforcing racial stereotypes, says Dr. Nadelson. A gay woman may not feel comfortable even with a woman therapist who does not share her sexual orientation.

By the same token, she notes, therapists may impose their own biased views on a patient's experiences, especially if these are gender-specific. Some studies do show that female patients show greater responsiveness to psychotherapy, more satisfaction and greater self-rated improvement with a female therapist. However, Dr. Nadelson stresses, when the experience of the therapist is considered along with gender, the more experienced the therapist, the better the outcome, regardless of sex. And most studies show little outcome difference between male and female therapists for short-term psychotherapy.

In fact, lingering gender stereotypes may play more of a role than the gender of the therapist, says Leah J. Dickstein, M.D., a professor of psychiatry at the University of Louisville School of Medicine. "Sex role socialization, stereotyping and women's experiences affect health and illness. They distort research and clinical practice," she remarks. "So men *and* women therapists must look into their own values and attitudes about gender before being able to adequately treat women patients."

Mental Health and Managed Care

Managed care entered the mental health arena around ten years ago and, for many people, it now determines the type and the *amount* of treatment they receive. An estimated 180 million Americans have mental health care through managed care firms. A traditional fee-for-service plan typically reimburses for mental health services at a much lower rate than for other medical services (for example, 50 percent for psychotherapy as opposed to 80 percent for medical procedures). Many insurers now reimburse for mental health services only after "managed behavioral care" consultants say that treatment is needed. A number of states, including Maine, Maryland, Minnesota, New Hampshire, Rhode Island and Texas, have passed "parity" laws, requiring insurers to reimburse equally for medical *and* mental health care. Members of Congress are trying to pass a similar federal law.

(continued)

Medicare pays 50 percent of its allowable charge for psychotherapy (which is relatively low), and requires that therapy be provided by mental health professionals who are licensed, or meet state or local requirements. (Contact your local Part B carrier for a list of qualified practitioners.)

Many HMOs limit patients to a maximum of twenty outpatient psychiatric visits and thirty hospitalized days a year. You may have to request a referral from your primary care physician (or "gatekeeper," in managed care lingo) before you can see a therapist or call an 800 number to talk to a "caseworker" who may or may not approve a referral. A growing trend is for HMOs and insurance carriers to work with (or own) a specialized company that either provides mental health services or advises on use of these services. You must pick therapists from the company's list; if you want to go "out of network," you have to pay more or bear all of the costs.

Managed mental health plans often require that therapists make a diagnosis and map out a treatment plan by the second therapy session, reporting periodically to the firm on the patient's progress. Some plans allow a patient to see a therapist only a few times (the average is three to seven sessions), then require the therapist to prove that the patient needs more treatment, or that treatment is working. Many therapists say this compromises patient confidentiality. While a majority of physicians have contracted with managed care plans, only about half of psychiatrists have done so. Many more psychologists and social workers have signed up.

Managed care plans are increasingly placing patients into limited programs, like day hospitals, instead of expensive psychiatric hospitals, reducing the expensive and dehumanizing institutionalization of severely mentally ill patients. Managed care plans have also been credited with helping to prove the efficacy of short-term therapies. But critics charge that managed care often provides inadequate and truncated mental health care.

On the plus side, many managed mental health care companies do offer people a source for referrals and services that might otherwise be hard to come by (such as in rural communities). Some companies not only offer medical and psychiatric treatment, but also stress management services, smoking cessation and treatment for eating disorders and substance abuse.

Unfortunately, many insurers routinely deny coverage, especially individual disability coverage, to people who have been in psychotherapy. If such people *do* obtain coverage, they are often charged higher premiums. Industry officials claim that people with chronic mental illness have a higher risk of becoming disabled, and that disability claims based on mental conditions have soared in recent years. Patients' rights advocates counter that recent studies show that people who seek psychotherapy cost *less* to insure because they don't use medical services as often.

THE BASICS OF PSYCHOTHERAPY

All psychotherapy involves talk therapy, but the goals can be very different. Long-term therapy is primarily aimed at gaining insight to improve personal functioning, while short-term therapies are designed to change thinking or behavior in order to help solve specific, current problems.

According to Michael L. Fleisher, M.D., a clinical associate professor of psychiatry at the NYU School of Medicine and an analyst in private practice, there are four basic types of psychotherapy: traditional *psychoanalysis*, *psychodynamic psychotherapy* (which is analytically based), *cognitive-behavioral therapies*, and *interpersonal psychotherapy*. With the exception of analysis and therapies grounded in specific schools of thought (such as "Jungian" therapy, based on the teachings of Carl Jung, a former student of Freud), most psychotherapies blend techniques from different disciplines, says Dr. Fleisher. Various forms of therapy may also be used in other settings such as group therapy, or family or couples therapy.

Psychotherapists also use a common language. Here are some frequently used terms that you should know.

- NEUROSES: Are any nonpsychotic symptom (such as anxiety), feeling or pattern of conflict causing undue pain or difficulty in a person's life. Neuroses are problems that are mostly self-generated rather than caused by life events, says Dr. Fleisher.

- TRANSFERENCE: Refers to the unconscious projection onto the therapist of one's needs, desires or feelings, and unconscious attitudes toward important figures from the past (including one's parents). Understanding transference provides useful insights for both therapist and patient.

- COUNTERTRANSFERENCE: Deals with feelings stirred in the analyst by an individual patient. Analysts examine these reactions for important information about the patient, which becomes part of the therapy.

- RESISTANCE: Is unconscious opposition by the patient to the therapist and the therapeutic process.

- THERAPEUTIC ALLIANCE: Is the positive working relationship, hopefully, that you build with a therapist, based on trust. A 1996 study found that this relationship was *just* as important to treatment outcome as the type of therapy and/or medication used.

WHICH TYPE OF PSYCHOTHERAPY IS FOR YOU?

The therapy you choose depends on the extent of a problem and on your own personal goals.

PSYCHOANALYSIS: Traditional psychoanalysis is based on theories originated by Sigmund Freud, which hold that the experiences of early childhood (real or imagined) and the unconscious mind strongly influence our psychic development and personality. Psychoanalysis explores these realms. "The goal of analysis is insight and restructuring of the self-injurious aspects of the personality," says Dr. Fleisher.

A complex and lengthy process, traditional analysis works at uncovering and understanding memories (or fantasies) of childhood experiences, our unconscious thoughts and our dreams, so we can become aware of how they shape the way we think and act.

In analysis, a patient lies on a couch, facing away from the analyst, and says whatever comes to mind. This is called "free association." The themes emerging from these seemingly random thoughts often reflect true feelings or desires we're unaware of. "Lying on the couch is like lying in bed when you're half-asleep; you allow random thoughts to run through your mind," explains Dr. Fleisher. "Face-to-face contact with the analyst can distract you from those thoughts, and you're more apt to censor what you say because you're speaking *to* another person. Without eye contact, you can focus inward on whatever is passing through your head."

Psychoanalysts also examine transference and resistance. The idea here is that transference represents a repetition of earlier patterns in life, usually the parent-child relationship or projections of fantasies; resistance is the patient's defensive reactions against revealing these to the analyst (again, a carryover from childhood). By exploring this push-pull relationship, one can understand and revise those injurious patterns of relating and problem solving.

"Analysis will benefit someone who has difficulties in just about every area of their life," says Dr. Fleisher. "These are people who can't form lasting love relationships, can't function optimally in a work or creative environment, have trouble with 'play,' relaxing, and have difficulties with self-esteem. But you have to be willing to work at self-exploration."

Analysis is intensive and expensive, requiring a major commitment of three to five visits a week over a period of up to six years. And, despite its decades of use, there is little good clinical data on its long-term effectiveness because it does not focus solely on isolated symptoms, like a phobia, but on the personality as a whole.

PSYCHODYNAMIC PSYCHOTHERAPY: This therapy is less *intense* than analysis, but is founded on many of the same principles and uses the same approaches. As with analysis, the goal is changing self-injurious thoughts and behaviors through personal insight.

A major concept of psychodynamic psychotherapy is that emotional well-being is upset by buried distortions in the way a person sees him or herself and the world around them, interfering with problem solving, says Dr. Veva Zimmerman, associate dean of the NYU School of Medicine, who is also a practicing psychiatrist.

In contrast with analysis, in psychodynamic psychotherapy individuals talk face-to-face with the therapist, recalling past experiences, and expressing feelings, until the significant unconscious information being sought can be shared and worked on. "The therapist plays a more active role than an analyst, listening and interpreting, pointing out ways an individual may be using defense mechanisms, such as denial or repression, to deal with problems," says Dr. Zimmerman. The goal is to educate the patient so that the work of treatment can be carried on in life after therapy ends.

Psychodynamic psychotherapy may be brief or long-term, with the frequency of session depending on goals set by the patient and the therapist. There's no definitive research on whether short-term or long-term psychodynamic psychotherapy has more lasting effects. Medication may or may not be used.

Psychodynamic therapy may be beneficial for people with personality disorders and chronic mental disorders who want to understand (and change) the ways their illness is affecting their life, says Dr. Zimmerman.

❧ *Caren's Story, Continued* ❧

"I have been undergoing cognitive therapy, and for me it works wonderfully well. . . . We videotape my sessions and I go home and I rewatch my session and . . . I also write about what I feel good about, what I feel bad about, and then I go back and talk about it with my therapist. . . . Like something will happen and I'll be blaming myself, and we work through that maybe it's not all my fault. . . . We look at other factors that could be at work. . . .

"In therapy you really look at yourself and how you're reacting to your everyday life . . . and slowly but surely that becomes your natural process of thinking, instead of your first response to everything being 'Oh, I goofed up, I'm not worthy, I'm not worth anything, so I'll just sleep through the next day.' . . . The cognitive therapy helps me really get in touch with what the real issues and emotions are."

COGNITIVE THERAPY: This is a short-term therapy in which a person learns to recognize patterns of negative thinking that cause problems, and changes how they think and react to events and people.

Cognitive therapy was first developed in the 1960s by Aaron T. Beck, M.D., now president of the Beck Institute for Cognitive Therapy and Research and professor emeritus of psychiatry at the University of Pennsylvania. Dr. Beck observed that many depressed individuals did not benefit from Freudian analysis of their unconscious so he decided to examine their *conscious* thoughts. He found that depressed people shared three major thought patterns: a negative view of themselves, a pessimistic outlook on their future and a negative interpretation of their experiences. These destructive thought patterns lead to emotional distress and maladaptive behaviors, especially when one is under stress. It's now believed that negative thinking may well interact with biological vulnerability to produce depression.

According to Judith S. Beck, Ph.D., director of the Beck Institute, located in suburban Philadelphia, cognitive therapy uses a variety of strategies: changing depressed thinking, active problem-solving, resuming activities abandoned due to depression, teaching patients to credit themselves for their achievements, and teaching them to break down overwhelming projects into small steps. Patients learn various skills in therapy sessions, such as evaluating and responding to their thoughts, and practice those skills daily at home.

Some patients, like Caren, may be sent home with videotapes or audiotapes of therapy sessions to review as part of their "homework." Other patients may be asked to keep a "Daily Mood Log," in which they record upsetting events and how they felt about them, then work with the therapist to analyze self-destructive thinking and work to change it.

"One of the big pluses to cognitive therapy is that it provides tools people can use throughout their lives, not just in overcoming a single episode of depression," says Dr. Judith Beck. (For tips on using the principles of cognitive therapy to avoid problems in everyday life, see Chapter 14.)

Cognitive therapy has been adapted for people in all age ranges, and is used in individual, group, couples and family therapy. Therapy can run from five to twenty sessions, depending on the severity of the problem. It has proven very effective in treating a wide variety of problems in addition to depression: anxiety disorders (including panic disorder, generalized anxiety disorder and social phobia), substance abuse and relationship problems. Preliminary studies show that cognitive therapy is also effective in treating eating disorders and personality disorders.

BEHAVIORAL THERAPY: This type of therapy is aimed at learning to modify destructive behavior patterns. The idea is that distressing psychological symptoms (such as panic) may be partly learned responses that you can modify or unlearn. And by changing a behavior, you can also change the feelings associated with it. A number of techniques are used, including *behavior modification*, which focuses on changing a single negative habit or behavior. (A good example is the techniques used to help people quit smoking.)

Desensitization uses a progressive series of exercises to teach people how to lessen or control specific fears. For example, "fearful flyers" may start out by watching videos of airplanes in flight, coupled with relaxation exercises to lessen feelings of anxiety, gradually building up to a short flight.

Relaxation training helps people control physical and mental stress. This can include "progressive relaxation," which involves sitting in a comfortable position with the eyes closed and relaxing muscles one by one, as well as visualization or meditation.

Exposure therapy involves gradually exposing a person to a feared object or situation. For example, an agoraphobic may be helped by a therapist to walk a short distance from her front door, progress to longer walks, then progress to outings in public places (while the therapist helps challenge unfounded fears), until her anxiety begins to ease. Exposure therapy may also be conducted in groups. "Virtual reality," computer-simulated experiences, is being tested in exposure therapy (see page 74).

Social skills training may be used to identify undesirable or feared behaviors, and to teach new ways of interacting.

Behavioral therapy usually involves less than twenty-five sessions, and is most often used to treat panic attacks, agoraphobia, obsessive-compulsive disorder and other anxiety disorders.

Between Doctor and Patient

Psychotherapists, whether analysts or psychologists, are required, both by the states that license them and by the professional organizations to which they belong, to adhere to strict codes of ethics. But sometimes they step over the line.

According to psychiatrist Arthur Zitrin, M.D., chairman of the Dean's Committee on Medical Ethics at the NYU School of Medicine, the most common ethical complaint against therapists involves those who engage in sexual intimacy with their patients.

"The best data indicate that about six to seven percent of psychiatrists have acknowledged having intimate, sexual or romantic relationships with their patients," reports Dr. Zitrin. "Even though some practitioners might contend that the sexual contact was consensual, that the patient initiated it, or did not object, this is the worst kind of exploitation of a vulnerable patient, and is strictly prohibited by the Principles of Medical Ethics established by the American Medical Association."

Therapists are also prohibited from employing or engaging in financial or business deals with current or former patients, among other boundary violations. Therapists also may not reveal patient records to *anyone* (except general progress reports for insurers), even after a patient's death or in court, says Dr. Zitrin. In 1996, the U.S. Supreme Court upheld that right to therapist-patient confidentiality in the courtroom.

The American Psychiatric Association reports that it suspends or expels about a dozen members a year for various ethics violations, most of them sexual. "When patients are ill, no matter how intelligent, educated or sophisticated they might be, they become dependent to some degree on their doctor or therapist. This puts the physician in a position of power, and there is the potential for abuse," comments Dr. Zitrin. "It's essential for practitioners to be alert for their own responses to patients, as well as patients' potential erotic transference, which may interfere with treatment."

The American Psychiatric Association's Committee on Ethics advises patients to be wary if their therapist:

- Begins to disclose personal problems, or discusses his or her personal life (including sexual experiences) in detail.

- Offers not to charge for sessions or greatly reduces the fee, even when payment is not a hardship for the patient.

- Offers to socialize with you outside the office.

- Begins to touch you in seemingly "comforting" ways during therapy, such as hugging, holding your hand or caressing you.

- Begins to regularly extend therapy sessions beyond the normal time by ten to fifteen minutes or more.

- Suggests a relationship beyond that of patient and therapist, such as offering you the chance to take part in business deals, or offering employment.

Patients who feel that a therapist has stepped over the line can file written complaints with their district branch of the APA, or other professional groups. You don't need a lawyer to do this.

"While expulsion or sanctions by the APA or other such groups will not bar a therapist from practicing, it can seriously damage their standing within the professional community," remarks Dr. Zitrin. The only body that can revoke a therapist's license is your state's board of medical or professional licensure.

You can also initiate a criminal or civil action against a therapist, depending on the laws in the state where you live. According to the APA, states that have laws barring therapist/patient sexual contact include California, Colorado, Florida, Georgia, Illinois, Iowa, Maine, Minnesota, New Mexico, North and South Dakota and Wisconsin. You'll need a lawyer to file this type of action, and statutes of limitations will apply.

The Public Citizen Health Research Group, based in Washington, D.C., can help you find out if a practitioner has ever been disciplined or sued for malpractice. (See Appendix I for information and listings of professional organizations.)

"All patients have the right to expect that when they come to a physician or therapist for help, they will not be harmed or exploited, and that practitioners will use all their expertise to alleviate the patient's problems," concludes Dr. Zitrin.

⊱ Faye's Story, Continued ⊰

"For me, therapy focused on my life and my family, my work and my relationships, figuring out what was causing me problems and what I could do to solve them. I believe therapy really helped me to resolve the underlying causes of my panic attacks.

"I think therapy was the key to getting rid of my panic attacks. . . . The medication controlled the symptoms, but to keep the attacks from coming back, I had to deal with a lot of issues in my life. . . . Was I being a good mother by working as much as I was? Which was more important to me? . . . I was a perfectionist, very success driven. And I couldn't face the possibility that I wasn't going to be the best in the world, that I might have to settle for less in some aspect of my life. . . . There was sort of a dissonance . . . what I was doing and what I wanted out of life, and the way my life was really turning out. . . . I had to figure out what it was I wanted, how to get myself in balance, or I wasn't going to get better. . . .

"Through therapy, I have also learned to be much more vocal in my life. . . . I will not take on more than I can handle. If I need something, I speak up. I have learned . . . not to hold myself to such a high standard. . . . And to be conscious of what my priorities are. That right now my family comes first. . . . When I see other people getting awards, I've learned not to eat myself up over it. I can't have it all. I've learned that's okay."

INTERPERSONAL THERAPY (IPT): This is a short-term therapy that focuses on improving relationships, helping individuals recognize their own feelings and needs, enhancing their interpersonal and communication skills, as well as treating depression.

IPT was developed in the 1970s by Myrna M. Weissman, Ph.D., of Columbia University and the New York State Psychiatric Institute, and her late husband, Gerald L. Klerman, M.D., formerly at Harvard and Cornell University medical schools. The idea behind IPT is that disturbed personal and social relationships can cause or contribute to depression.

IPT does not deal with past psychic origins of depression, but focuses on problems in the present, stresses Dr. Weissman. It is highly structured, with three distinct phases of therapy. The initial phase is diagnostic, evaluating clinical symptoms and deciding whether medication may be needed. "During this phase, an 'interpersonal inventory,' is completed, detailing what is going on in the patient's life, what their key relationships are, what the patterns and problems are, and what changes have taken place in their life," explains Dr. Weissman.

In the second phase, the patient and therapist work on one of four specific problem areas: grief reactions, inability to maintain relationships (or lack of social skills), role disputes (for example, a struggle with a family member) and role transitions (any major life change). In the third phase of treatment, therapists work with patients to consolidate what they've learned and develop ways of coping in the future.

IPT can range in duration from twelve to sixteen sessions, but may continue for longer periods (and may be combined with medications), particularly as a maintenance treatment for major depression. There is a manual to ensure consistency of IPT's use, and a patient book has also been written by Dr. Weissman, which helps the patient know what to expect from the therapy.

Interpersonal therapy can benefit women of all ages who suffer from dysthymia or chronic depression, women going through a divorce or career change and women who are dealing with a serious illness or a death. IPT can also help people who have trouble establishing relationships or interacting with others, and women facing problems as a caretaker to an elderly relative. Women with bulimia have also been helped by interpersonal therapy.

FEMINIST THERAPY: Examines a woman's experiences in the context of living in a male-dominated society (in any given culture), which is seen as devaluing and oppressing women. Among the goals of this woman-centered therapy are validation, empowerment and the establishment of egalitarian relationships. Therapy from a feminist perspective may be interwoven with other treatments, such as IPT, and may be valuable for women who see themselves as disenfranchised, such as lesbians, women of color or older women.

GROUP THERAPY: Brings together people with similar problems in a controlled setting and, with the help of a therapist-leader, allows them to observe how they interact with others and learn better ways of functioning. A variety of techniques may be used.

Culture, Ethnicity and Mental Health

The idea of going into psychotherapy for treatment for emotional problems is not one that is universally accepted. Our race, ethnicity, religion and cultural background can all affect the way we view illness; having a mental disorder still carries a shameful stigma among many groups. The *DSM-IV* now contains information on how different disorders manifest themselves in people of varying cultural backgrounds. While there are tremendous variations within large racial, ethnic and cultural groups, experts have found some general beliefs about mental disorders.

Within the African-American community, for example, therapy is often viewed as something for "sick" or "crazy" people. Black women, who are socialized to take on a caretaker role for a large extended family, believe that they must bear all burdens and be strong for their families, and may view psychotherapy as being for "weak" individuals, comments Dr. Freda Lewis-Hall, former Special Advisor to the Office for Special Populations at the National Institute of Mental Health. Black women may be more likely to seek help for a child than for themselves. African Americans, especially women, have traditionally drawn on their spiritual strength in times of trouble. "They may turn to their church and to prayer for emotional solace, rather than a white-dominated medical system they see as hostile and racist," says Dr. Lewis-Hall.

For many reasons, Latinos tend to utilize psychiatric services less than whites or blacks, says Silvia W. Olarte, M.D., chair of the American Psychiatric Association's Committee of Hispanic Psychiatrists. "There is still a lot of stigma in Hispanic culture for mental illness or visiting a psychiatrist, seeing those who do as *loco* ('crazy')," she explains. "Cultural factors tend to stigmatize those who suffer from depression, or what is called *ataques de nervios,* a sort of generalized anxiety disorder.''

In addition to a cultural fatalism, there is *marianismo,* which experts say focuses on the Virgin Mary as the ideal of womanhood: chaste, self-sacrificing and passive, enduring suffering for the good of family. Women are expected to be submissive to men and place prime importance on being a mother and caretaker. So they may deny their own needs, even in the face of unhappiness, a spouse's infidelity, or family violence. Within Latino culture, where religion plays a central role, emotional problems may also be viewed within a "spiritual context," and people may turn to the Church or to spiritual healers for help, rather than a therapist.

Experts say that Asian Americans may turn to mental health resources after all other traditional resources have failed. One reason is the belief that problem solving should take place within the family unit, and that disclosing an illness to an outsider may be seen as shameful. For many Chinese, mental health is achieved through the exercise of willpower and avoidance of "morbid" thoughts. Experts also say there are no equivalents for many mental health concepts in East Asian cultures or within Eastern medicine.

Among different religious groups, studies reported in *Ethnicity and Family Therapy* (Guilford Press, 1982) indicate that Jews may be more favorably inclined toward psychotherapy than Catholics or Protestants. Jewish Americans tend to value verbal ability as a by-product of learning, which is highly esteemed in Jewish culture. Experts say that ethnic groups and religions that regard suffering as a part of life (as Buddhism does), emphasize stoicism or have fatalistic views may be less likely to accept the notion that talking about problems helps to solve them.

Admittedly, these are generalizations made from studying large groups of people. However, most of us don't realize how much our cultural background influences our views and actions. So if you are experiencing emotional distress and are resisting the idea of going for help, you might want to examine just *where* that reluctance is really coming from.

WHICH THERAPIES WORK BEST?

It's hard to quantify the effects of therapy in the same way you measure symptom relief from a specific dose of medication. For one thing, the experience of therapy is highly subjective. Some people are receptive to psychotherapy, others are not.

However, the 1990 *American Psychological Association Task Force Report on Women and Depression* notes that cognitive, behavioral and interpersonal therapy may work best for women because they focus on "action, mastery and distraction from depressed rumination." In addition, the APA report said, interpersonal therapy may be especially helpful for women because it focuses on issues "central to the psychology of women. . . . For women, perhaps more than for men, social isolation, relationship loss and dysfunctional family relationships may precipitate, contribute to and/or prolong depression."

A recent study at the National Institute of Mental Health found that up to 69 percent of women with depression were symptom-free after a sixteen-week course of interpersonal therapy. (However, other experts argue that achieving lasting differences in behavior and social skills may take six months to a year.)

IPT has also had success in controlled clinical trials for acutely depressed outpatients. In cases of less severe depression, another major study by the NIMH comparing IPT, cognitive therapy and medication (*imipramine*) found that interpersonal and cognitive therapy were as effective as antidepressants. In more severe depression, the study found, antidepressants were most effective, with IPT coming in second.

IPT may help prevent depressive *symptoms* from turning into full-blown depression. "We have some evidence that interpersonal therapy can help prevent depression because it keeps people focused on their current interpersonal problems and trying to solve them. And it also focuses on interpersonal problems that might occur down the line, and trying to figure out strategies to prevent those problems," says psychologist Dr. Ellen Frank, director of the Prevention of Depression and Manic Depression Program at the Western Psychiatric Institute and Clinic in Pittsburgh.

For women who've had a previous episode of depression, preventing a recurrence may entail "maintenance" psychotherapy, as well as long-term medication. One randomized clinical trial at the University of Pittsburgh followed more than one hundred patients for five years, to see whether interpersonal therapy alone, antidepressant medication (imipramine) at the same dose used to treat the initial episode, or a combination of both, could prevent a recurrence of depression. The trial found that continuing medication was most effective in preventing recurrence of depression. People who received monthly maintenance with IPT did relapse, but had longer periods between depressive episodes.

✑ *Marcia's Story, Continued* ✑

"I've had years of therapy since I had my first episode of major depression, and I've had a wonderful therapist. I don't see her regularly, but I go in for 'tune-ups' when I'm feeling like I don't have a good perspective on things. Because she knows my history, she knows my issues. She saw me through a serious postpartum illness; she saw me get well.

"I use that, I use support groups, I talk to my friends and family. But it's always in the back of my mind. . . . I always wonder . . . is it going to come today or tomorrow? When you are well, it's not a pervasive thought, but it's there. . . .

"I actually have devised a list, I call it my 'contract for wellness.' It's the admission that I have an illness that may recur. The illness is not my fault . . . it happens. But it is my responsibility to seek treatment and to stay in treatment. If I choose not to be in treatment, then I can't expect people to stand next to me while I fall apart. My responsibility is to do as much for me as I can.

"It's also my responsibility to understand my markers, and to let people I love understand them, too. So they can help me get help if I can't make a good decision for myself. It is also my responsibility to take care of myself and to avoid people and situations that exacerbate my illness. What I learned in therapy to call 'toxic people' or 'toxic situations' . . . and surround myself with people who are going to be helpful. Whether that means seeing my therapist . . . or connecting with a good friend.

". . . I don't want any other woman to be as scared as I was. I want people to know that depression can happen, that it's treatable and that you're going to be okay."

―――

For patients with bipolar disorder, a 1994 study at the University of Pittsburgh found that manic episodes occurred less frequently and resolved more quickly among patients who underwent two years of therapy coupled with lithium, compared with those who only received medication.

For people who suffer from anxiety disorders, a number of studies have shown that a cognitive-behavioral therapy (including "exposure therapy") and/or medication can be effective in treating panic disorder, agoraphobia and social phobias.

Harder to treat is obsessive-compulsive disorder, which has a high relapse rate. An ongoing study conducted at three sites is comparing three weeks of daily intensive behavioral therapy (followed by home visits) with twelve weeks of the medication *clomipramine*, or a combination therapy of the two.

"To date, the response rate for behavior therapy appears higher than for clomipramine, which in turn is superior to placebo. Combined therapy is as good as behavior therapy, but not better in this study," reports Dr. Michael Leibowitz, director of the Anxiety Disorders Clinic at the Columbia-Presbyterian Medical Center. After three months of follow-up, most of those who took medication (and then discontinued) showed relapses, while those who responded to behavior or combined therapy appear to have maintained their gains after stopping treatment.

Treating people with personality disorders can also be difficult (especially borderline personality). But recent studies indicate that psychodynamic psychotherapy and newly formulated types of behavior therapy can be of significant help.

How *much* therapy you will need depends on the seriousness of the problem. A study by Northwestern University reviewed data from more than twenty-four hundred patients over a thirty-year period, and found that half of the patients showed measurable improvement by the eighth therapy session. After six months of once-a-week therapy, 75 percent had improved. It took longer for people with more serious disorders to get better. People with depression or anxiety responded to therapy by the twentieth session, while people with personality disorders took up to a year to show improvement.

But for *any* form of therapy to succeed, the patient has to be motivated to make changes, stresses Dr. Helen DeRosis. "All therapy is really self-cure. You have to want to get better, want to get something out of the experience. The therapist can help you to get started, but eventually you have to do the actual work of making the needed changes away from the therapist's office. Each person has the inner potential to change for the better."

CHAPTER 13

Medications—
What You Need to Know

As recently as the 1960s, people might have been hospitalized for years because of crippling mental ill-
ness. Today, except for the most debilitating cases, psychotropic drugs have
made it possible for many people with mental disorders to live normal, productive lives.

Use of medications has also helped to make talk therapy more effective.
A woman who is too depressed to even talk will not be able to benefit from
psychotherapy. The right psychoactive medication will enable her to participate fully in therapy.

In researching these medications, scientists have learned a great deal
about the workings of the brain and about the biochemical roots of mental
disorders. New insights have been gained into depression, anxiety, obsessive-
compulsive disorder, panic disorder and psychosis.

"Until recently, however, women have either been excluded from the major trials of psychotropic drugs, or sex-based analysis of clinical trials has not
been done. So gender differences in the effectiveness of psychotropic drugs
remain poorly understood," says Dr. Susan J. Blumenthal, U.S. deputy assistant secretary for women's health. "This is all the more disturbing because . . .
seventy percent of all psychotropic medications are prescribed for women.

"It *is* known that women have more side effects, and twice as many fatal drug reactions, from psychoactive drugs, as men do. These drugs act differently in women because they have different body composition than men, different cerebral blood flow patterns and different gastric emptying times than men. The use of hormones, such as oral contraceptives and replacement estrogen, can also affect metabolism of these drugs," she adds.

In 1993 the U.S. Food and Drug Administration (FDA) mandated that women be included in industry drug trials, and that all trials should examine gender differences. In addition, the National Institute of Mental Health is undertaking more research in this area, so more detailed information should be available in the coming years. Thanks to the generous assistance of several leading researchers, this chapter contains the most current information about psychotropic medications in women.

SOME BASIC FACTS

The length of time a woman must take medication depends on the problem. Women with panic disorder may take medication for six months. In more serious disorders, such as schizophrenia or manic-depression, long-term treatment may be needed.

Despite the recent hoopla over Prozac and other new antidepressants as being "personality pills," there's no evidence that medications can fundamentally change personality, stresses Dr. Robert Cancro, who heads the Department of Psychiatry at NYU Medical Center. "However, medications do have an impact on a person that may go beyond symptoms of depression, allowing them to experience their life differently.

"For example, if a person is sensitive to criticism and rejection because of an imbalance in brain chemistry, and you give them a medication that normalizes that chemistry, they may no longer be rejection-sensitive. Now they respond differently to the people around them, and people to them, and this is self-reinforcing. You cannot separate what was done pharmacologically and what was reinforced by experience. All you can accurately say is that the person feels better and is happier," says Dr. Cancro.

Here are some basic facts and terms you need to know.

- Most medications are given orally, and must first be broken down (*metabolized*) by the digestive tract; a good portion goes to the liver or kidneys to be metabolized and excreted.

- Break-down components (*metabolites*) of drugs are excreted in feces, urine, saliva, tears and breast milk. What's left binds to proteins in the blood, but as little as 10 percent of a psychotropic drug may actually reach the brain. New tests can measure a drug's effectiveness by the amount of metabolites present in blood or spinal fluid.

- A drug's *half-life* refers to the amount of time it takes for one half the drug's peak blood level to be metabolized and excreted. Drugs with a longer half-life take more time to reach therapeutic *steady-state* levels in the blood; they may also build up in the body, causing more side effects. Drugs with a short half-life are eliminated more rapidly and generally cause fewer side effects. *Potency* refers to the dose needed to achieve a therapeutic effect.

- Psychotropic drugs affect more than one neurotransmitter system, and their effects are not confined to the brain, so they can cause a wide range of side effects. A drug's *therapeutic index* is a measure of its safety or toxicity. A drug with a low therapeutic index may need careful monitoring for side effects.

- Medical diseases and even certain foods can affect the body's metabolism of psychoactive drugs, raising or lowering blood levels of the drugs, increasing side effects or causing dangerous reactions.

- Psychotropic drugs can interact with other medications, including birth control pills and over-the-counter preparations. Inform your physician about *any* other drugs you are taking.

- Some research suggests that hormonal fluctuations may affect the potency of some psychotropic drugs during different phases of the menstrual cycle (see page 280), so dosage may have to be adjusted accordingly.

- Psychoactive medications can pass through the placenta, and some carry a risk of birth defects when taken during early pregnancy. Where possible, experts say, alternative treatments should be tried during pregnancy. If a woman finds that she is pregnant while taking psychotropic drugs, she should immediately contact her doctor.

- Elderly people may metabolize and excrete drugs more slowly (these effects are often more pronounced in women), and often take other medications for chronic illnesses. Because there is an increased risk of side effects and drug interactions, older women often require lower doses of medication (see page 285).

Alphabetic Listings of Generic Medications

Source: U.S. Department of Health and Human Services

Generic Name	Trade Name
Antianxiety Medications	
alprazolam	Xanax
buspirone	BuSpar
chlordiazepoxide	Librax
	Libritabs
	Librium
diazepam	Valium
halazepam	Paxipam
lorazepam	Ativan
oxazepam	Serax
prazepam	Centrax
	Vestran
Antidepressant Medications	
amitriptyline	Elavil
amoxapine	Asendin
bupropion	Wellbutrin
clomipramine	Anafranil
desipramine	Norpramine
	Pertofrane
doxepin	Adapin
	Sinequan
dexfenfluramine	Redux
fluoxetine	Prozac
fluvoxamine	Luvox
imipramine	Tofranil
maprotiline	Ludiomil
mirtazapine	Remeron
nefazodone	Serzone

Generic Name	Trade Name

Antidepressant Medications

nortriptyline	Aventyl
	Pamelor
paroxetine	Paxil
phenelzine	Nardil
protriptyline	Vivactil
sertraline	Zoloft
tranylcypromine	Parnate
trazadone	Desyrel
trimipramine	Surmontil
venlafaxine	Effexor

Antimanic Medications

carbamazepine	Tegretol
lithium carbonate	Eskalith
	Lithane
	Lithobid
lithium citrate	Cibalith-S
valproate	Depakote
	Depakene

Antipsychotic Medications

chlorpromazine	Thorazine
chlorprothixene	Taractan
clozapine	Clozaril
fluphenazine	Permitil
	Prolixin
haloperidol	Haldol
loxapine	Daxolin
	Loxitane
mesoridazine	Serentil
molindone	Lidone
	Moban

(continued)

Generic Name	Trade Name
Antipsychotic Medications	
perphenazine	Trilafon
pimozide	Orap
risperidone	Risperdal
thioridazine	Mellaril
thiothixene	Navane
trifluoperazine	Stelazine
triflupromazine	Vesprin
Benzodiazepine Hypnotics (Sedatives/Tranquilizers)	
estazolam	ProSom
flurazepam	Dalmane
quazepam	Doral
temazepam	Restoril
triazolam	Halcion
Other Sedatives/Sleeping pills	
amobarbital	Amytal
ethchlorvynol	Placidyl
pentobarbital	Nembutal
seconbarbital	Seconal
zolpidem	Ambien

❧ *Sarah's Story* ❧

"I had lost my job, my husband's business had failed. . . . We had lost all our money, our nice lifestyle. . . . Suddenly we had nothing. . . . I was frightened, incredibly sad. I felt an enormous sense of loss . . . overwhelming hopelessness. I couldn't see anything getting better short of winning the lotto. . . . There was absolutely nothing that was going to make my life better. . . .

"The three of us moved into a tiny one-room apartment. . . . Some people we considered our friends seemed to avoid us after our financial picture changed. . . . I didn't have a life that had any joy left to it. . . . I love my husband. He's a wonderful, loving, upbeat person. No matter what happened, he never gave up. And we have a terrific, bright son. But when you feel so down, all of that doesn't mean anything.

"I'm now convinced that depression is an absolute medical illness. A life stress may provoke it, but then this chemical reaction occurs and . . . each thought makes you sadder. And the pain becomes almost unbearable. . . . You start thinking, you don't want to live, you just want to end the pain. . . . I had no interest in anything. . . . I didn't have any emotions. I just felt dead, like I had died inside. And I was engulfed in waves of sadness that came over me like a fog. You know how sometimes fog rolls in thicker, and sometimes it's a little bit lighter, and you can see the sun. Well, my whole life was enveloped in thick fog. When I got the right medication, it lifted that fog. . . . It was really amazing.

"My doctor tried me on two different antidepressants, but neither of them worked. One made me nervous . . . the other made me sick to my stomach. . . . Then we tried this new antidepressant, the smallest possible dose. . . . And I started getting better almost right away, maybe a week or so. . . . Now, with the medication I feel more on an even keel. . . . When something bad happens, I don't fold, I don't react the same way . . . I have some hope. I have my priorities together. I enjoy little things more. I can take great joy in a sunny day. I can appreciate my husband and child. . . .

"I really feel in my case that it was a chemical depression. Just like you might get indigestion from stress. And you're not going to get rid of it by talking about it, you need to take medication to make it better. . . . I have the same life that I had before, but without that mental indigestion. The medication is counteracting that. . . . And if I have to stay on medication for the duration, that's okay. . . . I'd love not to have to take anything. But I remember the agony I was in. I don't want to take a chance to see how I feel without it."

DO PSYCHOACTIVE DRUGS ACT
DIFFERENTLY IN WOMEN?

According to Jean A. Hamilton, M.D., director of the Institute for Women's Health at the Medical College of Pennsylvania and a leading researcher into sex differences in psychopharmacology, there are a number of reasons drugs act differently in women.

"Psychotropic drugs lodge in fatty tissue, and women have a higher proportion of body fat than men . . . over time, women can have a higher buildup of certain drugs in their bodies. Additionally, the action of estrogen and progesterone cause women's stomachs to empty much more slowly than men's, especially during the premenstrual period, reducing the amount of a drug that reaches the circulation. For reasons such as these, a woman may need different, higher or lower doses of certain medications," explains Dr. Hamilton.

Women may have lower blood volume than men, but they have higher blood flow to the brain. Women also secrete less stomach acid than men, so absorption is increased of benzodiazepines, tricyclic antidepressants and some antipsychotics, says Dr. Hamilton. Ovarian hormones slow the metabolism of some antipsychotics by the liver, the beta blocker *propranolol* and the antidepressant *clomipramine*. Medications are also eliminated more slowly in women, so women often have higher blood concentrations of drugs than men.

Five to 10 percent of women can have significant changes in drug metabolism premenstrually. In addition to lithium, recent reports suggest, women may show lower concentrations of the antidepressants *trazodone* and *desipramine* during the premenstrual period. (It's not known whether that is due to forgetting to take medication because of PMS symptoms or to physiological changes.)

The synthetic estrogen (*ethinyl estradiol*) in birth control pills may alter the absorption of psychotropic drugs. For instance, estradiol can slow the body's metabolism of tricyclic antidepressants and some benzodiazepines by the liver (increasing their effects), and hasten the metabolism of others (decreasing effects). Conversely, during pregnancy, hormonal changes may lessen the absorption and distribution of drugs. In addition, there is greater blood volume in which to dilute the drug, so the concentration is decreased.

Hormonal changes also cause drugs to be metabolized faster by the liver and excreted more quickly by the kidneys. So women usually need higher doses of some medications during pregnancy, a problem compounded by possible danger to the fetus. While most psychotropic drugs are not given (or are given with caution) during pregnancy, experts are reexamining their use in women with serious mental illness (see page 283).

As a woman goes through menopause, her ability to handle and eliminate medication also slows. Fatty tissue increases after menopause, raising the concentration of certain drugs. Liver metabolism is also slowed, and the kidneys excrete drugs more slowly. However, says Dr. Hamilton, less is known about effects at menopause than earlier in the life span.

Studies suggest that some drugs may be *less* effective in people of color. For example, 2 to 10 percent of African Americans and 15 to 25 percent of Asian Americans may have less (or none) of certain liver isoenzymes that metabolize tricyclic antidepressants and SSRIs. (Five to 8 percent of Caucasians are also poor metabolizers of these drugs.) Smoking can lower levels of tricyclics, and grapefruit juice also affects isoenzymes.

Questions to Ask Your Doctor

Most prescriptions for psychotropic medication are written by general practitioners, rather than by psychiatrists. Since your gynecologist or internist may not be up on the latest information about psychopharmacology, it's essential that you find out all you can about your medication. Useful sources include the *Consumer PDR*, published by Medical Economics Publishing, or *The Complete Drug Reference*, published by Consumer Reports Books.

The U.S. Food and Drug Administration and national mental health organizations suggest asking these questions before taking any psychotropic medications.

- Why is this medication necessary?

- What is it supposed to do? which symptoms will it relieve?

- What are the risks and the benefits of this drug?

- How long will it take to become effective?

(continued)

- What are the side effects of this drug, and what should I do when side effects occur?

- How and when do I take this medication? (For example, with or without food, or at bedtime.)

- What if I skip a dose, or accidentally take too much?

- Which foods, drinks, other medications or activities should I avoid while taking the medication?

- Will this medication affect my concentration, or my ability to work or to drive?

- Will it affect fertility or pregnancy?

FINE-TUNING DRUG DOSES IN WOMEN

All of these factors need to be taken into account when prescribing psychotropic drugs for women, stresses Kimberly Ann Yonkers, M.D., an assistant professor of psychiatry at the University of Texas Southwestern Medical Center in Dallas and frequent collaborator with Dr. Jean Hamilton. "We find that medications are better tolerated if they are started at a lower dose, and adjusted upward more slowly to account for the increase in plasma levels in women," says Dr. Yonkers. "With tricyclic antidepressants and lithium, we're able to check blood levels, so we have something to guide us."

The dose of certain drugs may sometimes be adjusted during different times of the menstrual cycle, according to whether a woman experiences an increase in symptoms premenstrually.

Some premenopausal women show decreased blood concentration of drugs premenstrually, so increased doses of up to 80 percent may be used in midlife to ensure steady-state drug levels.

The dose may also be adjusted if a woman is taking hormones. For example, the synthetic estrogen in birth control pills may increase side effects of some antianxiety medications by increasing plasma levels. For this reason, says Dr. Yonkers, "a woman should discuss the use of birth control pills with her physician. The strongest effects of the pill are seen with benzodiazepines, so women may be more prone to their sedating side effects." Women on the pill may require a two-thirds reduction in the dose of certain medications, such as imipramine.

Younger women taking estrogen in oral contraceptives may show greater effects than older women taking replacement estrogen. "It's almost as if hormone replacement restores metabolic activity to an equivalent in men," notes Dr. Yonkers. However, data show that the conjugated estrogen used most often (*Premarin*) does not have as pronounced effect on psychotropic drugs as synthetic estrogens in oral contraceptives.

WHICH DRUGS WORK BEST FOR WOMEN?

Some drugs probably work better in women, while others can cause unique side effects, some potentially serious.

Among antidepressants, SSRIs appear to be more effective in women: A recent study found a significant difference between active treatment with *paroxetine* (*Paxil*) and placebo in women, but not men. Paroxetine was more effective in women than in men. SSRIs also seem to work best for women with premenstrual depression or premenstrual dysphoric disorder (see page 203), possibly because severe PMS and PMDD appear to be related to low serotonin; these drugs boost levels of serotonin. Small doses of SSRIs may be used on a continual basis for women with PMDD.

"However, women with depression who are successfully treated may still have some trouble premenstrually," comments Dr. Norman Sussman, director of the Psychopharmacology Research and Consultation Service at NYU. "SSRIs may not necessarily eliminate all of premenstrual symptoms, such as irritability, which may be more hormonally mediated than serotonergic."

The atypical antidepressant *bupropion* carries an increased risk of seizures in higher doses, a risk that is slightly elevated in women, so doses must be monitored, notes Dr. Sussman. Because of a higher seizure risk, bupropion is not given to bulimic or alcoholic women. Bupropion can also cause menstrual irregularities in some women. Its use in pregnant women has not been studied, but since bupropion passes into breast milk, it is *not* used in pregnant or nursing women.

Lithium treatment in women can be hampered by thyroid disease. Women are more likely to have an underactive thyroid (which can cause depressive symptoms), and lithium can also cause hypothyroidism, says Dr. Ellen Leibenluft. (Thyroid hormones can also be affected by pregnancy, compounding bipolar disorder.) Tricyclics or other antidepressants may push vulnerable women into "rapid cycling."

Blood levels of the beta blocker propranolol, frequently prescribed for anxiety, menstrual migraines and social phobia, may decrease in the early follicular phase of the cycle.

In a report presented to the American Psychiatric Association in 1995, Drs. Hamilton and Yonkers write: "Given reports of premenstrual increases in anxiety, it would be beneficial to investigate whether changes in blood levels of drugs contribute to increases in symptomatology." Some physicians routinely tailor doses of antianxiety drugs and antidepressants to have a steady effect across the menstrual cycle.

In women, standard antipsychotics can trigger increased levels of the hormone *prolactin*, which can cause menstrual irregularity, breast swelling and production of breast milk. Women taking antipsychotic drugs may have difficulty conceiving a child because of menstrual irregularities. (Studies are under way regarding *bromocriptine*, which suppresses prolactin, to alleviate these symptoms.) Regardless of the drug they take, experts say, women with schizophrenia have lower levels of fertility.

The most serious consideration for women taking antipsychotics is the risk of *tardive dyskinesia* (*TD*), which can cause facial tics and involuntary movements of the arms and legs (see page 102). Women are at greater risk of developing TD than men, and the risk rises with age and the duration of drug therapy.

Antipsychotic medications can also lower libido, because they slightly reduce levels of the male hormone testosterone.

◅ Caren's Story, Continued ▻

"I was always used to thinking that a pill is all you need, take an antibiotic and you're well in ten days. . . . But all of a sudden I had a diagnosis that wasn't going to go away in a couple of weeks. . . . And to be told that I had to take a tablet every day, possibly for the rest of my life, was literally not an easy pill for me to swallow. . . .

"I also had trouble finding a medication that worked for me, which was difficult. . . . I went through four different types of drugs before they found one that really helped. And that process took a year. . . . Plus, I was going through the side effects of each one, constipation, diarrhea, dry mouth, sleep disturbances. . . .

"But today, I'm happy, I'm healthy, I have a future that is bright, promising. And if there's one thing I can get across to

other women. . . . it's that people with depression . . . are not crying every day, sitting in the chair, not being able to do anything.
. . . With medication and therapy, we can live normal lives. . . .
We're young, we're bright, we're articulate, we're smart, we're
funny, we're happy. . . . We have a diagnosis that makes life difficult sometimes. But it doesn't mean that we can't cope."

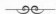

PSYCHOTROPIC DRUGS AND PREGNANCY

The possibility of birth defects and adverse effects on nursing newborns
restricts the use of many psychotherapeutic medications during pregnancy
or lactation. "However, we need to rethink treating pregnant women," says
Dr. Yonkers. "Stopping medication in women with a serious illness such as
bipolar disorder or schizophrenia may increase symptoms or trigger a relapse, which could endanger mother and child."

Since 1980, drugs have been categorized A, B, C, D and X by the FDA,
according to whether studies or case reports show risks to the fetus, such as
birth defects, and whether those risks outweigh benefits to the mother.

Category A drugs demonstrate no risks, while category X drugs are not
used during pregnancy. Many newer drugs (such as *bupropion, fluoxetine, sertraline* and *paroxetine*) fall into category B, for which no controlled studies
have been conducted in humans, but animal studies may or may not have
found problems.

There is some reassuring news about taking Prozac during pregnancy. A
1997 study comparing preschool children whose mothers had taken
fluoextine or a tricyclic antidepressant during pregnancy with children who
had not been exposed found no effects on IQ, language, or behavioral
development in those children whose mothers had taken antidepressants. An
earlier study found no significant differences in the rates of birth defects
between untreated women and those who took tricyclics or fluoextine.

Drugs in category C and D (including MAOIs, older tricyclics and anxiolytics, which have been associated with birth defects, are given *only* when
benefits to the mother outweigh the risks (although some studies have
shown that tricyclics do not cause birth defects and can be given safely).
Most antipsychotic drugs are in category C or D. While there are no birth
defects associated specifically with antipsychotics, their effect on the
developing brain of the fetus remains largely unknown.

Anxiolytics fall into class C and D. *Diazepam* and *alprazolam* have been associated with possible increased risk of cleft palate and limb malformations, as well as miscarriage. And while these problems generally occur at the same rate as in the general population, the literature "suggests caution when using these drugs in pregnant patients," write Drs. Hamilton and Yonkers. Benzodiazepines used in the third trimester may also cause withdrawal symptoms in newborns.

Lithium is generally not used during pregnancy. Bipolar women who want to become pregnant may be advised to switch to antipsychotics, since lithium taken in the first trimester has been linked to cardiac value abnormalities. However, in severe relapses, lithium may be given later during pregnancy.

USE OF MEDICATION DURING LACTATION

Experts are also taking a closer look at the use of psychotropic drugs right after delivery and during lactation, since this is a time of increased risk for postpartum depression and postpartum psychosis in vulnerable women.

Patients with postpartum disorders tend to see doctors after symptoms have become more serious, partly because there is a stigma attached to coming in with a new baby and seeking help for mental problems, notes Valerie Raskin, M.D., assistant professor of psychiatry at the University of Illinois College of Medicine in Chicago.

Unfortunately, many women may be given medication and automatically told to stop breast-feeding. "Some women who are having postpartum anxiety or depression say that nursing their babies is the one time they feel competent, like they have something to offer. It makes them feel like a good mother. So there may be some psychosocial benefits we have yet to measure in continuing nursing," says Dr. Raskin. "Medication may get a depressed woman back into feeling like her illness is not a sign of her inadequacy, that it's not proof that she wasn't meant to have children. But many times physicians feel it's easier to recommend the use of formula, rather than grapple with the issue of using medication."

Psychotropic drugs are excreted in breast milk, and nursing infants will absorb them. But given the benefits of breast-feeding to infants (including antibodies that help build immunity), and the risk of untreated major depression in the mother (which recent studies suggest can also cause developmental problems in her child), Dr. Raskin says, medication may be advisable in some cases. And since some mothers "supplement" breast-feeding with formula, it may be possible to time medication to minimize effects on the baby.

The American Academy of Pediatrics (AAP) classifies medications into four categories: contraindicated in lactation; unknown effect (no known adverse effect but may be of "concern"); should be given with caution; and compatible with breast-feeding.

The only psychiatric medication that is contraindicated by the AAP during breast-feeding is lithium. Drugs that should be given with caution include barbiturates. Antipsychotics like *clozapine* have been shown to accumulate in breast milk, as has fluoxetine. Benzodiazepines are secreted in breast milk and can cause sedation and slowed heart rate in newborns.

Medications considered compatible with breast-feeding include the anticonvulsants *valproic acid* (*Depakote*) and *carbamazepine* (*Tegretol*). As for tricyclic antidepressants, the AAP views the use of *imipramine* and *desipramine* with concern, although no adverse effects have been reported. Experts like Dr. Raskin feel that tricyclics can be compatible with nursing. But Drs. Hamilton and Yonkers comment that, while no direct toxic effects have been seen, the long-term behavioral consequences to the infant are unknown.

IF YOU'RE OVER SIXTY-FIVE

A woman over sixty-five may receive half the usual dose because of decreased drug clearance. For example, older women have been shown to retain higher levels of the tricyclic antidepressants *imipramine* and *desipramine*, leading to more side effects.

Studies suggest a relationship between benzodiazepine use and urinary incontinence, as well as hip fractures in mature women leading to placement in a nursing home, so behavioral management for anxiety might be tried before medication.

In women with schizophrenia, studies suggest that before menopause, estrogen may help lessen the severity of symptoms by suppressing levels of dopamine in the brain (just as some antipsychotic drugs do). But many women worsen after menopause, when estrogen levels decline. So postmenopausal women may need higher doses of antipsychotics compared with men the same age.

Older people tend to take several medications for chronic illnesses (including over-the-counter preparations), so the possibility of interactions is greater. This is especially true if both drugs act on the same chemical pathways and "compete" with each other for the same receptors in the brain. Many experts believe that medications like tranquilizers should be avoided by the elderly.

Women in general take more medications than men and are at greater risk of interactions, says Dr. Yonkers. So they and their partners (or caretakers) should be alert for any drug reactions.

Maintaining Mental Wellness

Although vulnerability to mental illness can be a matter of genes and biology, environmental and psychological factors play a major role. We can't eliminate all the stress in our lives, avoid losses or control the behavior of others. But we can be aware of risk factors (such as a family history of depression or other mental illness), know the red flags that signal trouble early on and learn to manage our own thinking and behavior.

By learning positive coping strategies to overcome blue moods, handle loss and anger, defuse stress, understand our personal "pressure points," and making time for ourselves, we may be able to avoid depression, anxiety, disordered eating and alcohol abuse (or other addictive behaviors).

Red Flags: Depression

Here are some warning signs that a bout with the blues is becoming more serious.

- Have you been feeling sad for some time, unable to bounce back? If you are in severe emotional pain and have been for more than a month, if such episodes keep recurring, or if you're unable to shake mild depression, you could have a problem.

- Have you experienced any changes in behavior that are unusual for you? If you usually sleep well, have a normal desire for sex and are able to concentrate on your work and those things change for a few weeks or more, it could signal depression.

- Do you have a feeling of constant fatigue that no amount of sleep seems to cure? That can be a key symptom of depression.

- Have you lost interest in work, family, friends, sex life? Normal mood swings don't usually prevent us from enjoying these things; clinical depression does.

- Are you drinking (or drinking more than usual) or using drugs to get rid of persistent bad feelings? Most of us don't turn to alcohol to ease a blue mood, but many people try to medicate the pain of depression with drugs or alcohol.

- Have you been feeling worthless and unlovable, and blaming yourself for bad things that happen? The blues make us feel down, but not down on *ourselves*. Depression usually erodes self-esteem.

- Have you had suicidal thoughts, or felt like just ending it all? This is a very important symptom. It's normal to feel rotten about losses in life, but feeling like killing yourself is not. If you have suicidal thoughts, get professional help *right away*. (For other suicide red flags, see page 310.)

BEATING THE BLUES

Experts say that by learning to cope with life's ups and downs, we may be able to prevent a blue mood from turning into major depression. (Although they note that biologically based, or *endogenous*, depression may not always be preventable.)

Depression almost always stems from a major stress or loss. According to a 1994 report titled *Reducing the Risks of Mental Disorders*, published by the Institute of Medicine (IOM), a division of the National Academy of Sciences, traumatic events; the loss of a job; death of a partner, parent or child; divorce; financial reverses; poverty and a history of childhood abuse and major losses in childhood are all risk factors for major depression. A string of negative events can chip away at self-esteem, and can foster a sense of helplessness, hopelessness and a feeling of not being in control of one's life, all of which can result in depression.

At the same time, the IOM report noted that the presence of close, intimate and supportive relationships may help to protect against depression. Good friends and family can provide a valuable support system when problems hit.

But our main protection from depression is emotional resiliency, which depends in large part on how we feel about ourselves, and how we handle problems.

All of us have had setbacks. We may lose a job or an important person in our lives; we may not achieve our goals; upheavals and changes in life may knock us for a loop. At such times, it's only natural to turn inward to lick our wounds, and marshal our resources so we can get on with life again.

Some people bounce back faster than others. Some of us don't. We all know people who seem to have "depressive personalities," putting a negative spin on everything that happens. Others are competitive, treating every situation as a win-or-lose proposition, where any setback is automatically a catastrophe. Some people are very sensitive, and one piece of criticism sets off an avalanche of negative thoughts.

Understanding *why* you react to events the way you do is important in developing more effective coping skills, says NYU's Dr. Helen DeRosis. "Your reactions to setbacks or criticism may originate in childhood if you came from a family where you were expected to be perfect and were criticized a lot for failing to meet those standards," she says. "You internalize that criticism. Then, when something 'bad' happens, *you* assume the voice of that critical parent. Such feelings can stay with you for a lifetime unless you learn to discard the need to be perfect."

Famed European psychiatrist Karen Horney originated the concept of "the tyranny of the shoulds," to which all of us fall prey at one time or another. These "shoulds" form compulsive standards, which can set us up for bouts of anxiety, depression and a host of self-destructive activities, explains Dr. DeRosis. "What's more, one's parents, upbringing, cultural attitudes and values all contribute to this internal inventory of how we believe we *should* think, act, look or do with our lives."

The trouble is, *none* of us can live up to the expectations of these "shoulds." And despite our successes, we can feel like a failure at times, or that it's somehow our fault when things go wrong. When we try to impose our "shoulds" on others, it can result in disappointment, resentment and frustration (for others are captives of their *own* "shoulds").

"One key to avoiding depression is to try to lessen the blame you heap upon yourself. Some things are under your control, others are not. Understanding that limitation is a key component of emotional resiliency," says Dr. DeRosis. "Two of the major ingredients of depression are guilt and anger, either at oneself or others. Both stem from all the 'shoulds' we pile upon ourselves and our partners."

Dr. DeRosis recommends sitting down and making a list of all your private "shoulds." "When you begin to understand how these unrealistic expectations are affecting your life, you may be able to better cope with them, or even gradually rid yourself of some of them. Once you stop being so hard on yourself, you will be better able to handle day-to-day stresses."

When you're blue, don't dismiss your feelings, but don't wallow in them, either, advises University of Michigan psychologist Susan Nolen-Hoeksema, who has done extensive research into how women cope with depression.

Dr. Nolen-Hoeksema has found that women are more prone to focus on depressive symptoms in a passive, non-problem-solving way. This "ruminative response" not only interferes with taking action to solve problems and overcome mild depression, but may lead to interpreting events in a more negative way, promoting and prolonging major depression. In other words, brooders get bluer.

"When confronted with a stressor or a problem, instead of focusing on how bad you feel, ask yourself, 'What are my options?' Once you see some choices, changes or possible solutions to a problem, your feelings of helplessness and hopelessness will greatly diminish. Depression feeds on hopelessness," she advises.

Dr. DeRosis has these other tips for beating the blues.

- Keep up your daily routines. It's more beneficial to get up in the morning at your usual time, get dressed, have breakfast and go to work or do daily chores, than to stay in bed with your unhappy thoughts. It will also keep your body's internal clock running smoothly.

- Try to get "out" at least twice a day, even for short periods of time. This can include taking a short walk, going window shopping at lunchtime, visiting the library or taking a coffee break or a meal outside.

- Don't neglect activities you enjoy. Depressed women often have too little pleasure in their lives; they're too busy doing what they think they "should" be doing, not what makes them happy.

- Stay in touch with family and friends as much as possible. Talk on the phone or, even better, pay short visits. If you find it hard to talk to people during a blue period, write letters or notes. Keep your lines of communication open.

- When you're feeling really down, let your partner know that this is not "business as usual," that you need some extra support and help. This goes for children, too. If you find it hard to ask for help, write notes.

- Avoid alcohol. Alcohol is a depressant, and while it may initially make you feel better, after a few drinks your mood will take a decided downswing. And, using alcohol as a tranquilizer can set you up for alcohol abuse.

- Don't try to eat your way out of a bad mood. This can increase your risk of disordered eating, not to mention expand your waistline (making you feel even worse).

- Most important, *get moving.* Exercise is one of the *best* ways to banish the blues. It acts as a natural antidepressant to some extent and helps reestablish the chemical balance of the brain, boosting mood-elevating neurotransmitters.

Exercise may also help us cope better with anxiety-provoking events. A workout can stimulate the body to rid itself of stress hormones, such as adrenaline and cortisol. Experts say regular workouts may "train" the body to react less intensely to these hormones. Exercise is also thought to boost levels of endorphins, the body's natural pain-reliever and feel-good chemical.

A recent study of seventy-four depressed men and women at the University of Wisconsin in Madison found that two 45-minute running sessions a week were just as effective in lifting depression as group therapy or meditation. Studies at California State University found that a brisk ten-minute walk was an effective way of beating the blues, providing more than an hour's worth of increased energy by revving up heart rate and breathing, reducing stress and muscle tension.

POSITIVE THINKING VERSUS NEGATIVE REACTION

Another mental health habit to help you avoid depression is positive thinking. It's no cliché: Positive thinking *is* powerful.

Many people suffering from depression have negative thought patterns that color every experience they have. "When people exaggerate the importance of each setback in their lives, it can set up a downward spiral that can end in major depression," warns Richard M. Wenzlaff, Ph.D., associate professor of psychology at the University of Texas, San Antonio.

A number of years ago, Dr. Wenzlaff conducted an experiment to see how our moods affect the way we react to failure and how negative thinking can snowball. Groups of volunteers were given a series of psychological tests. Some were told they did well, others that they scored poorly. People who had recently felt depressed reacted to bad scores by inflating the importance of the test and extending their feeling of failure to other areas of their life, becoming even more depressed. Those people who had not felt depressed reacted to their bad scores by seeing the test as less important, and said it didn't change their overall view of themselves. "Depressed people see one failure as indicative of their worth as a person and feel hopeless they can ever change. This tends to foster even more negative thinking," comments Dr. Wenzlaff.

According to cognitive therapists, common negative thought patterns include the following.

- All-or-Nothing Thinking: "If I can't have exactly what I want, I'll take nothing."

- Perfectionism: "No one will love me till I lose twenty pounds."

- Overgeneralization: "Nothing ever goes right." "Everything bad always happens to me."

- Catastrophizing: "I lost my job, I'll never get another."

- Minimizing: "I'm not talented enough to get a promotion."

- Comparative Thinking: "I'm not as successful as my friends." "Everyone makes more money than I do."

- Dismissing the Positive: "We had a great evening, but he'll never call again."

- Mind Reading: "I know my boss thinks I'm not doing a good job. How can I ask him for a raise?"

- Fortune-Telling: "I know what will happen, so why try?"

Recognize yourself?

You're not alone. We all tend to fall victim to distorted ways of thinking at one time or another. But when that becomes a habit, we leave ourselves vulnerable to major depression.

LEARNING TO THINK POSITIVE

It takes hard *work* to break the cycle of negative thinking. But you *can* do it by applying some simple techniques commonly used in cognitive therapy.

Keep a thought diary. Write down your thoughts and reactions to people and events, and review what you have written when you're in a relaxed mood. Or, review it with a close friend or your partner, letting them give you feedback on other ways you might have thought about or handled a situation.

Deal with the here and now, not the past. Regret is a common negative pattern of thinking. "One of the things that may be helpful to women is to take a more present- and future-oriented approach to dealing with life stress, and not ruminate on all the things they *should* have done," advises Dr. Ellen Frank, director of the Prevention of Depression and Manic Depression Program at the Western Psychiatric Institute and Clinic in Pittsburgh. "Women should focus on positive actions they can take now to improve a situation or reduce interpersonal stress, what they can do in the future to make things better and perhaps prevent similar problems from occurring. Decide what outcome you'd like to achieve and act on that."

Give yourself "time-outs" when you're under stress. The next time you start to react to a situation or criticism in a self-defeating way, stop and think. Tell yourself you are *not* going to fall into the same pattern of negative thinking.

Learn positive self-talk. This means unlearning all the negative things you tell yourself (again, that little voice that's been there since you were a kid), says Dr. Wenzlaff. Make a list of common negative words or phrases you use, and a list of new words or phrases to replace them with. Then memorize the lists. Every time you start to use one of the negative words on your list, consciously substitute a positive one.

Some tips for acquiring a new, positive vocabulary.

- Get rid of words like "everything," "nothing," "never," "always" and, of course, "should." These are all disabling words, which discourage us from moving forward with life.

- Stop saying, "I can't." For many of us, "I can't" is an excuse not to try, and implies that you have no control over your life. Say, "I could" instead.

- Take verbal charge. When you say, "It's not my fault," you also imply that you've lost control. Saying, "I'm responsible," you're taking control, even of a bad situation.

- Deep-six the self put-downs. Words like "fat," "unattractive" and "stupid" might be replaced by words like "voluptuous," "sexy" and "smart."

- Forget "win or lose," "all or nothing." Tell yourself that you can't lose, no matter what the situation, that you will gain opportunities to learn and grow.

- When you start feeling overwhelmed, tell yourself, "I can handle it." Instead of feeling helpless, you develop trust in yourself, believing you can deal with anything that happens.

It will take some practice to change your automatic negative thinking patterns, but cognitive therapists say it works! Other people react to how we feel about ourselves. If you adopt a positive, confident outlook, it will be self-reinforcing. Don't let one setback color your view of the future. Life has so many possibilities, don't be held back by a negative mind.

❧ *Caren's Story, Continued* ☙

"The hardest thing for me was learning how to deal with anger. Women are all taught that we're not supposed to have the emotion of anger, which, with depression, is one you have a lot. One of the biggest parts of depression . . . is poor self-image, worthlessness, helplessness feeling. That used to make me so angry. Because somewhere inside of me, I knew that wasn't true. I knew I wasn't worthless, I knew I wasn't helpless. But I couldn't get past it. And so you get frustrated and that frustration leads to more anger . . . anger that you have depression . . . anger that you have to take medication every day just to get by. . . . There's a lot of anger in just coping with those daily issues.

"I used to swallow all of that. Because I didn't have any good way to deal with it. Growing up, all I heard was being angry was not ladylike, it was not a Christian thing. . . . So I worked real hard on learning coping skills to deal with anger.

"The hardest thing I've learned . . . is to confront my anger straight up. Why am I angry? Who am I angry with? . . . I've worked very hard to find constructive ways to say, 'When you said thus and so, I felt very angry about that,' instead of 'you made me angry. . . . ' Anger is just an emotion you need to work through. . . .

"It doesn't work all that well with my family yet, but it does with some of my friends who've been through this with me. If I make them angry, or they make me angry, we've promised each other that we will talk about it. . . . The more you practice, the better you get at it, the easier you feel about it."

⎯☙☙⎯

HANDLING ANGER

Anger is a normal emotion. It's the way we *handle* anger that can be unhealthy, both emotionally and physically. Studies have shown that chronically hostile or angry people have five times the risk of heart attack, have high levels of stress hormones and blood pressure, and lower levels of the "good" HDL cholesterol.

Women are socialized to keep a lid on their anger, to be conciliators, sometimes at the expense of their own feelings.

Suppressing anger isn't healthy, either. It may lead to smoking, drinking, overeating and other unhealthy ways of self-medication. A 1994 study of five hundred women at the University of Tennessee, Knoxville, found that not only does suppressing anger lead to increased health problems, but so can venting anger. "Unhealthy" anger reactions (viewing provocations as deliberate or obsessing about quarrels) led to stress, depression and health problems. The study found that the anger reaction that had *health-promoting* benefits was discussing feelings. Understanding how *you* deal with anger, and correcting unhealthy reactions, may go a long way toward promoting mental and physical health.

People fall into six basic categories when it comes to maladaptive ways of dealing with anger, says Bonnie Maslin, Ph.D., a New York City psychotherapist and author of *The Angry Marriage: Overcoming the Rage, Reclaiming the Love* (Hyperion, 1995).

At opposite ends of the spectrum are "suppressors," who bury their rage, and "ventors," who express their anger with shouting, screaming, quarreling or even physical fights. "When a woman is a ventor, it has the effect of pushing her further and further away from what she needs. Anger is caused by the frustration of needs. But when she vents by screaming, she generally gets back more of the same, and that doesn't do anything to satisfy her needs. It just escalates tension," says Dr. Maslin. The problem with swallowing anger is that suppressors can shut down emotionally, and that can lead to depression.

In between are the "provokers," people who play opposing roles in relationships; for example, one person is angry and self-righteous, the other self-defensive. "Enactors" deal with anger by substituting behaviors such as having an affair or drinking. " 'Symbolizers' don't get mad, they get maladies," observes Dr. Maslin; they develop headaches or other physical ailments. "Displacers" take their anger out on others; they yell at the kids and coworkers, or kick the cat.

"Many people feel it's healthy to 'discharge' the tensions of their emotions by yelling, or by doing physical things like punching pillows. But if you discharge your anger instead of dealing with the emotions, you're not going to be able to identify the feelings and put them into words," contends Dr. Maslin.

Dr. Maslin stresses that everyone argues from time to time; arguing is not necessarily a sign that a relationship is in trouble. In fact, one report from the National Institute of Mental Health found that couples who know how to fight fairly have a 50 percent *lower* divorce rate than those who can't handle disagreements! However, when bickering and heated arguments become the norm, partners need to explore the feelings *behind* their anger.

"The most sensible and powerful strategy for handling anger is to be able to say, 'I feel,' and then to understand what you feel and what you need, and be able to communicate," she says.

Set aside regular times for talking when you can give each other undivided attention, without other distractions. Hear each other out, without raising voices, prohibiting emotional blackmail and other abusive behaviors. Try to get to the root of what's really bothering you, without hurling accusations.

Other tips for handling anger constructively.

- When talking about anger, avoid blame and generalizations. Say, "I felt angry when you said/did that . . ." instead of, "You always do that to me."

- Don't take cheap shots. Insulting a person or bringing up unrelated problems or shortcomings only assaults the other person's self-esteem and makes them feel angrier. Fight fair.

- Stick to the subject at hand. Don't drag in every past slight or injustice.

- Learn to *listen*. Rather than letting your anger blind you, tune in to what the other person is saying, not only with words, but with expressions and gestures. Take turns talking.

- Don't fight in front of other people; don't ask friends to arbitrate. If you and a partner need a referee for your fights, maybe what you really need is marriage counseling or couples therapy.

- Don't hang on to your anger. Nursing anger just allows it to fester. Try to resolve situations and restore goodwill. Don't take anger into the bedroom.

☙ *Caroline's Story, Continued* ☙

"I equated sweet, soft foods like pudding and ice cream with love. These were foods I was given as a child when I was sick, to make me feel better. Those are the foods I liked to binge on. . . . I had to find healthier ways to nurture myself, other than food.

"I also had to learn how to handle other people who equate food with love. Visiting my husband's family used to be really hard. There was real southern cooking: fried chicken, biscuits, pork roast, cookies. . . . I never knew how to turn them down without hurting someone's feelings. My husband's grandmother would tell us how she'd cooked for days. But I have learned that I don't have to eat to show someone I care. It's okay to say no.

"Perfectionism is part of the reason I developed an eating disorder. I was not satisfied with having an average body. . . . If our weight goals are unrealistic and our meal plans are too rigid, we are setting ourselves up for failure. . . . Food is just food. You can't build your life around dieting and watching what you eat and weighing yourself.

"You have to learn good eating habits, make them second nature and, this is very important, you have to like yourself, accept yourself, love yourself for what you are. Your appearance is not a true reflection of the inner you. We are *all* beautiful."

AVOIDING DISORDERED EATING

It's estimated that some thirty-one million American women are currently "dieting," limiting their food intake in hopes of miraculously changing the shape of their body. Unfortunately, a majority of people who go on drastic short-term diets eventually regain the lost pounds (and then some) and become trapped in a cycle of yo-yo dieting. And experts are still debating which factors add up to a "healthy" weight for an individual.

Millions of women develop chronic problems dealing with food, swinging back and forth between indulgence and denial, overeating and undereating, feeling guilty for indulging, their self-esteem riding on the ups and downs of the bathroom scale. "Women weigh themselves entirely too often. Everyone has normal fluctuations in weight; some people weigh more in the evening, some weigh less in the morning. Fluid retention can increase your weight temporarily, as can other conditions," says Dr. Melissa Ferguson of NYU Medical Center's Eating Disorders Program. "Women should weigh themselves once every two weeks, if that much."

People with disordered eating often label certain foods as "good" or "bad." "When you label a food as 'bad' and overly restrict that food, it makes you feel deprived, and you start to crave that food. Which sets people up for bingeing," adds Dr. Ferguson. "It's better to build small treats into your diet."

Also, be aware of foods that may "trigger" overeating. For some women it's sweets; for others it's carbohydrates. Cravings for carbohydrates and sweets (which often lead to bingeing) may have a biological basis, elevating mood by boosting serotonin levels. Studies show that women are more likely than men to have food cravings (and crave sweet foods). Rather than fighting cravings, eat a small amount to quiet the craving. If you do feel the urge to binge, delay eating the food in question for ten to fifteen minutes, until you feel more in control, or drink a glass of water.

Many of us use food as a tranquilizer in times of stress. We eat (and eat too much) when we're not really hungry, driven by a need for comfort. So avoid eating when you're upset or bored. Learn to *listen to your body*. Eat when you're *physically hungry*.

Stop "dieting." Concentrate on developing healthy eating habits. Increasing your activity and exercise level will do more to help control your weight than diets, and it can reduce symptoms of depression and PMS. If your physician says you need to lose weight for health reasons, investigate a supervised weight-loss program that teaches healthy eating habits.

Signs of a potential problem include: spending too much time thinking about what you should or shouldn't be eating; experiencing undue anxiety about food; hiding or hoarding food, sneaking food or refusing to tell what you're eating or spending on food. If you are exhibiting any of these behaviors, you may need professional help.

LEARNING TO ACCEPT YOUR BODY

What do you see when you look in the mirror? Do you see yourself as "fat" when others think you look fine? Do you avoid social situations because of your weight? Does your negative body-image prevent you from enjoying activities such as swimming because you hate being seen in a bathing suit?

Cognitive therapy to improve your body image may help. One new therapy program developed at the University of Vermont is aimed at helping chronically overweight women feel better about their appearance and stopping the self-recrimination and social embarrassment they feel about being overweight. The therapy, conducted in groups of four or five people, starts out by discussing a crucial experience that led to the women's negative feelings about their bodies (like being called "fatty" in junior high gym class). The women are helped to counter their negative body-talk and self-judgment ("I'm fat, people think I'm dumb").

The program also encourages the women to spend time alone looking at themselves in the mirror, slowly learning to look at big tummies or thighs without bad-mouthing their bodies. Those private exercises serve as a prelude to adopting freer and more attractive styles of dressing. For example, one woman who was obsessed with fat around her neck was able to start wearing blouses that did not conceal her neck, wearing jewelry around her neck and putting her hair up.

A study of the therapy program found that it was very effective in "remodeling" body image, no matter what the women weighed. The fifty-one participants ranged from those weighing more than 350 pounds to women who were only 25 pounds overweight.

Many of the volunteers were afraid that accepting their bodies would prevent them from losing weight (or cause them to gain even more weight). But that didn't happen, says James C. Rosen, Ph.D., a professor of psychology who developed the program. The women felt so much better about themselves they were less likely to overeat. The program also had an indirect effect on the women's level of fitness. Many who had avoided exercise (especially in public) felt free enough to join exercise groups, reports Dr. Rosen.

Some better body-image tips from Dr. Rosen's program.

- Don't keep putting your body down. Instead of making negative statements about your body, practice more forgiving, nonjudgmental self-descriptions. Instead of saying, "That sweater makes me look fat," say, "That red sweater is a good color for me."

- Learn to take a compliment. Other people are usually more objective and positive about your appearance.

- Be calm and objective when looking at yourself in the mirror. Take in the whole picture, not just "figure flaws."

- Put physical appearance in its place. Give yourself credit for other important things, like intelligence, sense of humor and special abilities at work and at home. Being overweight does *not* prove there's something wrong with your character!

- Develop a happier body-image by experimenting with different clothes and hairstyles.

- Face down frightening body-image situations that you avoid (like beaches or swimming pools), using positive self-talk to help conquer your fears. Tell yourself, "I'm going to enjoy the sun and the surf. No one is going to notice what I look like."

⇛ *Ruth's Story* ⇝

"I believe all addictions are the same, basically. You hurt, you're empty. You hate yourself. You need to escape. I got up in the morning and my only goal was oblivion. . . . You get high, then you forget and feel better. It's a vicious cycle. Because when that wears off you have to have more.

"Every addict is in denial. They are always having clean starts. Tomorrow I won't have a drink. Tomorrow I'll be sober, tomorrow I'll be on time for work. . . . But 'tomorrow' never comes.

"I blamed everyone else. . . . And I walked around with this attitude that it didn't matter because I was the only one who knew about my drinking. But it did matter. It finally occurred to me that drinking was my problem, that I was my problem.

"If you think you are teetering on problem drinking, see if you can do without it for thirty days. If the thought of going without alcohol for a weekend or a week makes you afraid, then you have a problem. It's not how much you drink, how much you smoke, how much coke you do, but what it *does* to you. If you can't live without cigarettes or booze, you have a problem."

AVOIDING PROBLEMS WITH ALCOHOL

Many people enjoy a glass of wine with dinner or a drink at a party. But when you can't seem to control *how much* you drink, or *can't go without* a drink, it could develop into alcohol abuse.

NYU Medical Center's Dr. Nicholas Pace, an expert on alcohol abuse and author of *Guidelines for Safe Drinking* (Fawcett-Ballantine, 1986), has a simple yardstick for measuring alcohol abuse. "If alcohol is interfering with any one of the major components of your life, your job, your relationships, your health, you have a problem," he says. "If you are *worried* that you may have a problem with alcohol, you probably do."

Dr. Pace stresses that if you want to avoid problem drinking, don't get into the drinking *habit*. "If you go out of your way to make sure there's wine with dinner every night, after a while that meal won't feel 'normal' without wine, and *you* won't feel normal without it. Don't fall into a habit of drinking after work each day to unwind. That can also get you into trouble."

Don't drink when you're under pressure, or when you're emotionally upset, or turn to alcohol to escape from marital or other troubles. "Alcohol may relax you for a while, you get an initial sedative effect for about an hour. But then it starts irritating the nervous system and you're going to want another drink. People believe alcohol helps depression, but alcohol is a depressant and they can become more depressed. Or they become irritable when they don't have a drink, which is a symptom of withdrawal. A person may drink more to combat their irritability. These are patterns that should set off alarms," says Dr. Pace.

Take the "CAGE" Test

The "CAGE" test is a simple questionnaire frequently used by mental health professionals. If you answer yes to any one question (especially E), you may have a drinking problem. Two (or more) yes answers indicate you may be abusing alcohol.

C—Have you ever felt the need to **cut down** on your drinking?

A—Have you ever felt **annoyed** by criticism of your drinking?

G—Have you ever felt **guilty** about your drinking?

E—Have you ever felt the need for an **eye opener** in the morning?

When you do drink, limit yourself to one to two drinks, then switch to non-alcoholic beverages, or alternate alcohol with nonalcoholic drinks. Try nonalcoholic wine, beer or drinks like wine "spritzers," which contain less alcohol.

Although light to moderate drinking may have some protective benefits for a woman's heart, experts say that if you don't drink, don't start. If you do drink, keep it on the light side. Light drinking for women is one to three drinks per week; moderate drinking is one drink per day. *Never* mix psychoactive medication with alcohol. For example, taking alcohol with antidepressants, anxiety medications or antipsychotics can result in respiratory depression, seizures, coma or death. *Remember, Dr. Pace cautions, there is* no *"safe" level of drinking for a woman who's pregnant. And, of course, don't ever drink and drive.*

AVOIDING BURNOUT

No one has to tell you that there aren't enough hours in the day. Women may no longer want to "have it all" as they did in the frenetic 1980s, but many of us are still *doing* it all: housework, office work, shopping, child care, cooking, caring for ailing partners or family members. The payback is often increased stress, depression, anxiety and a feeling of being "burned out."

A 1993 study by the Families and Work Institute found that between regular work hours, overtime, commuting, household chores and attending to children, the average person in a two-paycheck family puts in almost fifteen hours of work per day! Not surprisingly, 42 percent of people feel "used up" by the end of the workday, and 40 percent feel tired when they get up in the morning and have to face another day.

Burnout may feature all the signs of stress, but its main symptoms are exhaustion and feelings of hopelessness and apathy, says Reed C. Moskowitz, M.D., medical director of the Stress Disorders Medical Services at NYU Medical Center, and author of *Your Healing Mind* (Morrow, 1992).

According to one measurement scale, the components of burnout are: emotional exhaustion; no longer being able to contribute on a psychological level to a role, a job or relationship; depersonalization; lack of concern or cynicism about clients, coworkers or family; a reduced sense of personal accomplishment, to the point where a woman feels unhappy about herself and dissatisfied with her work or family role.

Burnout makes you irritable, fatigued, unproductive and just plain unhappy. It also makes personal and family relationships more difficult (not to mention your sex life). "Burnout is a progressive process, the end stage of struggling with stress. Your goal should be preventing daily stresses from taking that toll," says Dr. Moskowitz.

We need to recognize that some stresses are avoidable. An example of an avoidable stress is letting work pile up, or taking on too many commitments, so that you feel overwhelmed. Avoiding or changing situations that lead to those kinds of avoidable stress can help prevent burnout. Unavoidable stress can take the form of a traffic delay, an accident or a serious illness. By accepting the fact that some things are simply out of our control, we can help ourselves stay calm and do what we have to. "Knowing the difference between these two kinds of stress is a major key to problem solving. You won't waste time and energy spinning your wheels, feeling stressed out," says Dr. Moskowitz.

Other suggestions for avoiding burnout.

- Prioritize. Decide what's urgent and what can wait, what's important and what isn't. Make an "A" list and a "B" list (and even a "C" list).

- Delegate. Insist that partners (and children) take on an equitable share of household chores. Have the kids make their own school lunches, and make cleaning their rooms their responsibility.

- Organize. For example, cook in big batches and freeze in several containers for quick meals; post a list on the refrigerator door.

- Get extra help. If you can afford it, pay for hired help once in a while. Have the kids make extra cash by taking on major chores you haven't the time to do. If you are caring for a special-needs child, or an ill or an aged relative, investigate respite care in your area (see Appendix I).

- If you can, arrange for part-time or "flex-time" work arrangements to ease the juggling act between work and family.

- Downsize your duties. Don't be "guilted" by others into taking on more than you know you can handle.

- Don't push yourself too far, with work, with exercise, with any activity. Give yourself downtime to relax. Take a day off occasionally. Make time for *yourself*.

- Get enough sleep. For help, see page 307.

- Learn stress-reducing exercises so that you can avoid the long-term consequences of chronic stress.

⨈ *Marcia's Story, Continued* ⨈

"When I'm feeling good, feeling normal, I know what's important. Having dirty dishes is not as important as having your roof fall in, or your children getting hurt. But when you're depressed, everything is the same. A dust bunny under the bed can be as overwhelming as a child breaking an arm. There's no filter mechanism. You have no ability to . . . decide what's more important. So you're totally overwhelmed all the time. . . . What I've learned to do is prioritize. And that helps me avoid anxiety. . . .

"I've become very attuned to my danger signs. . . . When I'm getting sick, the first thing that happens is being unable to sleep. The second thing is that I start ruminating about horrible things. I really knock myself: 'I'm horrible, I'm bad, I can't do things right, whatever made me think I could do this? I'm incapable.' When I start thinking like this and my sleep becomes disturbed, that's a marker. And I always have a physical marker, almost an aura. A kind of darkness descends and I see things as if through very dark sunglasses. Things don't seem animated, don't seem lively. I have a feeling in my chest of tightness and anxiety, and I'm . . . very irritable and easy to tears. . . .

"I've had to find ways of counteracting those things when they start to happen. Making sure I get enough sleep, not letting little things get to me, doing positive self-talk, saying no to things I don't need to do and, if I need it, take medication."

LEARNING STRESS-BUSTERS

Some stress in our lives is actually healthy. It helps us meet deadlines and propels us to overcome obstacles. But letting stress constantly swamp us damages physical *and* mental health.

Stress can produce emotional symptoms such as nervousness, anxiety, crying, feeling on edge, angry, and under increased pressure. Stress can cloud our thinking, sap our creativity and make us forgetful, indecisive and unable to get things done. "Stress makes us feel drained, powerless, lonely, self-doubting and unhappy, all the ingredients for depression," says Dr. Moskowitz.

Chronic stress can also trigger a host of physical problems. They include headaches, stomachaches, muscle spasm (especially in the back and shoulders) and sleep difficulties. Recent studies indicate that stress lowers the body's immune responses; people under stress are more likely to catch frequent colds!

You can help neutralize the body's fight-or-flight response to stress with deep breathing, relaxation exercises, meditation or guided imagery, yoga or even tai chi (a mentally focused form of exercise from China). These activities reduce levels of stress hormones, lowering your heart rate and blood pressure and slowing breathing, calming you down, says Dr. Moskowitz. The increased oxygen to the brain enables us to think more clearly and make better decisions. Muscle tension drains away. Herbert Benson, M.D., director of the Mind-Body Institute and chief of Behavioral Medicine at the New England Deaconess Hospital in Boston, calls this the "relaxation response."

"The advantage to deep breathing and muscle relaxation is that they can be done anywhere, as opposed to going to exercise classes, which many people attend for a while and then drop because they're too busy," remarks Dr. Moskowitz.

Activities that produce the relaxation response utilize a mental focusing device such as repeating phrases, sounds, images or physical activities. They include:

DEEP BREATHING: To learn how to breathe deeply from your diaphragm, lie down and put your hand on your belly. When you're breathing from the diaphragm, your hand will rise and fall. Count slowly from one to ten as you breathe in and again as you breathe out. After you've mastered the technique, you can do it at your desk, in your car or in your kitchen. Taking the time to concentrate on your breathing during a stressful situation gives you time to compose yourself and gain control.

MUSCLE RELAXATION: Muscle relaxation exercises can be added to deep breathing. Close your eyes and with each deep breath imagine the tension draining away, one by one, from your head, your neck, your arms and so on. This technique is most effective if you are lying down in a quiet place, but you can do it in just about any setting, including at your desk.

MEDITATION: Meditation need not be more exotic than sitting or lying comfortably in a relatively quiet place, and focusing on breathing or muscle relaxation, while thinking soothing thoughts. Some people visualize a beam of bright light warming their body, dissolving muscle tension and negative thoughts. When you repeat a word or phrase during this process, it's called *transcendental meditation*, or *TM*. These repetitive phrases are called *mantras*, ranging from prayers to a single word.

Meditation has been used for thousands of years, in different forms, in different cultures and religions. Think of a Catholic saying the rosary in a quiet, darkened chapel or a Hindu doing yoga while soothing sitar music plays in the background.

YOGA: This is a form of exercise that combines gentle stretching with meditation that is focused inward on body sensations (the feeling of moving and relaxing muscles, sitting with proper posture, straightening and curving of the spine, for example). Yoga not only elicits the "relaxation response," but also provides some of the benefits of exercise. It can be used as a "warm-up" or "cool-down" along with conventional exercise.

GUIDED IMAGERY: Guided imagery takes the meditation process one step further: You use the time while you're relaxed to visualize positive images or even events.

GETTING A GOOD NIGHT'S SLEEP

Making sure you get enough sleep is extremely important, since studies show that upsetting your body's circadian rhythms may lead to depression and other problems.

Sleep disorders may overlap with symptoms of depression and anxiety, which is why they're listed in the *DSM-IV*. About 35 percent of people with chronic insomnia may actually suffer from an emotional disorder. Other sleep disorders with psychological underpinnings may include *hypersomnia* (sleeping too much), early awakening and disruption of normal sleep patterns. The symptoms of hypersomnia may also be caused by narcolepsy or sleep apnea (where a person literally stops breathing and awakens suddenly).

Women may be more sleep deprived than men. In women under forty, a recent study found, the number one cause of insufficient sleep was family responsibilities (working the so-called second shift). As many as 75 percent of menopausal women have symptoms such as hot flashes, which can interrupt sleep. More than half of people over age sixty-five have sleep problems. In older age, sleep patterns become disrupted, with people sleeping less soundly, awakening early and having a hard time getting back to sleep, explains Joyce A. Walsleben, Ph.D., director of the Sleep Disorders Center at NYU Medical Center.

Insomnia, and the psychological problems it brings, can be helped by learning "sleep hygiene," good sleep habits. Keeping regular hours, going to bed around the same time each night and waking up at a set time each morning help to keep your body's sleep-wake clock in working order.

"You can't tell yourself to go to sleep at a certain time. . . . But you can tell yourself to wake up at a certain time in the morning, with the help of alarm clocks, clock radios and such. If you do that on a regular basis, your body will adjust to that schedule," says Dr. Walsleben.

During the day, keep to a regular schedule of activities, eating breakfast, lunch and dinner at regular times. In the evening, relax in a quiet environment for an hour or so before bedtime, and keep your bedroom dark, cool and as free of noise as possible. "This way, you can structure your wake system to be awake when you need to be, and reinforce your sleep system so you can sleep when you need to," she explains. "If you're feeling depressed, it's helpful to maintain a normal sleep-wake cycle."

Regular exercise promotes deep sleep. But don't work out within three hours of bedtime, since it revs up the body.

Sleeping pills only help insomnia for about two weeks; after that the body develops a tolerance. Barbiturates, benzodiazepines and antihistamines can also be addictive, cause hangovers and, when taken in high doses for long periods of time, produce side effects that, in elderly people, can mimic dementia. Light therapy in the late afternoon can often help older people reregulate sleep patterns, if falling asleep too early is a problem.

Some other tips for good sleep hygiene.

- Use your bed only for sleeping and making love; if you pay bills or do work in bed, you may invite stress as your bedfellow.

- Avoid eating a full meal before bedtime; indigestion can ruin a good night's sleep. If you want a bedtime snack, keep it light. Better yet, have a glass of warm milk. Milk contains *tryptophan*, a natural amino acid that helps induce sleep.

- Avoid caffeinated beverages in the evening. Caffeine can linger in the body for up to six hours and rob people of sleep. If you still have trouble sleeping, eliminate caffeine totally.

- Avoid alcohol within four hours of going to bed. Alcohol disrupts regular sleep patterns. It may put you to sleep initially, but when your body finishes metabolizing the alcohol, a rebound effect will awaken you in the middle of the night.

- If you can't fall asleep after twenty minutes, get out of bed and go into another room for a quiet activity, such as reading, until you get drowsy. Tossing and turning only increase anxiety.

- If you work the night shift, make sure that you sleep in a completely darkened and quiet room during the day.

- Resist the temptation to stay in bed too long on the weekends; it can cause "Sunday night insomnia." Thirty minutes more than one's average amount of sleep every twenty-four hours should be enough to make you feel more rested.

☙ *Sarah's Story, Continued* ☞

"When I was depressed I was physically ill, not just mentally sad. My heart literally ached. It was a real, physical pain. . . . I had an overall sadness about life in general. Nothing seemed worth it. . . . I would read about a car accident or a terrorist bombing and I would wish . . . that I could have been killed instead of them. . . . It would be so simple and quick. . . .

"I would be driving, and I would have these thoughts about what would happen if I pressed the accelerator and put the car up to one hundred miles per hour and just drove straight ahead right into the seawall. I wasn't doing it. I just had thoughts of it. . . . The thing that scared me about it was that I didn't care what happened afterward, how my husband or child would feel. . . . I just wanted the pain to stop. . . . And that began to frighten me a lot. Because I do adore my husband and my son. I didn't really want to die. . . . I had always been an upbeat person. . . .

"What saved me was a chance meeting. We had gone to some event at my son's school and there was this local doctor I vaguely knew, and I asked him very casually if he knew anyone I could see for a problem I was having. And he said, 'Well, what's the problem.' And I told him, I'm depressed. And as I said the word 'depressed,' tears just started flooding down my cheeks. And he gave me the name of someone and told me to call them immediately. And I did call and went over to talk to him. . . . I told him, I don't know why I'm wasting your time. Because I want to kill myself, there's no reason for me to live. . . . And he said you don't have to feel like this. . . . Once he put me on the right medication, the pain went away. . . . The sadness and hopelessness lifted. And I was able to function. It was a terribly frightening thing to go through."

Red Flags: Suicide

As many as 1 percent of Americans die each year of suicide. While the rate of suicide has soared among young people aged fifteen to twenty-four, suicide remains most common among the elderly. While men (especially elderly white men) are more likely than women to kill themselves, two thirds of those who make suicide attempts are women.

Studies also show that suicide is more common among people who had a family member who attempted suicide. A history of major depression and bipolar disorder also increases risk, as can a serious medical illness.

The number one warning signs are suicidal talk, threats or plans for suicide or an actual suicide attempt. This is a medical emergency and requires professional help, either from a suicide hot line, physician or therapist. *If you have been thinking about suicide, find someone to talk to. Immediately.*

Other important red flags include:

- Suicidal gestures that seem designed to fail, such as "accidentally" taking too much over-the-counter medication.

- A preoccupation with death, either in remarks or in letters or diaries.

- Withdrawal from family, friends and normal activities.

- Giving away possessions, making wills.

- Persistent feelings of hopelessness and worthlessness; statements such as "Nothing matters anymore."

- An extreme reaction to a loss, where the person says they "can't go on."

- A sudden show of cheerfulness or calm after a traumatic loss or period of despondency.

- Sudden, radical changes in personality, sleep habits or appetite, or neglect of personal appearance.

- A decline in performance at work or school; neglect of everyday tasks.

- An increase in the use of alcohol, tranquilizers or other drugs. Drug or alcohol abuse can increase suicide risk fivefold.

⤳ Caren's Story, Continued ⤳

"I had really fallen into that woulda-coulda-shoulda trap. I would talk about something that happened with my family and I'd say, 'Well, I really should have done this. . . . ' And my therapist would say, 'Why should you have? Why are you responsible for everything and everyone?'

"The big thing I had to learn was that I am not responsible for the way anyone else feels. . . . I am responsible for how I feel. But more importantly, I am responsible for how I react to my feelings. Whether I react in a negative or positive way. And what may be positive for me may not necessarily be what is good for someone else. And that was hard for me to learn. . . .

"Now my first priority is that Caren takes care of herself. You have to make yourself first. It doesn't mean you're selfish. It doesn't mean you're self-centered. It just means that you know who you are, you're comfortable with your emotions and what makes you happy. You have to do that before you can let anyone else make you happy, before you can make anyone else happy.

"For so long we've been told to put ourselves last. . . . Once I learned that it was okay to put myself first, that gave me permission to say no. It meant I could say no to food, it meant I could say no to my family, it meant I could say no to men, it meant I could say no at work when I had too much. Sometimes it was a hard no, because maybe it was something I may have wanted to do. But if it kept me from taking care of myself . . . if it doesn't fit my life, then I don't do it. I am really learning to love myself and be who I am. And accept myself, and all the emotions and characteristics that are part of me. That acceptance is what will keep me mentally healthy."

―∽○∽―

KNOW WHO YOU ARE, WHAT YOU NEED

Like Caren, all of us need to focus more on ourselves. All too often, we pay more attention to the needs of our partners, our children, our parents and our coworkers. What happens is we get lost. That can be unhealthy.

"Many women, especially older women, have been brought up to think that it is their role to meet everyone else's needs and to take care of everyone else, and this often prevents them from doing things that they really like to do for themselves," says Dr. Ellen Frank. "One of the things that can be protective for women is figuring out what makes you feel good and improves your mood and doing it. It may be something very social, like going out with friends, or it may be very solitary, like gardening. Those are the things you need to do for yourself when you feel yourself slipping into depression."

Go to a movie, visit a museum, take a bike ride, go for a walk, set aside a "spa" day. Exchange baby-sitting services with friends. Find a "day care" program or senior center for elderly relatives. "Women who have a lot of caretaking responsibilities may feel that they can't do those 'selfish' things, but in fact, they become a more effective resource for others if they are functioning at the top of their program. And if what they need to function better is to take time for themselves, then they should do it. It's not selfish, it's health promoting," stresses Dr. Frank.

Paying attention to your needs means understanding your "pressure points," what drives you crazy, what stresses you out, which people cause your blood pressure to boil, and working out strategies for preventing those problems.

Paying attention to your needs also means being able to shift your emotional priorities when needed. "You have to maintain the flexibility to shift your emotional 'accounts.' Know when to say, 'This bank is closed, I have to put my money in a different bank and not leave it where it doesn't belong,' " advises NYU chief of psychiatry Dr. Robert Cancro. "For example, not trying to maintain a relationship that isn't working, not trying to hold on to something from yesterday that's gone, worn out or served its purpose. You have to know when to move on."

Remember, you have the inner strength to play whatever hand life deals you. Each challenge in life brings a chance to reinforce self-esteem and reverse worn-out negative thought habits. "Just because depression may be more common in women than men doesn't mean you're destined to be depressed. Women have natural strengths, and are in many ways more emotionally adaptive than men," observes Dr. Veva Zimmerman. "Women should take pride in being what they are, who they are, and develop a sense that they are valuable, unique and special."

While achievements and accomplishments are ego boosters, healthy self-esteem comes from within. Lack of self-esteem often comes from judging ourselves; focus on self-affirmation, what's *good* about you. That, plus an optimistic outlook on life, will enable you to handle just about anything.

Where to Go for Help

This appendix lists not only resources and support groups directly related to mental illnesses but services related to other issues that can affect women's mental well-being, including single parenting, infertility, death and dying and resources for lesbians and women of color.

GENERAL INFORMATION

National Institute of Mental Health (NIMH)
Information Resources and Inquiries Branch
5600 Fishers Lane, Room 7C-02, MSC
Bethesda, MD 20892-8030
http://gopher.nimh.nih.gov

The National Institute of Mental Health provides a wealth of information on every aspect of mental illness. A free catalog of publications is available.

Center for Mental Health Services (CMHS)
Office of External Liaison
5600 Fishers Lane, Room 13-103
Rockville, MD 20807
(301) 443-2792
http://www.mentalhealth.org./mhlinks/index.htm

The CMHS is part of the Substance Abuse and Mental Health Services Administration. CMHS runs a National Mental Health Services Knowledge Exchange Network (KEN), which provides information about mental health via a toll-free telephone number: 800-789-CMHS (2547).

National Mental Health Association (NMHA)
1021 Prince Street
Alexandria, VA 22314-2971
(800) 969 NMHA
http://www.worldcorp.com.dc-online/nmha

The oldest and largest volunteer mental health organization offers patient and family support services, material on depression and community outreach programs.

National Alliance for the Mentally Ill (NAMI)
2101 Wilson Boulevard, Suite 302
Arlington, VA 22201
(703) 524-7600
http://www.cais.net/vikings/nami

A grass-roots, self-help support and advocacy organization of families and friends of people with serious mental illness. Provides a variety of helpful booklets and referrals for support groups.

National Mental Health Consumer Self-Help Clearinghouse
311 South Jupiter Street, Room 902
Philadelphia, PA 19107
(215) 735-6367
http://www.med.upenn.edu/~cmhpsr/mhlinks.html

Mental Illness Foundation (MIF)
420 Lexington Avenue, Suite 2104
New York, NY 10170
(212) 682-4699

MIF was founded in 1983 by parents and relatives of mentally ill young adults. It raises funds for research grants and provides information and directories of services in New York City.

National Alliance for Research on Schizophrenia and Depression
(NARSAD)
60 Cutter Mill Road, Suite 200
Great Neck, NY 11021
(516) 829-0091
http://www.mhsource.com./narsad.html

Recovery, Inc.
802 North Dearborn Street
Chicago, IL 60610
(312) 337-5661

A self-help organization for former mental patients. Provides literature and sponsors group meetings across the United States, as well as in Canada, Puerto Rico, Ireland and Great Britain.

ADDICTION

National Clearinghouse for Alcohol and Drug Information
National Institute on Drug Abuse (NIDA)
5600 Fishers Lane, Room 15C-05
Rockville, MD 20807
(800) 729-6686 or (301) 468-2600
http://www.nida.gov/

Alcoholics Anonymous
P.O. Box 459
Grand Central Station
New York, NY 10163
(212) 870-3400
http://www.casti.com/aa

The original twelve-step program for recovering alcoholics. Staffed by nonprofessional volunteers who have "been there."

Al-Anon, Alateen and Adult Children of Alcoholics
Al-Anon Family Group Headquarters, Inc.
1600 Corporate Landing Highway
Virginia Beach, VA 23454
(800) 344-2666
http://solar.rtd.utk.edu/~al-anon

Help and fellowship for family members, friends and relatives of alcoholics. Will refer to local groups.

Cocaine Anonymous
3740 Overland Avenue, Suite G
Los Angeles, CA 90034
(800) 559-5833—National Referral Line
http://www.ca.org

National referral line provides individual state infoline listings for twelve-step self-help programs for recovering cocaine addicts.

National Association for Perinatal Addiction Research and Education
200 North Michigan Avenue, Suite 300
Chicago, IL 60601
(312) 541-1272

Parents Resource Institute for Drug Education (PRIDE)
50 Hurt Plaza, Suite 210
Atlanta, GA 30303
(404) 577-4500

Women for Sobriety, Inc.
109 West Broad Street
Quakertown, PA 18951
(215) 536-8026

Provides publications and referrals to self-help groups for women overcoming alcoholism and other addictions.

Gamblers Anonymous
P.O. Box 17173
Los Angeles, CA 90017
(213) 386-8789
E-Mail address (confidential): GAIOU@ix.netcom.com

Twelve-step, self-help program for compulsive gamblers.

National Council on Compulsive Gambling, Inc.
445 West 59th Street
New York, NY 10019
(800) 522-4700

Gam-Anon International Office, Inc.
P.O. Box 157
Whitestone, NY 11357
(718) 352-1671

Fellowship and self-help for families of compulsive gamblers.

Overeaters Anonymous
4025 Spencer Street, Suite 203
Torrance, CA 43229
(310) 618-8835
http://www.hiwaay.net/recovery

Sexaholics Anonymous
Central Office
P.O. Box 111910
Nashville, TN 37222
(615) 331-6230

Debtors Anonymous
P.O. Box 400
Grand Central Station
New York, NY 10163
(212) 642-8220

AGING AND MENTAL HEALTH

American Association of Retired Persons (AARP)
1909 K Street, N.W.
Washington, DC 20024
(202) 872-4700
http://www.aarp.org

Alzheimer's Association
919 North Michigan Avenue, Suite 1000
Chicago, IL 60611-1676
(800) 272-3900
http://www.alz.org

National Council on the Aging
409 3rd Street, S.W., 2nd Floor
Washington, DC 20024
(202) 479-1200

American Society on Aging
833 Market Street, Suite 511
San Francisco, CA 94103-1824
(800) 537-9728

National Institute on Aging
Information Office
Federal Building 6C12
Bethesda, MD 20892
(800) 222-2225

National Association of Area Agencies on Aging
1112 16th Street, N.W., Suite 100
Washington, DC 20036
(202) 296-8130

American Association of Geriatric Psychiatry
7910 Woodmont Avenue, Seventh Floor
Bethesda, MD 20814
(301) 654-7850

National Geriatric Psychiatry Alliance
1201 Connecticut Avenue, Suite 300
Washington, DC 20036
(888) INFO-GPA

ANXIETY DISORDERS

The Anxiety Disorders Association of America
6000 Executive Boulevard, Suite 513
Rockville, MD 20852
(301) 231-5484
http://www.users.interport.net/~lindy/adaa.html

TERRAP (Territorial Apprehensiveness)
648 Menlo Park Avenue, Suite 5
Menlo Park, CA 94025
(415) 327-1312

National network of treatment programs for agoraphobics.

CHILD ABUSE

Parents Anonymous, Inc.
The National Organization
675 W. Foothill Boulevard, Suite 220
Claremont, CA 91711
(909) 621-6184

A self-help group for parents who find themselves overwhelmed and are afraid they may harm (or have harmed) their children.

National Child Abuse Hotline
Childhelp USA
IOF Foresters
1345 El Centro Avenue
P.O. Box 630
Hollywood, CA 90028
(800) 4ACHILD (422-4453)
(800) 2ACHILD (222-4453) (TDD)
(213) 465-4016 (headquarters)

Crisis counseling for parents and referrals to professional groups that can help.

VOICES in Action, Inc.
Victims of Incest Can Emerge Survivors in Action, Inc.
P.O. Box 148309
Chicago, IL 60614
(312) 327-1500

Survivors of Incest Anonymous
P.O. Box 21817
Baltimore, MD 21222-6817
(301) 282-3400

DEATH/DYING/GRIEVING

National Hospice Organization (NHO)
1901 North Moore Street, Suite 901
Arlington, VA 22209
(800) 243-8728
http://www.nho.org

NHO provides information on hospice services and the names and addresses of hospices across the country.

Make Today Count
P.O. Box 6063
Kansas City, KS 66106
(913) 362-2866

Support for patients (and families) with terminal illnesses.

Compassionate Friends, Inc.
900 Jorie Boulevard
P.O. Box 3696
Oak Brook, IL 60522
(708) 990-0010

Self-help and support for parents who have lost a child.

DEPRESSION

Depression Awareness, Recognition, Treatment (D/ART) Program
National Institute of Mental Health
5600 Fishers Lane
Rockville, MD 20807
(800) 421-4211

NIMH's public education campaign provides free brochures and other materials in English and Spanish.

National Depressive and Manic Depressive Association (NDMDA)
730 North Franklin Street, Suite 501
Chicago, IL 60610
(800) 82-NDMDA

Clearinghouse for information on depression and bipolar disorder.

Depression After Delivery
P.O. Box 1282
Morrisville, PA 19067
(800) 944-4PPD

Publishes booklets and a newsletter for women who have experienced postpartum depression; list of experts in this area.

Postpartum Support International
927 North Kellogg Avenue
Santa Barbara, CA 93111
(805) 967-7636

National Foundation for Depressive Illness (NFDI)
P.O. Box 2257
New York, NY 10116
1-800-248-4344

Depressives Anonymous (Woman-only support group)
329 East 62nd Street
New York, NY 10021
(212) 689-2600

DOMESTIC VIOLENCE/RAPE/SEXUAL ABUSE

National Domestic Violence Hot Line
(800) 799-SAFE (7233)
(800) 787-3224 (TDD)

Launched in 1996 by the White House and the U.S. Department of Health and Human Services, the twenty-four-hour hot line offers specially trained, multilingual counselors and referrals to more than two thousand local services to help victims, from shelters to legal aid offices.

National Committee to Prevent Child Abuse (NCPCA)
332 S. Michigan Avenue, Suite 1600
Chicago, IL 60604
(800) CHILDREN (244-5373)
http://indy.radiologoy,uiowa.edu/Providers/ChildAbuse/NCPCA/
Ad.html

National Victim Center
2111 Wilson Boulevard, Suite 300
Arlington, VA 22201
(703) 276-2880
http://www.nvc.org

Resource center for violence and victimization provides referrals to eight thousand victim service organizations nationwide.

The National Organization for Victim Assistance (NOVA)
1757 Park Road, N.W.
Washington, DC 20010
(800) TRY-NOVA (879-6682)
http://access.digex.net/~nova

NOVA provides women across the country with information about shelters, hot lines and other services in their area.

National Coalition Against Domestic Violence
P.O. Box 18749
Denver, CO 80218
(303) 839-1852

National Council on Child Abuse and Family Violence
1155 Connecticut Avenue, N.W., #400
Washington, DC 20036
(800) 222-2000

National Displaced Homemakers Network
1625 K Street, N.W., #300
Washington, DC 20006
(202) 467-6346

Batterers Anonymous
8485 Tamarind Avenue, #D
Fontana, CA 92335
(714) 355-1100

National Coalition Against Sexual Assault
P.O. Box 21378
Washington, DC 20009
(202) 483-7165

National Clearinghouse on Marital and Date Rape
2325 Oak Street
Berkeley, CA 94708
(510) 524-1582

The Institute on Aging's Elder Abuse Prevention Program
1600 Divisadero Street
San Francisco, CA 94115
(415) 885-7850

National Center on Elder Abuse
810 First St., N.E., Suite 500
Washington, DC 20002
(202) 682-2470
http://www.ssp-ii.com/ssp/ncea

EATING DISORDERS

National Association of Anorexia Nervosa and Associated Disorders
(ANAD)
P.O. Box 7

Highland Park, IL 60035
(708) 831-3438
http://qlink.queensu.ca/~4map/anabhome.htm

Anorexia Nervosa and Related Eating Disorders, Inc. (ANRED)
P.O. Box 5102
Eugene, OR 97405
(503) 344-1144

American Anorexia/Bulimia Association, Inc. (AABA)
293 Central Park West, Suite 1R
New York, NY 10024
(212) 501-8351

Anorexia, Bulimia Care, Inc.
545 Concord Avenue
Cambridge, MA 02138
(617) 492-7670

Center for the Study of Anorexia and Bulimia
1 West 91st Street
New York, NY 10024
(212) 595-3449

National Anorexic Aid Society (NAAS)
Harding Hospital
1925 East Dublin Granville Road
Columbus, OH 43229
(614) 436-1112

Foundation for Education About Eating Disorders (FEED)
P.O. Box 16375
Baltimore, MD 21210
(410) 467-0603

Bulimia Anorexia Self Help, Inc. (BASH)
6125 Clayton Avenue, Suite 215
St. Louis, MO 36139
(314) 567-4080

Overeaters Anonymous
P.O. Box 92870
Los Angeles, CA 90009

(505) 618-8835
http://www.hiwaay.net/recovery

For more information on help for eating disorders in your area, check local hospitals or university medical centers for an eating disorders clinic.

FAMILY THERAPY

American Family Therapy Association
2020 Pennsylvania Avenue, N.W., Suite 273
Washington, DC 20006
(202) 994-2776

American Association for Marriage and Family Therapy (AAMFT)
1133 15th Street, N.W., Suite 300
Washington DC 20005-2710
To obtain referrals for your area, send self-addressed, stamped envelope to above address, attention Mr. Johnson. Reply will be sent in 2-3 business days.
http://www.aamft.org

Co-Dependents Anonymous (CoDA)
P.O. Box 33577
Phoenix, AZ 85067
(602) 277-7991

INFERTILITY

American Society for Reproductive Medicine
1209 Montgomery Highway
Birmingham, AL 35216
(205) 578-5000

Offers a series of patient information booklets, with topics ranging from endometriosis to IVF. Also maintains a list of infertility clinics nationwide.

RESOLVE
1310 Broadway
Somerville, MA 02144-1731

(617) 623-1156
(617) 623-0744 (help line)

National, nonprofit consumer organization established in 1974, offering information on infertility as well as referrals to its local chapter support groups.

LESBIAN HEALTH ISSUES

Association of Gay and Lesbian Psychiatrists
209 North Fourth Street, Suite D-5
Philadelphia, PA 19106
(215) 925-5008

National Gay and Lesbian Health Association
Lesbian Health Advocacy Network
1407 S Street, N.W.
Washington, DC 20009
(202) 797-3536

Gay and Lesbian Medical Association
211 Church Street
San Francisco, CA 94114
(415) 255-4547

Lesbian Health Project
8235 Santa Monica Boulevard, Suite 308
Los Angeles, CA 90099-5575
(213) 650-1508

National Latino Lesbian and Gay Organization
Leticia Gomez, Director
703 G Street, S.E.
Washington, DC 20003
(202) 554-0092

Lesbian Health Issues Newsletter
National Center for Lesbian Rights
870 Market Street, Suite 570
San Francisco, CA 94102
(415) 392-6257

MARITAL/SEXUAL THERAPY

American Association of Sex Educators, Counselors and Therapists
435 North Michigan Avenue, Suite 1717
Chicago, IL 60611-4067

AASECT will provide a list of sex therapists or counselors in your area.
Send a self-addressed, stamped envelope and $3.00.

Sex Information and Education Council of the U.S.
Department MM
130 West 42nd Street, Suite 2500
New York, NY 10036
(212) 817-9770

SIECUS will provide a catalog of publications on all aspects of sexuality.
Send a self-addressed, stamped envelope.

Impotents Anonymous
I-Anon (Partners of Impotent Men)
Impotence World Service
P.O. Box 5299
Maryville, TN 37802
(615) 983-6064

MENOPAUSE AND BEYOND

North American Menopause Society
c/o University Hospitals of Cleveland
Department of OB/GYN
11100 Euclid Avenue
Cleveland, OH
(216) 844-8748
http://www.menopause.com

Older Women's League (OWL)
666 Eleventh Street, N.W., Suite 700
Washington, DC 20001
(202) 783-6686

MISCARRIAGE/STILLBIRTH/INFANT LOSS

SHARE
c/o St. John's Hospital
800 East Carpenter Street
Springfield, IL 62769
(217) 544-6464

Support group network for people who have lost a newborn.

Pregnancy and Infant Loss Center
1421 East Wayzata Boulevard
Wayzata, MN 55391
(612) 473-9372

Information and support on miscarriage, stillbirth, newborn loss.

OBSESSIVE-COMPULSIVE DISORDERS

Obsessive-Compulsive Foundation
P.O. Box 70
Milford, CT 06460–0070
(203) 878-5669
(203) 874-3843 (infoline)
http://www.iglou.com.fairlight/oca

The Trichotillomania Learning Center
1215 Mission Street, Suite 2
Santa Cruz, CA 95060
(408) 457-1004

PATIENT ABUSE SUPPORT GROUPS

In Motion—People Abused in Counseling and Therapy
323 South Pearl Street
Denver, CO 80209
(303) 979-8073

PREGNANCY/POSTPARTUM

Depression After Delivery
P.O. Box 1282
Morrisville, PA 19067
(800) 944-4PPD

Publishes booklets and a newsletter for women who have experienced postpartum depression; list of experts in this area.

Postpartum Support International
927 North Kellogg Avenue
Santa Barbara, CA 93111
(805) 967-7636

Provides lists of professionals who can help.

Parents Care, Inc.
101½ South Union Street
Alexandria, VA 22314
(703) 836-4678

Support group for parents with newborns in intensive care.

PROFESSIONAL ORGANIZATIONS

American Psychiatric Association
1400 K Street, N.W.
Washington, DC 20005
(202) 682-6000
(202) 682-6325 (for psychiatric referral)
http://www.thebody.com/apa/apapage.html

American Psychological Association
1200 17th Street, N.W.
Washington, DC 20002
(202) 336-5500
PsychNET—http://www.apa.org

American Psychiatric Nurses Association
1200 19th Street, N.W., Suite 300
Washington, DC 20036
(202) 857-1133

American Association of Pastoral Counselors
9508A Lee Highway
Fairfax, VA 22031
(703) 385-6967

National Association of Social Workers
750 1st Street, N.E., Suite 700
Washington, DC 20002
(800) 638-8799

American Mental Health Counselors Association
5999 Stevenson Avenue
Alexandria, VA 22304
(703) 823-9800

American Association of Sex Educators, Counselors and Therapists
435 North Michigan Avenue, Suite 1717
Chicago, IL 60611-4067
(312) 644-0828

National Association of Private Psychiatric Hospitals
1319 F Street, N.W., #1000
Washington, DC 20004
(202) 393-6700

National Council of Community Mental Health Centers
12300 Twinbrook Parkway, Suite 320
Rockville, MD 20852
(301) 984-6200

RESPITE CARE

ARCH National Resource Center
National Respite Locator Service
800 Eastowne Drive, Suite 105

Chapel Hill, NC 27514
(800) 773-5433

Free national respite care provider locator service. Also helps find respite care for parents caring for special needs children.

THERAPIES

Association for the Advancement of Behavioral Therapy
15 West 36th Street
New York, NY 10018
(212) 279-7970

American Group Psychotherapy Association
25 East 21st Street, 6th Floor
New York, NY 10010
(212) 477-2677

National Association for the Advancement of Psychoanalysis
American Board for Accreditation and Certification, Inc.
80 Eighth Avenue, Suite 1210
New York, NY 10011
(212) 741-0515

The Beck Institute for Cognitive Therapy and Research
GSB Building, City Line and Belmont Avenues, Suite 700
Bala Cynwyd, PA 19004-1610
(610) 664-3020

The Center for Cognitive Therapy
University of Pennsylvania
133 South 36th Street, Room 602
Philadelphia, PA 19104
(215) 898-4100

SCHIZOPHRENIA

National Alliance for Research on Schizophrenia and Depression
(NARSAD)

60 Cutter Mill Road, Suite 200
Great Neck, NY 11021
(516) 829-0091
http://www.mhsource.com./narsad.html

SEXUAL HARASSMENT

Equal Opportunity Commission Hotline
(800) 669-4000

SINGLE PARENTS/STEPFAMILIES

Parents Without Partners, Inc.
401 North Michigan Avenue
Chicago, IL 60611-4267
(800) 637-7974

The Stepfamily Foundation
333 West End Avenue
New York, NY 10023
24 Hour Info Line: (212) 799-7837
Hot Line/Crisis Line: (212) 744 6924
http://www.stepfamily.org

Stepfamily Association of America, Inc.
215 Centennial Mall South, Suite 212
Lincoln, NE 68508
(402) 477-7837

SLEEP DISORDERS

American Sleep Disorders Association
1610 14th Street, N.W., Suite 300
Rochester, MN 55901
(507) 287-6006

Referrals to over two hundred accredited sleep centers across the U.S.

American Narcolepsy Association
P.O. Box 51113
Palo Alto, CA 94303
(800) 829-1933

WOMEN OF COLOR

National Latina Health Organization
P.O. Box 7567
Oakland, CA 94601
(510) 534-1362

National Black Women's Health Project
1237 Ralph David Abernathy Boulevard, S.W.
Atlanta, GA 30310
(404) 758-9590
Cynthia Newbille, Executive Director

The NBWHP is a national (and international) self-help and health advocacy organization incorporating 150 local self-help groups in thirty-two states. Publishes a quarterly newsmagazine, *Vital Signs*.

National Asian Women's Health Organization (NAWHO)
250 Montgomery Street, Suite 410
San Francisco, CA 94104
(415) 989-9747

WOMEN'S ISSUES

National Women's Health Network
514 10th Street, N.W., Suite 400
Washington, DC 20004
(202) 347-1140

National Women's Health Resource Center
2440 M Street, N.W., Suite 325
Washington, DC 20037
(202) 293-6045

Other World Wide Web/Self-Help Sites

HELP! A Consumer's Guide to Mental Health Information
http://www.io.org/~madmagic/help/help/html

Internet Mental Health (Canada)
http://www.mentalhealth.com

Mental Health InfoSource
http://www.mhsource.com

Mental Health Library
http://medhlp.netusa.net.mntlhlth.htm

Mental Health Net
http://www.cmhc.com

Online Psych
http://www.onlinepsych.com

Psych Central
http://www.coil.com/~grohol/

Additional Reading/Self-help

Caring for the Mind: The Comprehensive Guide to Mental Health by Dianne Hales and Robert E. Hales, M.D., Bantam Books, 1995.

It's Not All in Your Head: Now Women Can Discover the Real Causes of Their Most Commonly Misdiagnosed Health Problems by Susan Swedo, M.D., and Henrietta Leonard, M.D., Harper Collins, San Francisco, 1996.

New Passages: Mapping Your Life Across Time by Gail Sheehy, Random House, New York, 1995.

The New Personality Self-Portrait: Why You Think, Work, Love and Act the Way You Do by John M. Oldham, M.D., and Lois B. Morris, Bantam Books, 1995.

This Isn't What I Expected: Overcoming Post-Partum Depression by Karen R. Kleinman, M.S.W., and Valerie D. Raskin, M.D., Bantam Books, 1995.

Triumph over Fear: A Book of Help and Hope for People with Anxiety, Panic Attacks and Phobias by Jerilyn Ross, M.A., LICSW, Bantam Books, 1994.

The Courage to Heal: A Guide for Women Survivors of Child Sexual Abuse by Ellen Bass and Laura Davis, Harper Collins, 1994.

A Woman's Book of Grieving by Nessa Rapoport, illustrated by Rochelle Rubenstein Kaplan, William Morrow, 1994.

How to Go on Living When Someone You Love Dies by Therese Rando, Bantam Books, 1988.

You Mean I Don't Have to Feel This Way? New Help for Depression, Anxiety and Addiction by Colette Dowling, Bantam, trade paperback, 1993.

Winter Blues: Seasonal Affective Disorder: What It Is and How to Overcome It by Norman E. Rosenthal, M.D., Guilford Press, 1993.

My Name Is Caroline by Caroline Adams Miller, Doubleday, 1988.

Trusting Ourselves: The Complete Guide to Emotional Well-Being for Women by Karen Johnson, M.D., Atlantic Monthly Press, 1991.

All That She Can Be: Helping Your Daughter Maintain Her Self-esteem by Carol J. Eagle, Ph.D., and Carol Colman, Fireside, 1994.

Love and Sex After Sixty by Robert N. Butler, M.D., and Myrna I. Lewis, M.S.W., revised edition, Ballantine Books, 1994.

The Maria Paradox: How Latinas Can Merge Old World Traditions with New World Self-esteem by Carmen Inoa Vazquez and Rosa Maria Gil, Putnam, 1996.

The Columbia University College of Physicians and Surgeons Complete Home Guide to Mental Health edited by Frederick I. Kass, M.D., John M. Oldham, M.D., and Herbert Pardes, M.D., Henry Holt, 1992.

Your Healing Mind by Reed C. Moskowitz, M.D., Hearst Books, 1991.

Aging and Mental Health: Positive Psychosocial and Biomedical Approaches by Robert N. Butler, M.D., Myrna I. Lewis, M.S.W., and Trey Sunderland, M.D., National Institute of Mental Health, Merrill/Macmillan, 4th edition, 1991.

No Safe Haven: Male Violence Against Women at Home, at Work, and in the Community by Mary P. Koss, Ph.D.; Lisa A. Goodman, Ph.D.; Angela Browne, Ph.D.; Louise F. Fitzgerald, Ph.D.; Gwendolyn Puryear Keita, Ph.D.; Nancy Filipe Russo, Ph.D., American Psychological Association, 1995.

American Psychological Association Task Force Report on Women & Depression: Risk Factors and Treatment Issues edited by Ellen McGrath, Ph.D.; Gwendolyn Puryear Keita, Ph.D.; Bonnie R. Strickland, Ph.D., ABPP; and Nancy Felipe Russo, Ph.D., American Psychological Association, 1990.

Moderate Drinking: The New Option for Problem Drinkers by Audrey Kishline, See Sharp Press, 1994.

Guidelines to Safe Drinking by Nicholas A. Pace, M.D., with Wilbur Cross, Fawcett, 1986.

Self-help for PMS by Michelle Harrison, M.D., Random House, 1985.

Woulda, Coulda, Shoulda by Arthur Freeman, Ph.D., and Rose DeWolf, Harper Collins, 1990.

Our Health, Our Lives: A Revolutionary Approach to Total Health Care for Women by Eileen Hoffman, M.D., Pocket Books, 1995.

The Angry Marriage: Overcoming the Rage, Reclaiming the Love by Bonnie Maslin, Ph.D., Hyperion, 1995.

Emotional Intelligence by Daniel Goleman, Ph.D., Bantam, 1995.

Am I Thin Enough Yet? The Cult of Thinness and the Commercialization of Identity by Sharlene Hesse-Biber, Oxford University Press, 1996.

What Do You See When You Look in the Mirror? Helping Yourself to a Positive Body Image by Thomas Cash, Ph.D., 1995.

Emotional Weight: Change Your Relationship with Food by Changing Your Relationship with Yourself by Colleen A. Sundermeyer, Ph.D., Perigee, 1993.

Index